Guide for BHMS Students
PREVENTIVE
And
SOCIAL MEDICINE

Guide for BHMS Students
PREVENTIVE
And
SOCIAL MEDICINE

Dr. BALARAM JANA

B. JAIN PUBLISHERS (P) LTD.
USA — EUROPE — INDIA

GUIDE FOR BHMS STUDENTS PREVENTIVE & SOCIAL MEDICINE

7th Impression: 2014

Note from the Publishers
Any information given in this book is not intended to be taken as a replacement for medical advice. Any person with a condition requiring medical attention should consult a qualified practitioner or therapist.

All rights reserved. No part of this book may be reproduced, stored in a retrieval system or transmitted, in any form or by any means, mechanical, photocopying, recording or otherwise, without any prior written permission of the publisher.

© with the publisher

Published by Kuldeep Jain for
B. JAIN PUBLISHERS (P) LTD.
1921/10, Chuna Mandi, Paharganj, New Delhi 110 055 (INDIA)
Tel.: +91-11-4567 1000 • Fax: +91-11-4567 1010
Email: info@bjain.com • Website: www.bjain.com

Printed in India by
Printed at G.H. Prints Pvt. Ltd New Delhi

ISBN: 978-81-319-0022-2

In memory of my father
Late Beharilal Jana
(Freedom Fighter)

In memory of my father
Late Behanlal Jana
(Freedom Fighter)

CONTENTS

PREVENTION IS BETTER THAN CURE

[Page 2 to 6]

CHAPTER-I

PREVENTIVE AND SOCIAL MEDICINE

[Page 7 to 24]

PSM and its areas—7
Utilities of the study of PSM—9
Developmental history of PSM—11
Changing concepts of 'Hygiene' to PSM—14

Preventive Medicine and its main objects—15
Social Medicine and its main objects—16
Hahnemann's view on health and disease—19

PART-I

PHYSIOLOGICAL HYGIENE

CHAPTER-II

FOOD AND NUTRITION

[Page 26 to 98]

Food in relation to health —26
Balanced diet—29
Nutritional deficiencies—46
Vitamin deficiencies—48
Malnutrition and its Prevention (PCM/PEM)—58
Assessment of Nutritional status—68

Milk and Pasteurisation of milk—72
Preservation of food—87
Adulteration of food—88
Power of Food Inspector—91
Food Poisoning—91
Diseases from food—92
Dieto therapy—95

CHAPTER-III

AIR, LIGHT, SUNSHINE IN RELATION TO HEALTH

[Page 99 to 116]

Air and its importance—99
Composition of air—99
How air becomes impure—100
What are the effect of the changes of air on man—102
Overcrowding—103
Purification of air—105
Ventilation—106
Lighting—114
Sunshine—115

CHAPTER-IV

EFFECT OF CLIMATE

[Page 117 to 128]

Climate—117
Humidity—118
Temperature—119
Pressure—124

CHAPTER-V

PERSONAL HYGIENE

[Page 129 to 145]

Personal Hygiene and its main objects—129
Various health care—130
Cleanliness—131
Clothing—134
Food—135
Sleep and rest—137
Exercises—138
Health care and avoid able habits—142
Health Care of a house wife for maintaining her—144

PART-II
ENVIRONMENTAL SANITATION

CHAPTER-VI

ENVIRONMENTAL SANITATION

[Page 146 to 149]

CHAPTER-VII
ATMOSPHERIC POLLUTION

[Page 150 to 161]

Pollution—150
Various pollutants and their sources—150
Effect of pollution on health—153
Prevention of air pollution—157
Air borne diseases and their control—160

CHAPTER-VIII
WATER IN RELATION TO HEALTH AND DISEASES

[Page 162 to 217]

Properties of water—163
Biological importance of water—164
Uses of water—166
Quantity of water required—166
Quality of water—168
Sources of water—171
Water Supply of Rural Areas—181
Calcutta Water Supply—185
Impurities of water—190
Effects of impurities of water on health—191
Water borne disease—193
Purification of water—199
(In the cities 203, Villages—201)
Filteration of water—206
Hardness of water—210
Removal of hardness of water—212
Hydrological cycle—216

CHAPTER-IX
DISPOSAL OF HUMAN EXCREATA, REFUSE

[Page 218 to 259]

Disposal of Human Excreta in villages—218
Septic Tank—228
Disposal of refuse—248
Manure Pits—258

CHAPTER-X

DISINFECTION AND SANITATION OF A FAIR OR MELA

[Page 260 to 280]

Types of disinfection—260
Precurrent, concurrent and terminal—260
Various disinfactants—263
Insecticides—265
Larvicides—265

Practical disinfection in certain situations and particular cases like-smallpox, Tuberculosis cholera and typhoid—267
Sanitation of a fair or mela—272

PART-III

PREVENTIVE MEDICINE

CHAPTER-XI

EPIDEMIOLOGY

[Page 281 to 288]

Epidemic and Epidemiology—282
General Principles—284

Epedemic and its prevention and control—287

CHAPTER-XII

INFECTIONS

[Page 289 to 307]

Infection—289
Various methods of infection—292
Basic Principle for control and prevention of infectious disease—295
Notification—296

Isolation—296
Quarantine—296
Vector and vector control—300
Mechanical, biological and healthy carriers—300
Housefly and fly control—304
Arthopod's borne disease—307

CHAPTER-XIII

COMMUNICABLE DISEASES

[Page 308 to 393]

Communicable disease—309
How they occur?—310
Droplet Infection—312
Incubation period—313
Cholera—316
Gastro enteritis-Diarrhoea & Dysentery—322
Infective hepatitis—324
Hookworm—328
Soil borne diseases—333
Poliomyelitis—335
Polio vaccines—338
Tuberculosis—339
Housing—348
Smallpox and Chickenpox—349
Malaria—362
Filaria—372
Rabies—374
Leprosy—379
Endemic goitre—389
Beriberi—391
Pellagra—392

PART-IV

HEALTH FOR ALL BY 2000-AD

CHAPTER-XIV

[Page 394 to 430]

Immunity-Immunology prophylaxis—395
Immunity and immunization—395
Natural and artificial immunity—398
Immunization active and passive—402
Prophylaxis—412
Routine immunization procedure, recommended schedule—417

CHAPTER-XV

DEMOGRAPHY AND FAMILY PLANNING

[Page 431 to 454]

Demography—431
Population growth and demographic data—432
Contraceptive methods—441
Contraceptives, M.T.P. and sterilization—446

Various demographic features—435
Importance of population projects—437
Family Planning its definition and needs—437
Advantages of Family Planning—450
National Family Planning Programme and its organisational set up—451
Present attitude towards Family Planning—453

CHAPTER-XVI

MATERIAL AND CHILD HEALTH CARE

[Page 455 to 469]

Definations aims & its objectives—455
Under Five Clinics—464
Infant Mortality Rate—465
Antenatal care—458
5 Points Programme—463
Maternal Mortality Rate—465

CHAPTER-XVII

SCHOOL HEALTH SERVICES

[470 to 479]

Its need and main objects —470
Basic components of School Health Programme —471
Duties of Medical Officer as a member of school committee or Board—472

CHAPTER-XVIII

PRIMARY HEALTH CENTRE

[Page 480 to 486]

PHC's constitution and staff pattern and their activities—480
Functions of a Medical Officer Incharge of PHC's —484
Multipurpose worker scheme and community health worked scheme—486

(vi)

CHAPTER-XIX

MEDICAL STATISTICS

[Page 487 to 504]

Vital Statistics—487
Health Statistics—490

Population Census—492
Vital Events—493
Morbidity Statistics—493

CHAPTER-XX

INTERNATIONAL AND NATIONAL ORGANISATIONS

(Page 505 to 515)

W.H.O.—505
F.A.O.—510

U.N.I.C.E.F.—509
E.S.I.—511

HEALTH FOR ALL BY 2000 A.D.

(Page 516 to 519)

PART-V

QUICK REFERENCE CHARTS

(Page 520 to 536)

PART-VI

MULTIPLE CHOICE OF QUESTIONS

(Page 537 to 548)

PART-VII

PRACTICAL PART

[Page 549 to 581]

I. Demonstrations—550

II. Lesson—551

1. Information about community—551
2. Family & general health examination—555
3. Housing, disposal of refuse & sewage; water supply—561
4. Collection of water for chemical & bacteriological examination—565
5. Methods of chlorination—566
6. Nutritional assessment—568
7. Infact & underfive feeding & rearing—571
8. Growth & development of infant & "Underfive"—573
9. Maternal & child health & family planning—574
10. Case Presentations:

   Tuberculosis, Leprosy, Filaria, Fever/Malaria, Gastroenteritis, P.E.M. Goitre, Fluorosis, Caries, Rickets, Vitamin deficiencis, Measles, Infective hepatitis, Worm infestation. Anaemia, Skin diseases (scabies, ringworm, pyoderma,) Heart diseases, Diabetes, Whooping cough etc.—578
11. Guidelines for the Lessons—580

APPENDICES QUESTIONERIES & INDEX
(Page 582 to 601)

(viii)

Preface To The Second Edition

My sincere thanks are due to my students and to my fellow-teachers all over India for the appreciation with which the first edition of this book was received. In bringing out the second edition I have tried to meet the requirements of our patrons whom I thanks for their individual opinions expressed to me.

I hope that the present edition would satisfy the needs of our patrons.

Independence's Day   **BALARAM JANA**
15th Aug., 1990.

Centre of Advanced
Studies and Research
in Homoeopathic

30/4, Narasingha Dutta Road,
Howrah- 711 101,
West Bengal, INDIA

Preface To The Second Edition

My sincere thanks are due to my students and to my fellow-teachers all over India for the appreciation with which the first edition of this book was received. In bringing out the second edition I have tried to meet the requirements of our patrons, whom I thanks for their individual opinions expressed to me.

I hope that the present edition would satisfy the needs of our patrons.

Independence's Day
15th Aug, 1990.

BALARAM JANA

Centre of Advanced
Studies and Research
in Homoeopathy.

30/1, Narasingha Dutta Road,
Howrah-711 101,
West Bengal, INDIA.

PREFACE TO THE FIRST EDITION

The need for a compact and concise taxt book on *"Preventive and Social Medicine"* enabling the students to write their examination scripts correctly and easily has long been felt by the students and teachers alike. At the repeated requests of my beloved students and learned colleagues, I have humbly embarked myself on this arduous endeavour. While examining the answer papers of the students, I am constrained to feel that this is the most neglected subject by the majority of students, albeit a very important branch of medical science concerning public health. A through knowledge of the subject can help us in curbing and averting many maladies of the individual and the society at large, simply by observing certain norms of health and dietary habits.

As this book is written on a model of answers to questions of the important universities, boards and councils the reader can be guided well about the important and practical aspects of this subject matter. As far as possible most of the subject matters have been covered and written in a concise and simplified form according to the latest *syllabus for degree, graded degree and diploma courses as prescribed by the Central Council of Homoeopathy Medicine, New Delhi* (*1983*). To make it a standard help as well as text book in place of any standard text book the matter of this book has been derived from reference of different standard text books, research journals and papers on this subject, and are compiled in a compact and simplified form. The latest figures and other concepts of this subject have been incorporated whenever needed.

Finally, I would like to state that it would be too much to hope that the first edition should be entirely free of errors of omission and commission, and, in conclusion, I shall consider my efforts fully recompensed if the book serves the purpose for which it is written and published.

New year's day, 1986
Bengal Homoeopathic
Medical College & Hospital
Asansol, Burdwan
West Bengal, INDIA

BALARAM JANA

PREVENTION IS BETTER THAN CURE

"*All men are mortal*" is an universal truth. It is also equally true that men by their individual and collective endeavours can prolong the span of life, and can lead a comparatively disease-free life. Here medical science comes to our aid. It's two aspects-curative and preventive medicines, are the two faces of the same coin.

The object of curative medicines is the restoration of the diseased person to normal health, while preventive medicine aims at eliminating the causes of the malady that afflicts the community. The emphasis the former is on the individual and the later encompasses the community or society. The curative medicine deals with a sick person. Some of the diseases, such as is caused by stress and strain are generally of an individual in nature, while others, like cholera, smallpox, malaria etc. are of endemic and general in character.

Hygiene or preventive and social medicine imparts us knowledge how to fight out the general and epidemic diseases. It also teaches us to ascertain the causes and conditions of maintaining good health of the individual and the society at large.

To combat diseases successfully we must have to understand the causation of the malady. Before Hippocrates, the father of modern medicine, the primitive man used to believe that diseases were caused by wraths of dieties and demons, and in later days he used to feel that it was due to astronomical influences. The whole concept of medical science revolutionised with the knowledge of bacteriological theory. Moreover, modern medical science has further demonstrated another set of diseases known as deficiency diseases. Stress and strain are the causes of many more modern day's ailments.

Most of the preventive diseases are caused by environmental pollution and germs bacteria and viruses of such diseases are carried mainly either by air, water or insects. In any scheme of preventive medicine individual man is to be educated to know the value of sanitation for the benefit of the community and for his own self.

Primary prevention aims at averting the occurrence of a disease and the object of the secondary prevention is to limit the disability by early diagnosis and prompt treatment. The preventive medicine works before the patient goes to hospital.

Preventive medicine aims at the well-being of the society as a whole. Eradication and control of communicable and epidemic disease resulting from unhygenic environment are its main objects. Thus removal of unhygenic environment, control of pollution of air, water and earth are its main task. Its another major work is the production and administration of artificial immunity like cholera, enteric fever, smallpox etc. The other object of preventive medicine is the adoption of measures leading to prevention of diseases caused by the inadequate intake of proper food. To protect from accident and occupational diseases is also in its realm. Economic rehabilitation of the victims of social maladies is also its aim. Another important sphere of preventive medicine is the control of population for the welfare of the family and the community. Protection of the child and the mother before and after child birth is also in the dominion of social and preventive medicine.

The importance of preventive medicine is more pronounced for a developing country, like India but there are certain limitations in its application here fully. There is inadequate and poor infrastructural facilities, such as hospital accommodation, trained personnel and proper equipments needed to implement such a gigantic job due to poor economic conditions of our country. The government also cannot spare requisite fund for economic reasons.

The per capita income of our people is so low that a significant segment of it are unable to procure two square meals a day for them no to speak of any nutritious food to maintain their health in good condition. Moreover due to their extreme poverty they are forced to live in slums and unhygienic dwelling conditions. Even to day pure drinking water is not available to all our people. Two-third of our population being illiterate they do not know the scientific rules and principles for maintaining their health.

Moreover, the so-called religious beliefs and prejudices sometimes go against implementing preventive measures. Even to day many people refuse to take medicines during their smallpox attack in the name of "MA SITALA". Family planning measures which is most vital for general economic development and implementation of preventive measures are refused on many occasions on religious ground. Again due to their poor economic conception the illiterate and half-starved masses believe that large number of children, particularly male children are asset to the family. The whole problem is mainly rooted into the twin socio-economic problem of illiteracy and economic backwardness.

Any expenditure on social-medicine is really an investment on human resources a precions national wealth. It also helps the utilisation of human resources of the nation in a planned and fruitful manner. It is more economical as it corroborated the adage :

"*A stich in time saves seven.*" Thus, prevention is better than cure.

Role of Homoeopathy in preventing diseases.

Homoeopathy plays an important role in both preventive and therapeutics aspects. All men are born with some hereditary dyscrasis which are responsible for their increased pronchess towards certain diseases. This dyscrasia is further influenced after birth by environments, adaptation, disease producing agents and the susceptibility of the individual. This susceptibility is again modified by many factors e.g. age, sex, occupation, mode of living and so on. Immunity against disease depends on this susceptibility. Hypersusceptibity towards disease indicates less immunity and less susceptibility indicates strong immunity.

In order to prevent or cure a disease, we are to take care of both the disease producing agent and the susceptibility of the individual. Hygienic measures like water supply, ventilation, sunlight, sewage, drainage, mosquito control etc. take care of the disease producing agents and effective treatments, sufficient nourshing diet, mental peace and well regulated life take care of the susceptibility and thereby the, immunity.

Homoeopathy can correct this hereditary or acquired discrasia with the help of constitutional medicines and thereby susceptibility is reduced and a disease is prevented or cured.

Psycho-somatic make up of a man is his constitution. Homoeopathy believes in the individuality of a man. No two men are alike in this world. Hence, constitution varies from man to men in his physical appearance, mental development, intellectual capacity, reaction to external stimuli, likings and dislikings, sleep, dream etc. A person who is apparently healthy may show some deviation from others in the sphere mentioned above. Homoeopathic medicines were proved in different succh constitutions and thereby their capability of affecting the different types of constitutions have been ascertained. Any abnormal sensation or function in any type of constitution can easily be corrected by the judicious and time by administration of such constitutional medicines. This type of constitutional treatment is only possible in homoeopathy. Because, in other branches of medicine, as far as we know, a simple alteration in the sensation and function of a person is not generally considered as a disease unless some structural changes take place or a nosological name can be given to the condition. The only exception is the mental diseases or the so-called neuroses. Here also the approach is different and there is probably no specific effective treatment of them as yet. But homoeopathy considers the totality to the altered sensation and functions as disease. The medicines are selected on the totality of symptoms and their removal is considered as cure. Because, no disease, can be hidden in the interior. It must manifest as a symptom or sign perceptible to our senses including the instrumental or laboratory tests. As such the minor variations in the constitutions in early childhood are considered as disease-images of serious incurable conditions which may appear in future i.e. these symptoms in childhood are considered in homoeopathy as the fore-runners of many incurable diseases occuring in future life. Naturally if these minor deviations can be corrected in childhood with the help of constitutional medicines, most of the incurable diseases can be prevented long before they assume concrete shapes in the system of a living human beings. Thus tonsillitis, cancer, tuberculosis, leprosy etc. can be cured and prevented by constitutional treatment.

Even bronchial asthma, diabetes mellitus, spondylitis, lupus erythematosus, sickle-cell anaemia, thallaseaemia, leukaemia and many other diseases which are now considered as of genetic origin, may be prevented if the mothers are constitutionally treated during pregnancy and the children are treated immediately after their birth. Moreover, constitutional treatment increases the general immunity of an individual which makes him capable of fighting various constitutional diseases effectively. Even if newly married couple go to the homoeopathic treatment for their constitutional disorder before they want to have a child, the possibilities of genetic diseases may be averted. In case of epidemic disease like smallpox, cholera etc. Specific immunity against specific diseases may also be successfully effected with homoeopathic medicines in suitable potencies and repeated doses if applied in time before the outbreak of such an epidemic. Even after the outbreak of such an epidemic, the disease may successfully be controlled from not being spread amongst the unaffected persons. Homoeopathic medicines are cheap and easy to apply and as such mass scale immunization can easily be performed at a very low cost.

So, homoeopathy can play an important role in the National Health Service, specially in materialising the rural health programmes provided the Government of India and other State Government take active interest in this system of medicine and the homoeopaths spare no pains to qualify themselves upto the standard necessary for proper utilisation of all its resources.

CHAPTER-1

PREVENTIVE AND SOCIAL MEDICINE (P.S.M.)

DISCUSSION FOR LEARNING

I. Preventive and Social Medicine and it's arena.
II. Utility of the study of Preventive and Social Medicine.
III. Development history of Preventive and Social Medicine.
IV. Changing concept of "Hygiene and Public Health" to "Preventive and Social Medicine".
V. Preventive Medicine and it's main objects.
VI. Social Medicine and it's main objects.
VII. Hahnemann's view on Health and Disease.

I. PREVENTIVE AND SOCIAL MEDICINE AND IT'S ARENA

Q1.1. What is meant by Preventive and Social Medicine ?

Preventive and Social Medicine is that branch of science which treats the promotion and preservation of health i.e., which contribute to the most perfect development of the body and mind, renders life more vigorous, decay less rapid and death more distant. It embraces various influences operating upon the physical and mental condition of individuals and communities, whether in promoting material good or preventing their deterioration. It consists essentially in the prevention of disease by the removal of its avoidable causes (biological, physical, social etc.) and consequently involves legislative control, that the safety of the whole may be protected against the errors of the few. In its widest sense, the term *"Preventive and Social*

Medicine implies rules for the perfect culture of the body and mind of individuals, family, group and community."

Q1.2. What are it's areas ?

Preventive and Social Medicine includes the following:-
(A) Impersonal services, and
(B) Personal services.

(A) IMPERSONAL SERVICES

1. Epidemic diseases controled by

a) Quarantine,
b) Epidemiological services,
c) Public Health,
d) Contract tracing,
e) Vector control, and
f) Eradication measures.

2. Sanitary Hygiene

a) Sewage disposal
b) Prevention of social pollution
c) Water supply,
d) Food hygiene,
e) Housing,
f) Atmospheric pollution,
g) Light, heat and noise control,
h) Temperature and humidity control (Air condition),
i) Sanitation in industry, and
j) Radiation hazards.

(B) PERSONAL SERVICES

1. Preventive Medicine

a) Immunisation,
b) Preventive Health Examination,
c) Health Education,
d) Nutritional measures,
e) Carrier prevention,
f) Vital and Health statistics, and
g) Epidemiological studies of infectious and non-infectious diseases (heart diseases, diabetes, high blood pressure)

2. Social-cum-Preventive Medicine

a) Infant health,
b) Child and adolescent health,
c) School health,
d) Maternal health and,
e) Mental health.

3. Preventive Medicine-cum-Social Hygiene

a) Tuberculosis control,
b) Veneral disease control,

PREVENTIVE AND SOCIAL MEDICINE

c) Leprosy control,
d) Accident prevention.

4. Curative Medicine or Medical care

a) Hospitals,
c) Dispensaries
e) Clinics (paying/free).
g) Maternity homes,
b) Nursing homes,
d) Sanatorium,
f) Private clinics,
h) Convalescent care.

5. Social Medicine

a) Health centres,
b) Health promotion in hospital practice (Hospital and social service),
c) Health promotion in general practice,
d) Industrial health,
e) Rehabilitation of the sick, handicapped, neglected children, and the aged groups,
f) Rehabilitation of social casualities, illegitimate progenies and problem families,
g) Social surveys,
h) Social welfare, including social insurance, health insurance etc.
i) Population control, and
j) Family Planning.

II. UTILITIES OF THE STUDY OF PREVENTIVE AND SOCIAL MEDICINE (PSM)

Q1.3. Why we should study P.S.M. and what are it's utilities ?

PSM can be defined as the science and art of preserving and improving health. It embraces all factors which contribute to healthy living and preventing disease either in the individual or in the community as follows:

1) It imparts knowledge of maintaining good health, and to take necessary action to improve the quality of life physically as well as mentally.

2) It teaches us the art and science of maintaining, protecting and improving the health of the people through organised community efforts, which is known as Public Health. *Public Health* is concerned with the control of communicable diseases in the community and furnishes medical service to special groups of people.

3) Through *sanitation* we come to know all the efforts

towards the maintenance of—
a) Safe drinking water, free from pollution and harmful organisms,
b) Controlling the disposal of sewarage,
c) Conducting inspection of sanitary conditions of food supplies,
d) Enforces housing regulations,
e) Supervising the control of rats, flies, mosquitoes, and other intermediate sources of disease transmission.

4) Through *Social\Hygiene*, we come to know the problems of sex and from the health point of view we can adopt various measures for the control of veneral diseases.

5) *Maternity and Child Welfare* branch of PSM advise the mothers during pregnancies. These advices relate to proper diet in order to protect their children from deficiency diseases. To give immunisation to the children against the prevalent specific diseases such as smallpox, poliomyelities, diphtheria, whooping cough etc.

6) *Industrial Hygiene* gives us knowledge to promote and maintain the highest degree of physical, mental and social well-being of workers in all occupations and also to prevent and protect health from the various industrial hazards.

7) *Mental Hygiene* teaches us not only the rules and regulations to maintain normal mental health but also to prevent any mental disorders.

8) From *Social Medicine* we come to know the epidemiology of diseases, as epidemiology extends over the entire range of human disease taking into consideration the physical and social environments and constitutional factors which determine individual reactions to the environment.

9) Now, *PSM* also includes:
    a) Restorative Medicine,
    b) Conservative Medicine and Genetics,
    c) Socio-Medical Demography,
    d) Socio-Medical Anthropometry, and
    e) Socio-Medical Pathology.

a) *Restorative Medicine* gives us knowledge about the occupational rehabilitation of the patients. Generally it includes orthopaedics, plastic surgery, prosthesis, physiotherapy and all other methods by which the vocational and mental retaining can be effected and is assisted by welfare services including employment rehabilitation.

b) *Conservative Medicine and Genetics* are also included under PSM from which we come to know the best method of keeping the invalids and old people in the best possible physical and mental condition.

c) *Socio-Medical Demography* demonstrates before us the difference of reactions and behaviors of different classes and communities to the forces of birth, death and illness.

d) & e) *Socio-Medical Anthropometry* and *Socio-Medical Pathology*—The former reveals the inequalities in the physical and intellectual characteristics of these classes and the latter is elucidated by the joint observation of doctors, medical and social workers depicting the part played by the various social factors in the origin and progress of diseases.

*Besides these the study of **genetics** (heredity), **gerontology** (science of old age and the peoples), **geriaties** (the branch of medicine concerned with the treatment of old people), **demography** (the science of population growth), **psychology** (the science of mental function), **social science**, **social work** and **social services** etc., which work their contributions to establish new medical sociology i.e., Social Medicine gives us knowledge about the promotion of health, prevention of disease, diagnosis, treatment and social rehabilitation of the people. Even *family planning* also becomes an important branch of **PSM** which teaches us various family planning methods for enjoying our life also.

III. DEVELOPMENTAL HISTORY OF *PSM*

Q1.4. How *PSM* developed?, Or describe the developmental history of *PSM*?

Man like all other animals is the product of nature and is subjected to the influences of biological, physical and social environment. But because of his superior intellect and dynamic thinking and action he is constantly creating an artificial environment and exposing himself to far greater and frequent risk of damaging his health and body through diseases and injury than the animal kingdom. Thus arose the necessity of adopting certain steps against injuries and diseases inspite of these appearing mysterious to him.

1st Stage : In fact the primitive man, having no knowledge of how disease was caused and how it spreaded, so he was depending more on preventing disease than on cure. For instance, he was avoiding things proved to be harmful, he sought fresh and wholesome food and exposed himself to fresh air and sunshine and kept himself vigorously in sports and hunting. So the stage comes nearer to living on timely hygienic life than his civilised descendents of the present time or despite and latter's boasted civilisation.

2nd Stage : As the idea and knowledge improved the second stage of preventive medicine which he/she undertook with good effects was called *personal/hygiene*, as depicated in *Manu's Law of Health and Mosaic Codes*, incorporated with religious practice.

So religion in prevention of disease held the field for many centuries till a new orientation was given by the Greek Priest Physician Hippocrates in the 4th century B.C.

3rd Stage : Hippocrates followed the simultaneous search for causes and remedies which led to the study of anatomy, physiology, pathology and biochemistry for the better understanding of the disease process and to evolving progressively improved methods of diagnosis and treatment i.e. *clinical medicine and therapeutics.*

4th Stage : The position improved further with the discovery of microscope and other physical instrument in aid of diagnosis and of vital statistics during the 17th and 18th centuries. This combined with the industrial revolution in the western countries, the Preventive Medicine took the shape of Public Health, epitomised by the discovery of vaccination against small pox by *Edward Jenner in 1798.*

5th Stage : But the greatest landmark of *PSM* is the discovery of microbe in the 19th century and its final establishment as an agent of causation of large number of the prevalent diseases by Pastur in the seventies of the century

(1870). Then followed a plethora of discoveries such as specific microbes causing different diseases, the smallest being the ultramicroscopic viruses and knowledge of infection and immunity in man and animal.

Final Stage : So towards the last public health era of preventive medicine the host, the agent and the environmental factors of disease received full consideration. But it was soon realised that this was not enough for dealing with epidemic diseases like Tuberculosis, Leprosy, Veneral diseases, man made Malaria, Cholera, Diarrhoea and Dysentery. The social, cultural and socio-economic factors of disease were often found to play very important role in their perpetuation. Nutritional disorders, cardiac complaints and even mental disorders, arise from social disorders. The Western countries achieved better health and higher expectation of life by improvement of socio-economic condition, and later by preventive medicine. According to the famous scientist BERNAL "an overwhelming majority of diseases throughout the world are due to direct or indirect lack of primary necessities, such as, food, shelter etc. and many of the remainder are attributed to bad working condition."

There was thus need to supplement preventive medicine by the study of social factors i.e, *Preventive Medicine* has to be further modified, so as to be more rational and radical in its approach in dealing with human illness including treatment into *PSM.*

According to his concept the disease connates an impairment in the physical, mental and social well being of the individual and of the society at large and *PSM* is the science and art of preserving and improving health embracing all factors which contribute to healthy living and prevention of disease either in the individual or in the community.

•Developmental stages of PSM.

1st Stage	4th Stage
[Primitive stage : Avoidance of harmful things, seeking of fresh air, sunshine and wholesome food, maintenance of	[Origin of *Public Health* and discovery of Vaccination of smallpox by *Edward Jenner.*]

health by hunting or by sports.]

2nd Stage
[Maintenance of personal hygiene by various religious practice.]

3rd Stage
[Origin of Clinical Medicine and Therapeutics by *Hippocrates*.]

5th Stage
[Discovery of microbes i.e., causation of diseases, discovery of ultramicroscopic viruses, knowledge of infection and immunity.]

6th Stage
[Consideration of the disease as caused by various social factors. Finally origin of Preventive and Social Medicine.]

IV. CHANGING CONCEPT OF "HYGIENE AND PUBLIC HEALTH" TO "PSM"

Q1.5. Subject "Hygiene and Public Health" has become the subject "PSM"—Discuss why such change has taken place ?

Subject *"Hygiene and Public Health"* has changed to *"PSM"*, so the common question is why such type of change occured.

First of all *Hygiene* has been defined as the science of health as personified in the Greek goddess *Hygiea* and embraces all factors which contributes to healthful living by preventing disease either in the individual or in the community. When different measures are applied for the wellbeing of the community as a whole in an organised manner, it is known as *Public Health*. So the main object of *Hygiene* was to teach the individual to take necessary action to improve the quality of his life physically and mentally for buoyanting health through out his life and *Public Health* was originally concerned only with environmental sanitation.

But at present *Public Health* has different fields of activities and this is now concerned with the control of communicable diseases, in the protection of the community and with furnishing medical service to special groups of persons. It is also concerned with maternity and child welfare, school hygiene, epidemiology and vital statistics, health education, industrial hygiene, and mental hygiene etc. So besides environmental sanitation as these are included under Hygiene and Public Health, they are considered under the heading of Preventive Medicine.

Secondly, it is considered that the disease is an abnormal state which results from harmful effects of processes, injurious substances or accidents and illness is not necessarily due to disease but due to several other factors such as environment, housing, malnutrition, bad effects of industry, bad economic conditions and ways of life etc. Recently as these factors are included under Social Medicine, or as the Social Medicine has the role of studying these factors which are indirectly effecting the person and the disease process and it places emphasis on man's consideration in relation to its environment and the prevention of non-infective diseases such as peptic ulcer, myocardial infraction and accidental injuries etc., the subject *Hygiene and Public Health* take up the new heading *Preventive and Social Medicine (PSM)*.

Recently LEAVELL and CLARKE consider that *Public Health* is only a division of *PSM* as it involves only that part of the discipline which requires organises community effort or action.

V. PREVENTIVE MEDICINE AND IT'S MAIN OBJECTS

Q.1.6. What is meant by Preventive Medicine?

According to BOYD, Preventive Medicine may be defined as the branch of applied biology which seeks to reduce or eradicate disease by removing or alternating the responsible and associated etiological factors.

GALDSTON defines it as consisting of two sections namely, *Personal Preventive Medicine and Community Preventive Medicine*. The later is the province largely of sanitary engineer, chemist, epidemiologist and public health officer while the former is principally the domain of the medical practitioners dealing with the individual practice and the Communal Preventive Medicine is the main domain of health officer.

SIMILIE defines Preventive Medicine as the activities that are catered to individual in family as unit, and Public Health is representing community responsibility which are carried out for community benefit.

WINSLOW (accepted by WHO) defines Preventive Medicine as, "It is the science and art of preventing disease, prolonging life, promoting physical and mental health and efficiency, through organised community efforts for the sanitation of individual in the principle of personal hygiene, the organisation of medical and nursing services for the easily diagnosis and preventive treatment of disease and the development of social machinery which will ensure to every individual in the community a standard living adequate for the maintainance of health."

Main Objects : According to BOYD its main objects are Hygiene and Sanitation. Hygiene is the proper care of the various organs and tissues while sanitation is the proper cleanliness of the environment i.e., health of the individual and health of the community.

Generally, *Preventive Medicine* includes environmental sanitation, control of communicable or non-communicable diseases, degenerative diseases, accidents, good health habits, maternity and child care, child guidance, genetic counselling, health promotion and adequate health services for the individual, healthful environment at the place of work.

VI. SOCIAL MEDICINE AND IT'S MAIN OBJECTS

Q.1.7. What is meant by Social Medicine and what are it's main objectives?

According to RYLE who started the first Institute of Social Medicine at Oxford in 1942 states that Social Medicine embodies the idea of Medicine applied to the service of man as *socius*, as fellow or comrade, with a view to better understanding and more durable assistance of all his main and contributory troubles which are inimical to active health and not merely to removing or all eviating a present pathology. It also embodies the idea of medicine applied to service of socialists for the community of man a view to lowering the incidence of all preventable diseases and raising the general level of human fitness.

Social Medicine emphasises on man and endeavours to study him in relation to both physical and social environment i.e., diet, housing, clothing, air, sunlight, working conditions, leisure and other factors including habits and way of life. It considers that disease is an abnormal stage which results form harmful effects of proceses, injuries, substances or accidents. The illness is not necessarily due to disease but due to several other factors such as environment, housing, malnutrition, bad effects of industry, bad economic conditions and ways of life etc. It is also concerned with all diseases, including cancer, hypertension, heart disease, psychoneuroses, accidents etc., all of which have their epidemiological co-relation with social and occupational conditions.

In hospital practice, Social Medicine stresses upon man as a whole and involves medical, social work, social diagnosis, social pathology, social therapy, aftercare, rehabilitation and readjustment of lives of individual and families. Among other contents may be mentioned medical aspects (health, happiness and efficiency) of human and social biology and human ecology. According to professor Crew, the laboratory of social medicine is the organised community in which the problems of social physiology, pathology and theraphy are clearly to be seen. Biostatistics and health education are the two pillars of both medicine and social science constituting Social Medicine.

Def : Social Medicine is a branch of medicine which deals with the preservation or eradication of disease with the promotion of general level of human fitness, physically as well as mentally and spiritually along with the studying of his total environment i.e., physical, biological, psychological and socio-economical relationship.

So, in the practice of Social Medicine, the physician is therefore interested in the man in disease and not merely in the disease in man. He sees the individual not only as a patient entity but also in his relationship to his family, work place and the community as an aggregate. This idea of Social Medicine has been advocated by Hahnemann about 200 years ago by the words "we treat the patient but not the disease."

Main Objects :

a) Studies of health and disease in the context of the individual family and community in relationship to heredity, personal and impersonal (environmental factors);

b) Determination from such studies of methodology, programmes and procedures by using all necessary medical as well as non-medical measures by which

i) Health can be promoted, protected and preserved;

ii) Disease can be prevented or eradicated, cured or ameliorated;

iii) Patients can be rehabilitated socially, economically and mentally.

c) Concerning itself with the social policy and action for organisation of the measures for social application of the methods suitable for the purpose, for the benefit of the individual, family, community, nation and humanity.

d) Also Social Medicine has two main facets:

i) *Academic Discipline* and

ii) *Social Service.*

i) As an academic discipline, it comprises of the medical and social science. The medical sciences are clinical medicine along with other basic and biological sciences. It also includes epidemiology and biostatistics. The social science comprises of behavioural sciences e.g., anthropology, sociology and social psychology and other social sciences e.g., economics, political science, history etc.

ii) As a *social service,* it is involved in social action for the organisation of health and welfare services in the service of the people at various levels by the state, community organisation or voluntary agents.

PREVENTIVE AND SOCIAL MEDICINE 19

As such, Social Medicine becomes a branch of social science and a field of social service applying practically every basic science directed towards comprehensive programme of community health for the purpose of promotion of health, maintenance of health by preventive and curative measures, and social and economic rehabilitation.

Q.1.8. Why we will study Social Medicine, or what are the utilities of the study of Social Medicine?

We should study social medicine as it secures the health of the population and it's tasks are:

a) to assess the health status of the population and its development;

b) to assess the sanitary condition of the environment;

c) to work out methods and means leading to the promotion of the health of the people and the prevention of disease, disability and infirmity;

d) to organise medical care and rehabilitation for the whole population;

e) to control sanitary conditions in the environment; and

f) to control the birth rate in order to secure the harmonious development of the population.

[N.B. Also see to the last part of the Answer of the Q. No1.7 (d)]

VII. HAHNEMANN'S VIEW OF HEALTH AND DISEASE

Q.1.9. What is Health? Describe the Hahnemann's views regarding health.

OR

What are the basic constituents which determine the quality of health?

According to World Health Organisation (WHO) "health is a state of complete physical, mental and social well-being and not merely the absence of disease or infirmity."

But it is difficult to achieve complete physical, mental and social well-being in our worldly life which is constantly being impinged upon by a host of forces and factors, and health can not be conceived as a fixed quantum.

So a clear definition of health is—"Health is a flexible state of body or mind which may be described in terms of a range within which a person, due to the operation of internal or external stimuli-physical, chemical, physiological, psychological or socio-biological (Bio-PSYCHO-Socio GEN) may sway from the conditions wherein he is at the peak of enjoyment of physical, mental and emotional experiences, as influenced by his genetic constitution, environment, age, sex and socio-biological characteristics, and can regain that position without any external aid."

Therefore the raw materials or the constituents which determine the quality of health are:

1. Biological Constitution

a) Genetic inheritance;
b) Adaptability to climatic change;
c) Adaptability to resist privation, bacterial infection, toxic agents and adaptability time;
d) Physiological normality and vigour.

2. Mental or Emotional Constitution

a) Behaviour pattern;
b) Stability of mind (normality);
c) Capacity for control and discipline;
d) Choice of recreation.

3. Social Constitution

a) Adequate food and drink;
b) Adequate living conditions;
c) Occupation (employment);
d) Right consciousness, spiritual and moral standard;
e) Standard of education and knowledge;
f) Level of medical and health care.

The negative concept of health defines health as an avoidance of disease i.e., prevention of disease, but the positive concept is the promotion of health, which in turn demands the improvement of working and living conditions. Thus health promotion can be achieved by higher standard of living viz. good food, proper housing, adequate working facilities, etc. and according to positive concept, health has been defined as "a state of feeling well in body, mind and spirit, together with a sense of reserve power, based upon normal functioning of tissues, a practical understanding of principles of healthy living, a harmonious adjustment to the environment (physical and phychological), is a means to rich life of service."

Hahnemann's View

Dr. Hahnemann says about health in the 9th aphorism of the *Organon*, "*In the health condition of man, the spiritual Vital Force (autocracy), the dynamis that animates the material body (organism), rules with unbounded sway and retain all parts of the organism in admirable, harmonious, vital operations, as regards both sensation, and functions so that our indweling, reason gifted mind can be feely employ this living, healthy, instrument for the higher purposes of our existence.*"

Thus, Dr. Hahnemann gives to health the quality of moral power without which health is not possible. He would not call a dacoit a healthy person, because he is devoid of the moral will power so essential for the health.

Health depends on the following conditions :

1) Healthy parents.
2) Training and pursuing of healthy habits.
3) Nutritional and wholesome food.
4) Sanitary environment and residence.
5) Precautions from polluted air, water and food in order to prevent infectious diseases.
6) Preventive measures against communicable diseases, and
7) Supply of deficiencies as and when they occur during life.

So health is the highest virtue and every person must keep in mind that happiness depends in a large measure upon the personal health and the health of his near and dear ones. Physical exercises, pranayam and exercises for the development of nervous system and control of mind have been recognised from ancient times as very useful for the achievement of health and peace of mind.

Q.1.13. What is Disease? Describe the Hahnemann's view regarding disease. What are the factors that are responsible for disease?

Disease is an abnormal state of the body and mind that arises out of maladjustment with external and internal environment due to the operations of socio-biological, physical, chemical, physiological or psychological stimuli (Bio-Socio-GEO-GENS) on man, operating beyond the scope of physiological recovery on the part of the subject, resulting in an alteration of his normal activities or reduction of efficiency by causing modification or damage to the body cells or of systems of cells or their substratum, and leading to an unpleasant state of body and mind and other associated phenomena (signs and symptoms), and ending in recovery, chronicity or ultimately to death.

The factors which are considered for the disease prevalance, are:

i) host factors and (ii) environmental factors.

I. HOST FACTORS

a) Genetic, heredity and diathesis.
b) Racial factors and herd structure—blood groups and other ethnic and anthropological characters.
c) Adaptability.
d) Anatomical and physiological status—constitutional defects, endocrine disorder.
e) Diet and nutritional standards.
f) Over exertion, fatigue and exposure.

II. ENVIRONMENTAL FACTORS

A. Biological

i) *Causative agents:* Microbes, toxins, persons, injuries, physical and chemical agents.
ii) *Transmisson factors—reservoir*—man, animal and soil,
Insect vectors: mosquito, fly flea, ticks, mites etc. —.
Water, milk, food, drinks, fruits, vegetables, fingers, human and animal excreta.
iii) state of artificial immunisation against various diseases.

B. Socio-Economic

i) *Population:* Urban and rural, density and distribution, rate of growth, age and sex structure.
ii) *Standard of living:* diet and nutrition, housing and sanitation, clothing, occupation, income and expenditure.
iii) *Cultural:* literacy and standard of education, outlook on food and on causes and prevention of disease, intra and extra familial relationship, attitude towards community.

iv) *Religious customs and superstition:* marriage, custom, tradition and superstitious beliefs.
v) *Human activities*: movement, aggregation and dispersal etc.
vi) State of disabilities and addiction.
vii) Communication facilities.
viii) Standard of medical care and public health service.

C. Geo-Physical Condition

i) *Climate:* Latitude and longitude, temperature and humidity, rainfall, barometric pressure, sunshine and cloudiness, wind direction and radiation, seasonal changes;
ii) *Soil characteristics:* Laterite, alluvial, granite, sandy clay etc.;
iii) *Relief:* plains, mountains, seaside, plateau, desert;
iv) *Hydrography:* rivers, canals, lakes, irrigation channels;
v) *Terestial:* Magnetism, radioactivity;
vi) *Biogeographical:* Vegetable, animal life in water and on land, parasitism in human beings and animals;
vii) *Natural calamities:* storm, earthquake, flood, draught and famine;
viii) Prevalent diseases,
A balance between man (host) and environment centre-Connotes health, and imbalance beyond certain limit-disease and gross imbalance leads to death.

Hahnemann's View:

Disease means dis-ease or when a person does not feel at ease. There are some abnormal sensations and functions which deny him the ease felt during health.

Dr. Hahnemann says in aphorism 12 of the *Organon*, "It is the morbidly affected vital force that produces disease" and in aphrosim 11 of the *Organon* he says, "when a person falls ill, it is only this spiritual, self-acting (automatic) vital force everywhere present in his organism that is primarily deranged by the dynamic influence upon it of a morbific agent inimical to life; it is only the vital force, deranged to such an abnormal state, that can furnish the organism with the disagreeable sensations, and incline to the irregular processes which we call disease; for, as a power invisible in itself, and only cognisable by its effects on the organism, its morbid derangements only make itself known by the manifestation of disease in the sensations and functions of these parts of the organism exposed to the sense of the observer and the physician that is, by morbid symptoms, and in no other way can it make itself known.

The difference between homoeopathic and allopathic conception of disease is that a homoeopath considers the phenomenon of disease of the sickness of a particular individual vitally connected with his life, whereas an allopath considers disease as an independent and universal phenomenon, each disease has its seperate existence in nature; any change from the normal, from biochemical structural and functional findings in the different systems, organs, tissues, cells and fluids of the patient is regarded as disease from the pathological point of view. This is essentially a materialistic view of disease.

PART I

PHYSIOLOGICAL HYGIENE

"we eat to live"

CHAPTER-II

FOOD AND NUTRITION

DISCUSSION FOR LEARNING

I. Food in relation to health.
II. Balanced diet.
III. Nutritional deficiencies.
IV. Vitamin deficiencies.
V. Malnutrition and it's prevention (PCM/PEM).
VI. Assessment of nutritional status.
VII. Milk and pasteurisation of milk.
VIII. Preservation of food.
IX. Adulteration of food.
X. Powers of Food Inspector.
XI. Food poisoning.
XII. Diseases from food.
XIII. Dieto-therapy (Diets in diseases).

I. FOOD IN RELATION TO HEALTH

Q.2.1. What is food and what is nutrition?

What we eat is not food. *Food* signifies substances of either animal or vegetable origin, containing different nutrients like *protein, fat, carbohydrate, mineral* and *vitamin* which are utilised in the human body for the purpose of (a) liberation of heat and energy, (b) building up of body tissues for growth and repair of wear and tear, and (c) protection of the body against infection and disease.

Nutrition is the process of assimilating food. The study of nutrition is the study of foods and their use in diet and therapy. The word nutrition is derived from *nutrious* meaning to suckle at breast, and it is a dynamic process in which the food is consumed and is utilised for nourishing the body.

FOOD AND NUTRITION

Q.2.2. Why food is required?

(a) Life is practically synonymous with *activity* or *work* and work demands *energy* or the *vital force* and the source of this energy is the metabolism of food. So basically food is essential for life to supply *energy*

(b) An animal without food must live on its own resources for certain period. After that it would ultimately die for want of food. So *food is essential for repair and growth and maintaining long life.*

(c) For various life processes, such as in the mechanism of transformation of food stuff into substances suitable for utilisation, certain temperature of the medium is essential, what is known as the *body temperature* or *the body heat* which remains nearly at a constant level (97°- 98.4 F) throughout life in health. So to maintain this heat certain food factors, particularly the carbohydrates and fats are the essential fuels.

(d) To maintain the equilibrium of carbon and water in the body, metabolism of the food constituents carbohydrates and fats is essential.

(e) The proteins are also required as food as they replenish the wear and tear of the tissues and for the formation of specific tissues proteins and the various secretions are essential.

(f) Vitamins and minerals protect the body from various types of disease and are essential for secretions of enzymes and growth promoting substances for maintenance of health.

Q.2.3. What are the main functions of food?

The main functions of food are:
- a) Provision of energy,
- b) Provide nutrients for:
  - (i) Body building and repair, wear and tear,
  - (ii) Maintenance and regulation of body temperature, water balance and growth, and
  - (iii) Development and formation of specific tissue substances like enzymes and hormones.
- c) Protection of the body from various diseases and infections.

Q.2.4. What would be our food or what will be the essential constituents of our diet?

The ideal food is a platable mixture of substances to satisfy the cravings of living organisms for maintenance of form and energy. This craving is the natural demand to replenish the wear and tear of the body and supply the fuel for the ever-present fire so necessary for the activities of life as also for growth. A living body is not a man-made machinery; and the needs of life present a variable factor—an individual problem, not even of class/order. For instance, the food of one animal may be poison for another, and again the food of any one season or age could not be the food for all the time and all ages. So one has got to study him from all points of view—his taste, his habits of life, his daily excretion, and above all his tolerance. We can only at best give a general scheme of food or diet to recast and redisbursed according to individual craving and requirement. So the normal diet or essential constituents of our diet should be:

a) An adequate proportion of different energy forming food stuffs like *carbohydrate* and *fat* to provide calories for the requirement of the body under the normal condition or the muscular work.

b) It must contain the tissue forming substances like *proteins and minerals* (calcium, phosphorus, iron etc.) and essential amino acids to compensate the loss of substances of the body as a result of the wear and tear of the tissues in the process of metabolism and due to work and age.

c) It also must contain the accessory food factors like *vitamins* to provide energy for ensuring proper growth, nutrition and tissue cell activities and for the prevention of health from the disease.

The body of a young adult human male weighing 65 kg consists of some 11 kg of protein, 9 of fat, 1 of carbohydrates, 4 of minerals and 40 of water.

Q.2.5. What is meant by proximate principles of food?

The chemical compounds which are present in the food are mainly responsible for carrying out all the functions of food and are known as proximate principles of food.

FOOD AND NUTRITION

Generally the normal diet contains:
- i) *Carbohydrates* ii) *Proteins* iii) *Fats*
- iv) *Minerals (essential or trace elements)*
- v) *Vitamins and* vi) *Water*

These are known as the proximate principles of food. The first three of these are for energy production, growth and maintenance of tissues and the last three are essential for chemical mechanisms i.e., for the utilisation of energy synthesis of various metabolities viz. enzymes, hormones etc.

II. BALANCED DIET

Q.2.6. What is meant by balanced diet?

A diet is said to be balanced one if it contains different food items in proper amount, quality and proportion, so as to carry out the following three basic functions in the body:

- i) Energy giving function,
- ii) Body building function,
- iii) Protective function.

Moreover, a balanced diet should be cheap, nutritious and within the economic means of the people, catering to their liking and taste and should contain enough of roughage materials to promote peristalsis.

Q.2.7. What is protein?

The word protein is derived from the Greek work *proteus* which means "of first importance". Moulder in 1840 suggested this terminology, as protein can be considered as the food of great importance. Proteins are one of the basic constitutents of our diet and mainly consists of *Carbon, Hydrogen, Oxygen, Nitrogen,* sometimes *Sulphur* and *Phosphorus.* Proteins are built by amino-acids. So the protein molecule is a polymer of *amino-acids* joined in *peptide linkage.* It has high molecular weight, the average molecular weight is 36,000. The properties and characterstics of proteins are determined by the *amino-acids* composition in the protein molecule and arrangement in which they are placed within it. The value of the protein depends on its amino-acid content. Generally 23 amino acids are known of which on an average, 20 different amino acids occur in most proteins. When we eat protein, it is digested as amino acids and then they are absorbed in blood. Some types of amino acids can be pepared in our body (non-essential aminoacids). But some types of amino acids cannot be produced in our body. To get these amino acids, we must eat food containing these amino acids and these are called essential amino-acids. They are mostly present in animal protein i.e., meat, fish, egg, and milk and hence these animal proteins are called superior proteins or proteins of high biological value. The proteins from the vegetable kingdom like pulse, gram, wheat, nuts etc. lack of one or more of these essential amino acids, and so vegetable proteins are called inferior proteins or proteins of low biological value. Our diet usually consists of 20 amino acids and out of these 10 are essential amino acids. The essential amino acids for man are *tryptophane, lysine, methonine, leucine, isoleucine, valine, phenylalanine and threonine. Arginine* and *histidine* are essential for rats but not for men.

Non-essential amino acids are also essential for life, but they can be synthesized within the body from other amino acids, viz *cystine, tyrosine, alanine, glycine* and *asparatic acid* etc.

The biological value of protein is the percentage of protein digested and utilised to replace protein (generally it is 60% or less).

UTILITIES

Q.2.8. (a) What are the utilities of proteins?

Protein cannot be stored in the body. After the intake of necessary amount of protein for growth and repair, the excess protein is broken down to urea, uric acid, creatine etc, and during this process heat and energy is liberated to the body. One gram of protein gives out 4.1 calories of heat. One gram of protein is required per 1 kg of the body weight.

FOOD AND NUTRITION

Normally a person required about 75 grams of protein a day. However, children and pregnant women require more protein. Generally proteins are changed to carbohydrate during starvation.

By eating less protein, the growth of the body will not be proper. Children suffer from malnutrition, Kwashiorkor's disease due to protein deficiency. By eating more protein we suffer from constipation, high blood pressure, gout etc.

FUNCTIONS

Q.2.8.(b) What are the functions of proteins?

Dietary proteins are mainly utilised in the body for carrying out specific functions which cannot be done by other food constituents; such as:

a) Building up of body tissues, and maintaining growth,
b) Repair of wear and tear of tissues,
c) Specific dynamic action,
d) Formation of enzymes and hormones,
e) Formation of antibodies,
f) Maintenance of fluid balance, and the neutrality regulation of the blood and tissue fluids,
g) Regulation of osmotic pressure, and
h) about 60% of protein can be transformed into carbohydrates during starvation and in certain conditions it can synthesis fat.

FATS

Q. 2.9. (a) What are fats?

Fats are normally esters of fatty acids with glycerol and commonly known as tri-glycerides. They are also one of the basic constitutents of our diet and consist of hydrogen, oxygen and carbon, of which hydrogen and oxygen ratio is other than 2:1. Fats may be from animal or vegetable kingdom. The animal fats are saturated fats and they remain solid at room temperature. Fish fat is unsaturated and remains in liquid form. Vegetable fats are unsaturated fats and remain in liquid form. Only coconut oil is saturated fat and may be in solid form.

The saturated fats are hard for digestion. The unsaturated fats are easily digestible. Animal fats contain Vitamins A,D,E,K. The vegetable fats do not contain vitamins A and D.

Only carrot has carotein which is converted to vitamin A. Vitamin E is present in vegetable oil.

Unsaturated fat can be made saturated fat by the process of hydrogenation. It becomes solid at room temperature and is called "Vanaspati". In Vanaspati 700 I.U. of vitamin A and 50 I.U. of vitamin D are added per ounce.

Q. 2.9 (b) What are the uses of fat in our body?

i) Fats are called a source of reserved energy of the body. In case of starvation of carbohydrates, fats change to carbohydrate and glucose and then supply energy to the body. Generally 1 gram of fat will give 9.3 calories of heat.

ii) Fats are said to be protein sparing food as fat diminishes protein metabolism. If only protein is given, then the body will require large amount of protein. If fat is added in the food, then the protein demand is considerably reduced.

iii) Essential fatty acids are the acids that cannot be produced by the body. They must come through food. They are in the unsaturated fatty acids. They keep the skin smooth and healthy. They also keep the blood fat (i.e. cholesterol) low, and thereby prevent the hardening of the arteries and ultimately, the thrombosis of the blood vessels are low. (Linolic acid is a such type of essential fatty acid).

iv) The sub-cutaneons fat acts as a non-conductor.

v) Animal fats contain fat soluble vit. A, vit. D. Generally skin fat (ergosterol) becomes vit. D by the rays of the sun and prevents rickets.

*Fat from the body cannot be reduced by less intake of fat. That can be reduced by exercise. About 60 grams of fat is necessary for a normal person daily. If fat intake is less, the reserved energy will be less. If fat intake is more, then the person may suffer from indigestion, dyspepsia, flatulence, and become fatty and susceptible to thrombosis of blood vessels.

FOOD AND NUTRITION

CARBOHYDRATE

Q. 2.10. What are carbohydrates?

Carbohydrates are one of our basic constituents of diet and consist of carbon, hydrogen and oxygen, of which hydrogen and oxygen ratio is 2:1. Carbohydrate gives energy to the body, and maintains the body heat. Starch, rice, wheat, vegetables, cane sugar, fruits etc. mainly contain carbohydrates. All carbohydrates are digested to glucose and then absorbed in the blood.

Glucose is stored in liver and in muscles of the body as glycogen. Excess of carbohydrates may be converted into fat and stored under the skin. Fat also consists of carbon, hydrogen and oxygen. So fat can be changed to carbohydrate and carbohydrate can be converted to fat. When carbohydrates in the muscles are oxidised, CO_2, H_2O are formed and during this process, energy is liberated. One gram of carbohydrates give 4.0 calories of heat. Normally a person requires 400 grams of carbohydrates a day. During starvation, the body protein is broken down to produce glucose, and maintain the glucose level in blood. By eating more carbohydrates we may suffer from flatulence or become fatty or diabetic.

Q.2.11. What is meant by Specific Dynamic Action (SDA) of proteins?

The basal metabolism increases with the metabolism of every kind of food but it was noticed that proteins in excess would raise metabolism to greater degree without doing any external work. Rubner called it as the Specific Dynamic Action of proteins. Mitchels, Lusk and others recently suggested the alternative term *calorigenic action of food stuffs* and this drug like stimulation of metabolism is probably due to carboxylic residues which are left after deamination of the amino acids. Rubner found that proteins utilised for growth exert very little specific dynamic action, but amino acids, such as glycine, alanine, leacine, glutumic acid, tyrosine and phenylalanine, are mostly responsible for the production of the specific dynamic action—the proteins actually metabolised for energy contribution.

Direct human calorimetry has confirmed that each gram of protein is capable of producing 4.1 calories of heat and specific dynamic action does not involve extra production of the calories out of the proteins. Every type of food stimulates metabolism but protein stimulates most. While proteins contribute 36% above the basal work, fats 12% and carbohydrates 6%. An animal fed on 100 grams of protein only, would yield heat energy to the extent of 410 calories only, never more but this ingestion of assimilable proteins would increase general metabolism in the tissues. The total energy output in a given time would show 36% above the basal. Thus if 1500 calories was the basal quota, 100 grams of proteins would, while being metabolised, give rise to 2040 calories, i.e. 36% above the basal unit. Calorimetry shows that 100 grams of protein should contribute 410 calories only and the excess of 130 calories becomes the quota of extra amount of heat energy, due to the specific dynamic action of the proteins effecting extra general metabolism.

Q.2.12. What is the most important inorganic component of human body?

It is water. The total body water constitutes 50% to 70% of adult body weight; the values are somewhat lower in women than in men and decrease with increase in age.

The total body water is distributed into two main compartments *water within cells* (intra-cellular fluid) and water outside cells (extra-cellular fluid). The intra-cellular and extra-cellular spaces or compartments contribute about 50% and 20% of the body weight respectively. The extra-cellular fluid is further divided into (a) plasma water or inter-vascular fluid (water circulating in the blood vessels constituting 5% of the body weight); and (b) interstitial fluid (water as extra-cellular fluid present outside the blood vessels constituting 15% of the body weight).

Q.2.13. What are the functions of water in our body?

OR

Why water is necessary for human body?

The water for human body is of an utmost importance to perform the following specific physiological functions:

FOOD AND NUTRITION

1) It acts as solvent for the secretary and excretory products,
2) It acts as a carrier of nutritive elements to tissues and removes waste materials from them;
3) Water is a solvent for electrolytes. It helps to regulate electrolyte balance of the body and maintain a healthy equilibrium of osmotic pressure exerted by solubles dissolved in water. A state of good health is possible as long as the osmotic pressure exerted by the solubles remain constant; and
4) It is a regulator of body temperature; evaporation is the main way of conducting heat to outside and dissipating it. The latent heat of evaporation of water is high, so the loss of a small amount of water in evaporated sweat means a relatively greater loss of heat.

*Besides these water is more important than food. Deprivation of water brings about death much more quickly than that of food. Loss about 10% of body water causes illness and a further loss of about 10% may cause death. It is also seen that if water is given but food is not, the individual may survive for several weeks by utilizing the body fat and 50% of the tissue protein. Sometimes much water is lost from the body, such as in the case of diarrhoea accompanied by vomiting leading to dehydration. If not controlled immediately, it may lead to death. It is controlled by giving water with salt orally or glucose solution parenterally. This fact also suggests the necessity of water.

Q.2.14. (a) What are the essential factors to be considered to make a good diet chart?

The factors which are essential and to be considered for making a good diet are as follows:

1) The diet must meet the total caloric requirement of an individual depending upon age, sex, physiological condition, height, weight, build, occupation and work etc.

2) It must contain required amounts of all food articles like carbohydrates, proteins, fats, minerals and vitamins.

3) The protein and fat should be derived from both animal and vegetable sources.

4) Vitamins and minerals should be present insufficient quantities in assimiable form and the food should contain enough roughage to promote peristalsis.

5) The diet must be cheap so as the person can buy it easily.

6) The food articles must be easily available in the locality for long continued use.

7) The food should be socially acceptable i.e., religious and social factors are most important.

8) For a non-vegetarian, there should be supplementation of the vegetable proteins from more than one sources i.e., from pulses, atta, rice, soyabean etc. instead of one. Milk or milk products, fruits are four times richer than that of meat and pulses to be considered.

9) Absorbility of food is to be considered. A food that is easily digested may not necessarily be completely absorbed and vice versa. Carbohydrates are more completely absorbed than the proteins and fats, and more readily absorbed than the vegetable ones.

Q.2.14 (b) How we will make a good diet chart?

OR

How we can prepare a balanced diet chart? Explain with examples.

To prepare a good diet chart or balanced diet chart the basic consideration is the selection of food items and their quantities per day, according to the availability of foods, purchasing power, food habit of an individual and keeping in view the over all total requirement of nutrients i.e. requirement of an individual per day.

Generally energy for physiological process is provided by the combination of carbohydrates and proteins. The daily energy requirement or the daily caloric need is the sum of the basal energy demand pluse that is required for the additional work of the day.

FOOD AND NUTRITION

The energy is quantitatively expressed as unit of heat which in this case is the kilo caloric (K cal.).

So the quantity of food will be proportional to total energy requirement of the individual. The total energy requirement can be calculated from the following data:
i) Basal Metabolic Rate (B.M.R.)
ii) Nature of work done.
iii) Allowance for growth, and working hours.

Examples

If the average height of an Indian male adult is 5ft ½ inch i.e. 164 cm, normal weight is 75 kg, and total surface area is 1.8 sq. meters, the total caloric requirements in 24 hours is 3000 *K calories* (at the rate of B M R 40 K cal per hrs. per sq. meters of surface area of a person).

Basically this amount of heat derived by the oxidation of proteins, fats and carbohydrates, and the amount of heat yields by these three are 307.5 K cal, 199.5 K cal and 697.5 K cal respectively.

As one gram of carbohydrates liberates 4 K cal heat, one gram of protein liberates 4.1 K cal heat and one gram of fat liberates 9.3 K cal heat, so the total amount of carbohydrates, proteins and fats required to make a good diet or balanced diet chart of an Indian male adult are :

$$Carbohydrates = \frac{199.5}{4} \text{ gms} = 498.7 \text{ gms (500 gms approx)}$$

$$Proteins = \frac{307.5}{4.1} \text{ gms} = 75 \text{ gms, and}$$

$$Fats = \frac{697.5}{9.3} = 75 \text{ gms}$$

Q.2.14.(c) What is the composition of an balanced diet of an Indian adult man and women doing moderate work (vegetarian and non-vegetarian)

The following is the composition of an ideal balanced diet suitable for an Indian normal adult male and female, vegetarian and non-vegetarian, which is recommended by the I.C.M.R. Nutrition Expert Committee.

Balanced diet for Indian Adult Male and Female doing moderate work.

Items of food	Male adult Quantity (gms per days) Veg.	Male adult Quantity (gms per days) Non-veg.	Female adult Quantity (gms per day) Veg.	Female adult Quantity (gms per day) Non-veg.	Additional allowances preg-nancy	Additional allowances Lactation
1. Cereals (rice wheat, maize etc.)	475	475	350	350	50	100
2. Pulses	80	65	70	55	x	10
3. Green leafy vegetables	125	125	125	125	25	25
4. Other vegetables	75	75	75	75	-	-
5. Roots and tubers	100	100	75	75	-	-
6. Fruits	30	30	30	30	-	-
7. Milk	200	200	200	100	125	125
8. Fats and oils	40	40	35	40	x	15
9. Fish and Meat	x	30	x	30	-	-
10. Eggs	x	30	x	30	-	-
11. Sugar and Jaggery	40	40	30	30	10	20

N.B. 1. For vegetarian, 15 gms. of pulses and 100 gms. of milk should be increased.

2. Quantity of cereals will vary according to the geographical area.

3. In fat and oils, one third of the fat should be from animal origin.

Q.2.15. (a) What is the composition of a balanced diet for Indian children and adolescents ? (for school and college going students).

The following is the composition of a balanced diet of Indian children and adolescents as recommended by the Nutrition Expert Committee. See table 2.15(a).

For Balanced diet for Indian Children and Adolescents. I.C.M.R. 1981

Items of Food	Pre-school going children				School going children				Adolescents (School & College going students)			
	1-3 years age		4-6 years age		7-9 years		10-12 years		Boys 13-18 years		Girls 13-18 years	
	Veg	Non veg	Veg	Non veg	Veg	Non veg	Veg	Non veg	Veg	Non veg	Veg	Non veg
1. Cereals	150	150	200	200	250	250	320	320	450	450	350	350
2. Pulses	50	40	60	50	70	60	70	60	70	50	70	50
3. Green leafy Veg.	50	50	75	75	75	75	100	100	100	100	150	150
4. Other Veg.	30	30	50	50	50	50	75	75	75	75	75	75
5. Root Veg.	x	x	x	x	x	x	x	x	100	100	75	75
6. Fruits	50	50	50	50	50	50	50	50	30	30	30	30
7. Milk	300	200	250	200	250	200	250	200	250	100	250	150
8. Fats & Oils	20	20	25	25	30	30	35	35	45	50	35	40
9. Meat & Fish	x	30	x	30	x	30	x	30	x	30	x	30
10. Eggs	x	x	x	x	x	x	x	x	x	30	x	30
11. Sugar, Jaggery	30	30	40	40	50	50	50	50	40	40	30	30
12. G. nuts	x	x	x	x	x	x	x	x	50	50	x	x

N.B. An additional 30 gms. of fats and oils can be included in the diet in place of groundnuts.

Q.2.15.(b) What should be the components of our diet?

OR

What are the different classes of foods?

Food can be divided into nine classes :

1. Cereals and cereal products,
2. Starchy roots,
3. Pulses and legumes,
4. Vegetables and fruits,
5. Sugars, preserves and syrups,
6. Meat, fish and eggs,
7. Milk and milk products,
8. Fats and oils, and
9. beverages.

Each of these contributes some of the nutrients essential for the make up of a good diet.

Q.2.16. Why extra calories of food are required for children and students?

Children as a rule require excess of energy for their body processes especially to promote growth. The average rate of growth in children from 11 to 16 years is about 4 kg of weight per year, which shows that for the normal growth, they would require about 30 extra kilocalories daily.

For school going children the calories requirement is same as that of an adult i.e., 3000 k calories. But as the active growth is going on, the protein requirement is more i.e., about 2.5 gms/kg of body weight per day. This does generally come from milk, meat, fish, egg etc. for non-vegetarian and from milk and pulses for vegetarian. About 20-30% of the total energy come from fats, so he must take about 100 gms of fat per day. This generally comes from

N.B. The above diet will supply 2615 calories,
Total amount :   Protein—82 gm.
Fat—43.7 gm., and
Carbohydrate—469 gm.

DIET OF INFANTS

A new born baby, weighing 5½ to 6 lbs., should be on a sufficient supply of milk for its life and growth to gain 50 gms., or 1 ounce weight a day, for the first thirty days. Its average diet will be 6 calories per hour or 150 calories per day. The average Bengalee mother's milk yields about 18 calories per 1 ounce. Thus, a new-born baby should get 8 to 18 ounces of milk from the mother and this quantity will gradually go up with growth. A child of one month would require 8 to 10 calories per hour or 250 calories per day, and would require 15 to 20 ounces of milk. A child of 6 months would require 500 to 600 calories or 30 ounces of milk. Breast milk is unquestionably the best food for the baby, but to ensure proper and good supply of mother's milk, the food given to the mother must needs be good and sufficient. When mother's milk is insufficient, it has to be supplemented by artificial feeding. But this involves cost, apart from the risk of infection and the possible lack of some of the biological elements of vitamins etc.

USE OF MOTHER'S MILK AND ITS SUBSTITUTE OR ARTIFICIAL FEEDING

Q.2.17.(a) How we will use mother's milk or its substitute?

1. **Mother's milk** can be given to a baby up to 1 year. It should be started as soon as it comes in the mother's breast for 3-5 minutes in each breast, up to 8 minutes at a time, at the interval of 4 hours. It can also be given as per schedule, viz 6 a.m., 10 a.m., 2 p.m., 6 a.m., and 10 p.m.. Mother must prepare herself mentally and physically for the breast feeding.

FOOD AND NUTRITION

2. Cow's milk. In absence of mother's milk, and or prolonged illness of the mother, *Cow's milk* can be given after proper boiling. No dilution with water is necessary after 3 month, up to 3 month it should be diluted in the proportion of:

0-15 day = 1:1 (milk : water),
2.6 weeks = 2:1 (milk : water),
1½ -3 months = 3:1 (milk : water).

with one teaspoonful of sugar. The quantity of cow's milk required for such feeding, is about 2½ ounces per lb. of the baby's weight. But the **Goat's milk** is a near approach to mother's milk, so sugar and or cream should not be added. Goat's milk is very much useful than cow's milk. Buffalo milk contains nearly double the amount of fat (8.8 percent) and for this reason many babies do not tolerate buffalo milk. So it is advised to remove fat partially and dilution of the milk before use. From the 3rd month onwards along with milk, vegetable soup, dal, boiled fish, should be added. Rice should be introduced in suitable from 6 *months or on wards*. Fruit juice like orange, grapes, tomato etc. should be started from 3rd month. But fruit juice should not be added with warm or boiled water as it destroys the Vit C content. Traditional sago and bearley water should not be given to infants.

Some times in developing countries like ours, introduction of solid food like boiled and mashed potato, boiled papya, yellow portion of egg, etc. should be introduced earlier (at 3 months) to prevent malnutrition. But the basic rule is that "no starchy food (rice) should be given to a baby before the teeth are cut, for the starch-digesting ferments do not appear sufficiently in their digestive juices before the sixth or seventh month."

Bengal, Assam, Tamil Nadu, Bihar and some other southern states of India mainly consists of rice, dal and vegetables which contain too much carbohydrates but lack in other essential elements. *Rice* which is staple food is generally used without its nutritive parts, as it is husked and polished and also when reject the gruel after cooking the nutritive part go out. *Pulses,* which are the chief sources of protein, are lacking most of vitamins and the protein quality is also of second class.

It is also noted that the cost of the composition of the diet as recommended by the Nutrition expert committee is very high and beyond the economic means of majority of our people, so they are taking low price diet which generally lacks nutrient.

So the *basic defects of Indian diet* are that:
   i) the diet is unbalanced and of low calorie value.
   ii) undue preponderance of cereals and very small amount of proteins and that too second class proteins.
   iii) less amounts of fat.
   iv) deficient in minerals and vitamins.

Suggestion for fulfilling the deficiencies:

1. Diet must contain proper protein. Generally, animal protein of high biological value like meat, fish, egg and milk are best if economical condition permits, otherwise it can be procured from rich vegetable protein sources like soyabean, pulse etc. For a vegetarian, more milk to be added in place of meat and fish.

2. Diet must contain ghee, butter, vegetable and hydrogenated oil, milk and animal fat, as it is required for filling up the fat deficiencies.

3. The bulkiness of the diet is mainly due to much intake of rice. It not only causes fermentation but also prevents absorptions of proteins and vitamins contained in other diet like pulses. So the amount of rice should be reduced by taking one meal of the day with rice and an other by atta.

4. Over and all the food stuffs will be adjusted in such a manner that it must yield required amount of energy for a normal person i.e about 2500 Kcal daily.

Q.2.19. What is meant by deficiency diseases?

Deficiency diseases are those which are produced due to lack of sufficient and balanced diet for a normal growth and development of a body. Or when the food taken does not contain adequate supply of proteins, carbohydrates, fats, minerals and vitamins, they produce different abnormal manifestations (signs and symptoms) over a large part of the body are known as deficiency diseases.

IV. VITAMIN DEFICIENCIES

Q.2.20. What are the causes of vitamin deficiency in a body?

The main causes of vitamin deficiency in a body are:-

i) When the food taken does not contain enough vitamins, they produce deficiency symptoms, and are generally seen in infancy, pregnancy and lactation and also in prolonged illness.

ii) *From failure of the gastro-intestinal tract to absorb sufficient vitamins from the foodstuffs*, as happen in case of patients suffering from achlorhydria gastritis or diarrhoea. These prevent absorption of vitamin B complex, while prolonged use of liquid paraffin produces avitaminosis by preventing absorption of carotene which is dissolved and excreted with faeces.

iii) In obstructive jaundice vitamin-K is not absorbed due to absence of bile.

Q.2.21. What is vitamin?

Vitamins are complex organic compounds without any energy value, but whose presence in trace amounts in the food are absolutely necessary for the normal health and growth, as well as prevention of diseases.

Vitamins do not supply any calorie, but they act as a

FOOD AND NUTRITION

component of the important enzyme system and as catalysts by which proteins, fats and carbohydrates are metabolised. They are generally designed by the letters of alphabet i.e. *Vit. A, Vit. B, Vit. C, Vit. D, Vit. E,* and *Vit. K.* All the vitamins are under the groups of (a) *fat soluble vitamins*, and (b) *water soluble vitamins.*

Vit. A, D, E and K *are fat soluble*, where as *Vit. B-complex* (B_1, B_2, B_3, B_6, B_{12}, pantothenic acid, biotin, folic acid, cheline, inosital, para amino benzoic acid etc.) and *Vit. C are water soluble*. But this method of nomenclature is being replaced as the vitamins becomes known by their chemical names viz Retinol (Vit. A), Calciferol (Vit. D), Tocopherol (Vit. E), Phyloquinon (Vit. K), Thiamin (Vit. B_1), Riboflavin (Vit. B_2), Niacin, Pyridoxine (Vit. B_6), Pantothenic acid, Cyanocobalamin (Vit B_{12}) & Ascorbic acid (Vit. C).

Q.2.22. What are the differences between fat soluble vitamins and water soluble vitamins?

The main differences of these two groups of vitamins are:-

Character	Fat soluble group	Water soluble group
1. Solubility	1. Soluble in fat solvents, e.g. benzene, chloroform etc.	1. Soluble in water.
2. Absorption	2. Takes place along with dietary fat which depends on a number of factors and complex.	2. Absorption is quick, simple and complete.
3. Storage	3. Capacity for storage is enough and can sustain even upto 1 year.	3. Capacity for storage is limited and can sustain for 2-3 months only.
4. Excretion	4. Being insoluble in water it cannot be excreted in urine.	4. Being water soluble it is easily excreted in urine
5. Excessive intake	5. Causes toxic effect being locked up in the system by the body as is excreted in urine within 48 hrs.	5. Causes no risks as the extra amount not required.

Q.2.23. What is meant by antixeropthalmic or anti-infective vitamin? What are its sources of functions and deficiency of signs and symptoms?

OR

Name a fat soluble vitamin. What are the sources of it? Mention its functions and deficiency diseases.

Vitamin A is known as growth promoting antixeropthalhmic or anti-infective vitamin. Because of its presence in our daily diet, it promotes bodily growth, maintains a healthy state of the ectodermal tissues, prevent xerophthalmia and consequently increases the resistance of the body to infections. Also it is a *fat soluble*, thermostable but early oxidised vitamin.

SOURCES

Animal kingdom—butter, ghee, eggs, milk, fish-oils, cod-liver and shark liver oils etc.

Vegetable kingdom-carrot and green leafy vegetables, turnips, and shoats of vegetables and fruits like tomatoes, mangoes the in the form of carotenoids B carotene called pro-vitamin A, converted into vitamin A by the liver, at the rate of 3.1.

FUNCTIONS

1) Maintains the normal integrity of epithelial cells all throughout the body, particularly of stratified epithelium and prevents hyper-keratinization. It prevents infection and hence called anti infective.
2) Helps in the formation of rhodopsin in the retina, essential for vision in a dim light (dark adaptation of eyes).
3) Stimulates growth of skeleton.

DEFICIENCY SIGNS AND SYMPTOMS

Vitamin A deficiency is fairly widespread in India, more in the preschool and school going age and comparatively less in the adults. The various signs and symptoms of vitamin A deficiencies are.

1. OCULAR (in the eye)

(a) Lachrymal glands atrophy causing cessation of tear secretion.

(b) Corneal epithelium becomes red, dry winkled and known as *Xeropthalmia*. *Bitot's spots* are always seen in this condition.

If it remains untreated the cornea becomes necrosed and soften with concomitant of secondary infections ultimately cornea is destroyed and sloughted out. This is known as *Keratomalacia*. This leads to blindness unless the process is stoped before ulceration.

(c) Effects on retina-poor dark adaptation is the earlysing, leading to night blindness *(Nyctalopia)*.

2. DERMAL (Skin)

(a) *Xerosis of skin*—due to hyper keratinisation of the stratum corneum of the epidermis and the skin is dry and rough.

(b) *Toad skin*—formation of thorny nodules on the elbow, knee and buttock due to blockage of the mouth of the follicles by keratinized plugs.

3. DIGESTIVE TRACT

(a) The *salivary glands atrophy* and they stop secretion due to proliferated duct epithelia blocking the lumen.

(b) The epithelia of the tongue and pharynx also show metaplastic change.

(c) Swelling of the gums are also seen.

4. RESPIRATORY

Metaplasia of the lining cells of the mucous membrane of the nasal cavity, nasopharynx, trachea and bronchi leading to the different respiratory infections like common colds, bronchitis etc.

5. URINARY

Epithelia of renal pelvis, ureter and bladder also show metaplastic changes forming phosphatic claculi.

6. SKELETAL

Over growth of bones occur and more predominant changes are seen in the cranium and vetebral column.

7. FOETAL

During pregnancy it leads to the production of congenital malformation in the off spring.

8. RESISTANCE TO INFECTIONS

It drastically lower the resistance against disease and men are prone to secondary infections which ultimately cause death.

Daily requirements:

Adult—5000 International Unit (I.U.).
Child (3-6 years)—2500 I.U.
Pregnant women—6000 I.U.
Lactating women—8000 I.U.
(1 mg. of pure vit.-A = 3300 I.U.).

Q.2.24. What are the main symptoms of Vit.-A deficiency? Mention them with their causes and tissues involved.

Symptoms of Vitamin A deficiency.

Symptom	Causes and tissues involved
1. Loss of appetite	1. Taste bud degeneration.
2. Retardation of growth.	2. In adequate in take and utilization of food, intestinal obstruction etc.
3. Nervous disorder.	3. Defective myelinization, abnormal growth of bone.
4. Follicular hyper keratosis.	4. Epithelial keratinization.

Symptom	Causes and tissues involved
5. Defective reproduction.	5. Testicular degeneration, foetal resorption, hormonal abnormalities.
6. Night blindness.	6. Loss of rhodopsin.
7. Xerophthalmia.	7. Defects in corneal epithelium, tear duct obstruction infection.
8. Blindness.	8. Rod and cone cell destruction, corneal repture etc.
9. Generalized infection.	9. Immunological defects, reduced mucus secretion, keratinization of larynx and trachea.
10. Death.	10. Infection, volvulus, urinary blockage.

Q.2.25. What is meant by antirachitic vitamin? What are its sources and functions. Describe the condition produced due to its deficiency in early and chronic stages.

Vitamin D is called antirachitic vitamin because it contains the whole group of substance which has antirachitic property i.e. prevents ricket in children, osteomalacia in adults and dental caries in young individuals. It is a fat soluble vitamin and belongs to a group of compounds known as sterols. The synthetic name of vitamin D is CALCIFEROL or VIOSTEROL.

SOURCES: Animal kingdom

Vitamin D mostly presents with vit. A, in egg yolk, milk, butter, cheese, ghee and fish-liver oils. It has been established that by the action of ultraviolet rays of the sunlight i.e. exposure of sunlight, converts ergosterol in the skin to calciferol, a pure form of vitamin D, where as the natural vit. D derived from 7-dehydrocholesterol present in the skin.

Plant kingdom:- Irradiation of ergot by ultraviolet rays leads to the production of 'irradiated ergosterol' or calciferol having anti-rachitic properties. This can be produced on commercial scale at cheaper cost. Both ergosterol and 7-dehydrocholesterol are called provitamin-D.

Functions

i) helps in absorption of dietary calcium and phosphorous from the intestine;

ii) helps to maintain the optimum concentration of calcium in the extracellular fluids around the growing ends of bones;

iii) helps the process of degeneration of the cartilaginous bands at the growing ends of the bones prior to osisfication.

iv) helps in the formation of teeth.

DEFICIENCY DISEASES

Lack of vit. D causes defective calcification of bone. This lead up to a condition which clinically known as RICKETS in growing children and OSTEOMALACIA in adults. Osteomalacia usually affects females who often bears children and do not get sufficient sunlight and good nourishing diet. In India, because of frequent exposure of our children to radiant sunlight of typical ricket is much less except in the valley areas of Punjab and Kashmir where access to sunlight is limited and children are not generally left bare bodied in open. It is more common among muslims because of the pradah system. However, mild and moderate cases of vit. D deficiency are not uncommon.

In human rickets the following signs and symptoms generally occur—

I. In Early Stage—Delayed development of the milestone is the early sign of vit-D deficiency. Generally turning in bed sitting, standing, walking will be delayed. When the child begins to walk, be walks with wadding gait. There may be delayed dentition, closure of fontanelle and a relatively large head compared to the chest circumference and also significant flabbiness of muscles and hyper extension of joints. Increase in level of serum alkaline phosphatase is an indication of early D deficiency.

II. Last State—Development of typical rickets characterised by boxhead, bowlegs and rickety rosary, pot-bally appearance and toneless muscle are common in India. These are due to the fact that when vit. D is lacking the

FOOD AND NUTRITION

epiphyseal cartilage expands several times, but bone is soft and it becomes deformed under the weight of the body. Also muscles are poorly developed so causes pot-bally appearance i.e. the abdomen is distended due to increase gas formation in the intestine which causes bulging of the abdominal wall.

OSTEOMALACIA

Osteomalacia generally affects the pregnant women, as her calcium is further depleted by the inexorable demand of the foetus, leading to softening and bending of the pelvic bones and consequently parturition becomes difficult. There may be general weakness, gridle pain and tetany.

Daily requirement : Adults—400 I.U.

Children (0-2 Years)—800 I.U.

Pregnant—400-600 I.U.

Nursing mother—800 I.U.

Q.2.26. Give an example of a water soluble vitamin or a vitamin found in citreus fruits like lemon, oranges etc. What are its sources, functions and deficiency symptoms?

OR

Describe the sources, functions and deficiency signs and symptoms of antiscorbutic vitamin. Or Ascorbic acid.

Vitamin C is a water soluble vitamin and also found in citreus fruits like lemon, oranges, amla, tomatoes etc. Chemically it is known as *ascorbic acid.* It is also known as antiscorbutic vitamin as it prevents the occurance of the disease *scurvey.*

SOURCES

Animal-freshly killed meat is a good sources but milk contains little of it. Vit. C of the milk is destroyed by pasteurisation, heating or dying, and cooking in utensils made of copper and iron.

Vegetables—Fresh citreus fruits like oranges, lemon,

margarine, grape, guava, amlaki and green vegetables like tomato lettuce, cauliflour, cabbages and germinating cereals are good sources of vit. C.

FUNCTIONS

i) Helps in the proper formation and maturation intracellular matrix and there by, strengthen the collagen material in the capilary wall;

ii) Helps in the absorption of the dietary iron by reducing ferric iron to ferrous iron;

iii) Helps in the process of repairing wounds;

iv) Raises the body resistance against infection;

v) Takes part in the detroxication some drugs and heavy metals;

vi) It is possibly related to the production of steroids in the adrenal cortex.

DEFICIENCY DISEASE

Vitamin C deficiency can occur only in man and other primates but not in any other animals excepts guinea-pig. Moulds, fungi, higher plants and most animal except primates, man and guinea-pig can synthesize this vitamin. This is the reason why most animals do not suffer from symptoms of deficiency due to this vitamin.

The deficiency of vitamin C leads to a disease known as scurvy a condition characterised by *gingivitis with bleeding gums and petechial haemorrhage on the skin.*

Sign and symptoms (of scurvy) of *vit-C deficiency:* In the early stage of vit. C deficiency i.e. in gingivitis the gum margins are swollen, oedematous and tender followed by recession of the gum margin. Bleeding may be spontaneous or on the application of slight pressure. Haemorrhagic spots also appear on the skin on pressures or scratching, signs of anaemia is also present.

In adults—Before the above signs are developed there is often premonitary like weakness, lassitude, irritability and loss of weight.

FOOD AND NUTRITION 57

In infants—It develops between one to one and half years. The child loses appetite and weight. He becomes irritable and cries when he is handled by limbs due to tenderness in the muscles. In infants born of mothers deficient vitamin C, scurvy may occur as an acute *(Infantile scurvy)* and may lead to death unless promptly treated with doses of vitamin.

Generally haemorrhage is common specially under the periosteum of long bones, in the gums, skin and mucus membrane. There is enlargement of costochondral junctions and radiogical changes showing periosteal haemorrhage and stoppage of osteogenesis are valuable signs.

The changes due to deficiency of vitamin C is reversible because as soon as vit C is administered these signs and symptoms disappear.

Daily Requirement : 50 mg/day or if required more.

Q.2.27. What is meant by ariboflavinosis? What are its signs and symptoms?

Ariboflavinosis is a disease which occurs due to deficiency of riboflavin i.e. vitamin B_2.

Signs and symptoms : This is common in all age groups but children, pregnant women and lactating mothers are specially vulnerable. The manifestations i.e. signs and symptoms of this disease generally occurs in (a) Ocular (b) Oral (c) Dermal and (d) Nurological area of man.

1. OCULAR

(a) Formation of a congested ring of capilaries surrounding the cornea manifested as *circum-corneal injection.*

(b) *Corneal vascularisation*—Invasion of the corneal tissue by the newly growing capillaries from the limbic plexus followed by devitalisation of cornea-infection ulceration-and loss of eye sight.

2. ORAL

(a) *Angular stomatitis*—Cracks in the corners of month which may extend to the inner side of the cheek or to the outer surface as a very chronic condition.

(b) *Cheilosis*—Inflammatory condition of the lips with cracking, and crust formation associated with pain and tenderness.

(c) *Glossitis*—It causes a magenta-coloured flaby tongue with hypertrophy of the papillae in the early stage and atrophy at the late stage. There are cracks and fissures on the surface of the tongue with or without patchy ulceration.

3. DERMAL

Irritation of the sebaceous glands lead to hypersecretion of sebaceous material which accumulates on the surface of the skin in the form of small hard white crystals. These lead to irritation and inflammation of the surface epithelium producing desquamation, exudation, crust formation and pigmentation. The common sites are alae nasi, outer canthus, behind the ear, mid-sternal and mid scapular regions and over the genitalia. This condition is known as *"Seborrheic Dermatitis"*.

4. NEUROLOGICAL

Damage of optic nerve has been reported in few cases.

Functions: vit. B_2 has a function in amino acid oxidation and it is intimately associated with cell respiration, as well as dehydrogenation of glucose and lactic acid.

Daily requirement: 1.5 mg/day for adult,

2.1 mg/day for nursing mother.

V. MALNUTRITION

Q.2.28. What is meant by Malnutrition?

Malnutrition means a pathological state of the body resulting from a relative or absolute deficiency or excess of one or more essential nutrients. This is nearly always due to several deficiencies in the diet, such as inadequacy of available calories, proteins, vitamins, minerals and other factors.

FOOD AND NUTRITION

Excess of total calories and fat leading to obesity and causing atheroslerosis may also be considered in this respect.

Generally malnutrition is divided into 4 heads:

(a) *Under nutrition,*

(b) *Over nutrition,*

(c) *Imbalance, and*

(d) *Specific deficiency.*

(a) *Under nutrition* is the condition which results, when insufficient food is eaten over an extended period of time. In extreme cases it is called starvation.

(b) *Over nutrition* is the pathological state resulting from the consumption of excessive quantity of food over an extended period of time.

(c) *Imbalance* is the pathological state resulting from a disproportion among essential nutrients with or without the absolute deficiency of any nutrient, and

(d) *Specific* deficiency is the pathological state resulting from a relative or absolute lack of an individual nutrient.

Q.2.29. What are the causes of malnutrition?

The important causes of malnutrition in India, are:

A) *Imbalanced and faulty diet i.e.*

    i) The caloric value is too low;

    ii) The total amount of protein is often insufficient.

iii) Animal protein is often scanty and sometimes entirely absent.

iv) The total amount of fat is frequently too low and animal fat is scanty or lacking.

v) Carbohydrates, rice staples—particularly rice or wheat, usually form 80 to 90% of diet, which therefore contains too much starch in proportion to other essential elements.

vi) Deficiency of one or more of mineral elements, particularly calcium and iron, is frequent.

vii) One or more of the vitamins is frequently deficient, particularly, in diet, of which the staple article is polished rice or tapioca or a mixture of both.

viii) Pure vegetarian diet is bulky, less easily digested and due to bulkiness ferments. It is also deficient in animal proteins.

B. *Ecological factors:*

JELLIFFE (1966) listed various factors like geographical, climatic, environmental, cultural, socio economic, food production etc. which are under the head of *'ecology of malnutrition'* related to malnutrition. Generally these are:-

i) Rapid growth of population,

ii) In adequately agricultural food production due to lack of irrigation facilities.

iii) Prevalance of parasitic and infection diseases like hookworm, ascariosis, dysentery etc. Generally these diseases are responsible for decreased intestinal absorption. Lack of proper work and lack of hygienic conditions are generally responsible for these diseases.

iv) Religious and cultural food fads also causes malnutrition as it make some people not to use the local available nutritious foods.

v) General illiteracy and ignorance about importance of balanced diet is the main cause of malnutrition.

vi) Over and all proverty i.e. lack of capacity to purchase sufficient food is the main cause of malnutrition in India.

Q.2.30. What are the disease generally occur due to malnutrition?

Generally malnutrition diseases are divided into 2 broad heading according to etiological factors:-

I. Disease caused due to the deficiency in the diet of certain nutrients, and calories, and

II. Disease caused due to the consumption of certain types of foods and excess of certain nutrients and calories.

FOOD AND NUTRITION

Common Malnutrition Diseases or Disease Due to Deficiency and Excess.

Types	Clinical Name	Probable Chief causes
A. Deficiencies		
1. Starvation diseases or protein energy or protein caloric Malnutrition. (PEM/PCM).	a) Dietetic Malnutrition. b) Kwashiorkor. c) Famine oedema.	Deficiencies of calories proteins.
2. Vitamin deficiency diseases.	a) Xerophthalmia and night blindness. b) Ariboflavinosis c) Beri beri d) Pellagra e) Scurvey f) Rickets and osteomalacia g) Multiple vitamin deficiency	Deficiency of vit-A. Deficiency of Riboflavine. Deficiency of Vit B Deficiency of Nicotinic acid Deficiency of Vit C. Deficiency of Vit D. Deficiency of several Deficiency vitamins.
3. Mineral deficiency diseases	a) Endemic Goitre b) Dental caries. c) Nutritional anaemia	Deficiency of Iodine Deficiency of Fluorine. Deficiency of Iron
B. Excesses		
4. Excess of food	a) Obesity b) Athero-sclerosis	Excess of fat, and lipids.

Q.2.31. How we can prevent malnutrition?

Prevention of malnutrition can be done by.
1) Increased food production by scientific cultivation.

2) Infants, pre-school children, pregnant women should be protected. Mid-day meals for the school students should be provided.
3) Fortification of the flour with protein and calcium will help a great deal.
4) Improvement of environmental sanitation to prevent the parasitic infections.
5) Nutrition education to the public.
6) Applied nutrition programme should be extended to all the affected areas.
7) Prevention of unnecessary loss of foods in the storage, transport and cooking.
8) Steps to be taken to improve the socio-economic condition of the people.

** *Cal. phos., Cal. carb., Nat. mur., Acid phos.* etc. in low potencies are used in homoeopathic treatment for malnutrition diseases. Correcting of constitutional defects, which produce malnutrition symptoms, are also essential for such treatment.

Q.2.32. What is meant by Protein Caloric Malnutrition (P.C.M.) or Protein Energy Malnutrition (P.E.M.)?

Protein Caloric Malnutrition (or Protein Energy Malnutrition) means the disease caused by inadequate and disproportionate consumption of dietary calories and protein which is particularly manifested in children of 1-5 years age group.

Q.2.33. What are the main causes of P.C.M. ?

The main causes of PCM's are (i) non availability of protein rich diet, (ii) faulty feeding habits, owing to customs, superstitions and ignorance of the mother, and (iii) poor, socio-economic and environmental conditions of the community causing infection, and worm infestation of the child population. (iv) Generally in early infancy, breast milk provides adequate protein, but after the weaning, the replacement of breast milk by sago, barly waters etc., result

FOOD AND NUTRITION

protein deficiency, due to inadequacy of protein content of such diet.

Q.2.34. How can we diagnose a case of P.C.M. ?

OR

What are the clinical features of P.C.M. ?

We can easily diagnosis a case of P.C.M. by the help of following clinical manifestations:

i) Retardation of growth, and

ii) Depigmentation of hair and skin are generally seen in the children.

iii) The black hairs are converted into reddish and silky, with change of texture.

iv) There is peeling of the skin characterized by exposure of (non infective type) raw surface,

v) Oedema of legs, or dependent parts may take place, owing to hypo-proteinaemia.

vi) The liver is enlarged soft and tender due to fatty infiltration.

vii) Diarrhoea.

viii) Mental retardation.

ix) The child is more irritable and apathetic.

x) The child looks pale due to anaemia and this is a common feature in rural area due to hook-worm infection.

xi) Other signs and symptoms are like that of vit-A vit-B complex deficiencies.

Q.2.35. What are the various types of PCM ? Describe them in brief.

PCM are generally divided into two main types, viz; *Kwashiorkor and Marasmus*. Although the combinations of these two types may also take place, viz., marasmic kwashiorkor.

1. KWASHIORKOR

If the diet fed to an infant is markedly deficient in protein but slightly deficient in calories, it produces the kwashiorkor type PCM. It is a serious disease causing gross damage to most of the vital organs of the body. It is most prevalent between 1 to 5 years of age and female children are said to be most vulnerable, though definite sex distribution has not been recorded. In India the incidence of frank kwashiorkor is 1% in the pre-school age group (1-5 years) and ten times that number of cases of mild-moderate kwashiorkor is visible in the community.

CAUSES

The etiology of kwashiorkor is a complex one. Mother affected with malnutrition and having inadequate lactation fail to provide enough breast milk to their infants beyond 4 to 5 months after child birth, resulting in the need for supplementary feeds. Prompted by ignorance, superstition and faulty feeding habits these poor mothers usually select a cheap locally available starchy food particularly devoid of protein. Sago, tapioca, rice, ripe banana are used in different parts of India. Therefore, at the crucial age of the infant, when the daily protein requirement is as high as 2 to 2.5 gms./kg. of body weight, these babies are made to thrive on a protein free starchy gruel. Solid foods are not started at the proper age of 5 to 6 months of the infant but most of them are left on any of the starchy diets, mentioned above, till the age of 1 to 1½ years. So the death rate among children between 1 to 5 years in the developing countries, is 10 to 40 times higher than in countries with good diets.

Main characteristics for Kwashiorkor :

A typical case of 'Kwashiorkor' characterised by retarded physical growth, wasting of muscles but retention of subcutaneous fat, psychomotor changes, oedema, discolouration of the hair, flaky paint dermatosis, anaemia, enlarged liver and recurrent attacks of diarrhoea. They become highly susceptable to infectious diseases.

2. MARASMUS

Nutritional marasmus is the other type of PCM where the diet fed to the infant is inadequate in quantity and

FOOD AND NUTRITION

markedly deficient in protein as well as calories. Marasmus is most frequent between ages of 1 to 2 years and the incidence is 2% in the age group of 1 to 5 years.

Main charactristics of Marasmus:

Marasmus produces a picture of starvation or semi-starvation reducing the child to bone and skin. There is marked wasting of muscles, loss of subcutaneous fat, loosening and winkling of the skin, retarded physical growth and the face resembles that of an old man. In marasmus, the pathological changes in the internal organs are not so severe and widespread as in kwashiorkor.

3. Marasmic Kwashiorkor

In the diet fed to the infant is markedly deficient in protein but moderately deficient in calories, then it produces few sign of kwashiorkor as well as few sign of marasmus producing there by a mixed syndrome.

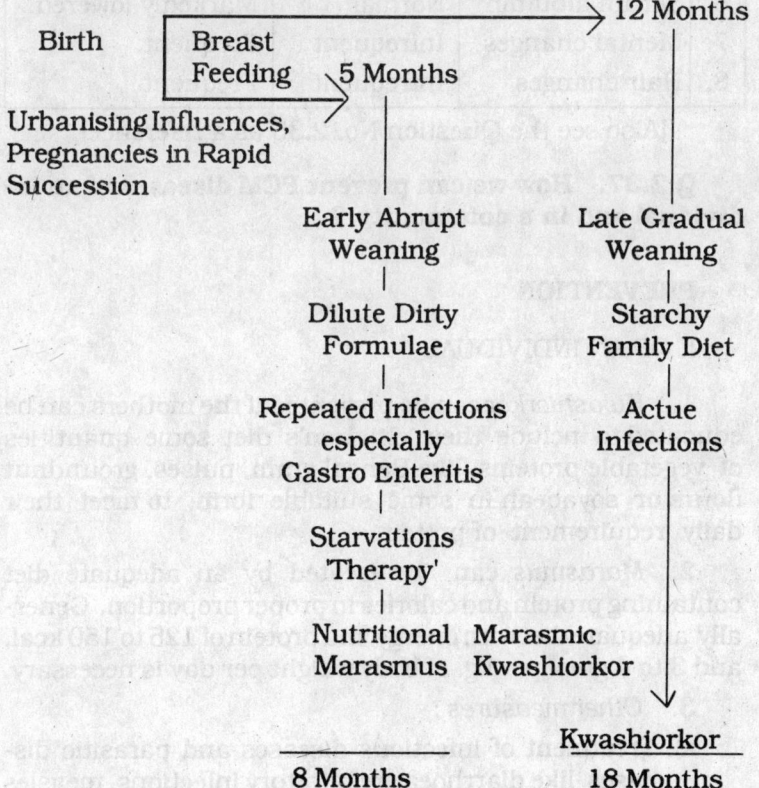

Paths leading from early weaning to nutritional marasmus and from protracted breast feeding to kwashiorkor.

Q.2.36. What are the differences between marasmus and kwashiorkor?

Main differences between marasmus and kwashiorkor are as follows:

No.	Clinical Feature	Marasmus	Kwashiorkor
1.	Age of incidence	6-18 months	12-18 months.
2.	Emaciation	+ + +	+
3.	Oedema	Absent	+ + +
4.	Fatty liver	Absent	+ + +
5.	Skin changes	Infrequent	Frequent.
6.	Serum albumin	Normal	Markedly lowered.
7.	Mental changes	Infrequent	Frequent.
8.	Hair changes	Infrequent	Frequent.

[Also see the Question No. 2.35 as a reference]

Q.2.37. How we can prevent PCM diseases of an individual and in a community ?

PREVENTION

I. OF AN INDIVIDUAL

1. *Kwashiorkor* can be prevented if the mothers can be educated to include their children's diet some quantities of vegetable proteins, like Bengal gram, pulses, groundnut flours or soyabean in some suitable form, to meet their daily requirement of protein.

2. *Marasmus* can be treated by an adequate diet containing protein and calories in proper proportion. Generally adequate diet with energy and protein of 125 to 150 kcal. and 3 to 4 gms. per kg. of body weight per day is necessary.

3. *Other measures* :

a) Treatment of infectious diseases and parasitic diseases like diarrhoea, respiratory infections, measles

FOOD AND NUTRITION

and intestinal worms are also necessary to control P.C.M.

b) Health education of parents and knowledge of adoption of other preventive measures of its relapse is very need ful.

II. OF A COMMUNITY

There is no simple solution to the problem of P.C.M. There are many types of measures to prevent P.C.M. but 8th F.A.W./W.H.O. *Expert Committee on Nutrition* has recommended the following measure's to prevent P.C.M. in a community.

A. For Health Promotion

1. Measures directed to pregnant and lactating women—education and distribution of supplements.
2. Promotion of breast feeding.
3. Development of low cost weaning foods—the child should be made to eat more food at frequent intervals.
4. Measures to improve diets, like, use of Bengal gram, groundnut flours, soyabean etc. in the diet of vulnerable groups.
5. Nutrition education—promotion of correct feeding practices through group teaching in well baby clinic and M.C.H. clinic etc.
6. Home economics, like increase use of kitchen-gardens in rural area, for the production of beans, peas etc.
7. Instruction about family planning and spacing of births, to reduce the size of family, and family environment.
8. Increase production of animal protein food, viz. milk, fish, skimmed milk etc. for the consumption vulnerable groups.
9. Increase production of vegetable protein containing essential amino-acids viz. leans, peas etc.

B. For Specific Protection

1. The child's diet must contain protein and energy rich foods like milk, eggs, and other protein containing vegetables.
2. Schedule immunization.
3. Fortification.

C. Early Diagnosis and Treatment

1) Periodic surveillance.
2) Early diagnosis of any lag in growth.
3) Early diagnosis and treatment of infections and diarrhoea.
4) Development of programmes for early rehydration of children with diarrhoea.
5) Development of supplementary feeding programmes during epidemics.
6) Deworming of heavily infested children.

D. Rehabilitation

1) Nutritional rehabilitation through well baby clinics, M.C.H. programmes and School Health programmes etc.
2) Hospital treatment services, and
3) Follow up care.

Thus PCM is not a problem which is to be solved by medical personnel alone. It involves joint efforts of various disciplines.

VI. ASSESSMENT OF NUTRITIONAL STATUS

Q.2.38. What is meant by nutritional survey ? How we can asses the nutritional status of a group of population in India ?

Nutritional Survey means to asses quality, as well as, quantity of the diet consumed by a sample of population and thereby to judge the diet of the whole community. So this includes, diet survey and nutrition *assessment survey*.

FOOD AND NUTRITION

Assessment of Nutritional Status

Just a diagnosis of a disease in an individual is essential before instituting proper treatment, so also, in a community, assessment or survey of the nutritional state of a group of population is a prequisite for planning out any comprehensive nutrition programme in an area. In India, malnutrition being widely prevalent, so it is often required to carry out nutrition surveys among groups of population at various levels.

The methods for the "Assessment of Nutritional Status" are of 6 types, namely -
1. Clinical,
2. Anthropometrical,
3. Laboratory and biochemical,
4. Dietary,
5. Vital statistics, and
6. Ecological.

1. Clinical Method

With the idea of making the method of nutrition assessment and surveys more practical and useful method is field work. The NAC (Nutrition Assessment Committee) of ICMR evolved a revised Nutrition Assessment Schedule in 1963 in which individual card method has been adopted and the grading process has been eliminated. In this process a person is examined clinically for the presence or absence of a set of known signs of malnutrition and the presence of one is indicated by putting a cross (x) in the square ([]) marked against the sign.

2. Anthropometric

It is concerned with the measurement of the variation of the physical dimensions and the gross composition of the human body at different levels and degrees of nutrition.

Anthropometric indices commonly recommended in the assessment of nutritional status include:

(a) Standing height,
(b) Sitting height,
(c) Weight,

(d) Chest circumference (Midpoint of)
(e) Mid-arm circumference,
(f) Head circumference,
(g) Skin fold thickness.

Anthropometric measurements are more useful and significant in growing children because of the rapid increase in the different dimensions expected in a normal healthy child. Sitting height is measured to find out any disproportionate growth between the trunk and the lower limbs. Head and chest circumferences provide some clue to the existence of protein caloric malnutrition in an infant. At birth, in a normal infant the head circumference exceeds that of chest but they equalise at the age of six months and there after the chest circumference exceeds that of the head. Mid-arm circumference gives an idea about the growth of the bone, muscles and fat at that region. Of course, the amount of subcutaneous fat can be measured directly by a skinfold caliper at two convenient point e.g. Infra scapular region and back of the arm. All these measurements should be done in duplicate and the menu taken by the same person as far as possible.

3. Laboratory and Biochemical Method

In routine nutrition survey, clinical and anthropometric data are also supported by few laboratory investigations, like, haemoglobin estimation, stools and urine examination etc. Recently bio-chemical investigations are also very useful and generally these are done to assess nutritional status in early cases of under-nutrition and malnutrition, when clinical signs have not yet appeared i.e. the patient is in the sub clinical stage.

For a nutritional assessment of a large group of population biochemical studies are also done only in a representative percentage of the total sample.

4. Dietary Examination

The nutritional assessment is also enhanced when it is supplemented by diet survey. A diet survey provides information about the people and bring out dietary inadequencies as judged by the available standards. A diet survey generally carried out by one of the following methods:

a) Weightment of raw foods,
b) Weightment of cooked foods and
c) Oral questionaries method.

FOOD AND NUTRITION

Then the data that is collected by the diet survey is analysed:

i) for the mean intake of foods in terms of cereals, pulses, vegetables, fruits, milk, meat fish and eggs, and

ii) for the mean intake of calories, proteins, fats, carbohydrates, vitamins and minerals per adult man value or consumption unit.

5. Study of Vital Statistics

The study of vital statistics provides an indirect means of nutritional assessment of human groups. The rates used for this purpose are the *infant mortality rate, neonatal mortality rate, still birth rate, perinetal mortality rate, mortality in the age group of 1-4 years and life expectancy.*

Because these rates are influenced by nutritional status. It is well known that these rates are low in well nourished populations. Hospital statistics relating to kwashiorkor, marasmus, keratomalacia, parasitic infestations etc. also help to assess nutritional status of a person or population.

6. Assessment of Ecological Factors

For any nutritional survey, it is necessary to collect certain background information of a community in order to make the assessment complete. A study of ecological factors related to malnutrition are done and they are comprise of:

(a) *Conditioning influences* e.g., Bacterial, viral and parasitic agents.

(b) *Cultural influences* —Food habits and attitude to food, infant feeding practices, feeding of pregnant and lactating women, cooking practice etc.

(c) *Food production* — Customs relating to methods of cultivation, animal husbandry, food storage and distribution.

(d) *Socio-economic factors* — Family size, occupation, income, education, housing etc.

(e) *Health and educational services*—Numbers of hospital and health centers, distribution of health personnel, preventive, promotive and curative services, mass-media of communication.

NUTRITIONAL DATA BASE
History
Previous weight curve.
Dietary intake by retrospective recall and prospective diary.
Alcohol intake.
Socio economic and family status, including income.
Anorexia, vomiting, diarrhoea.
Blood loss.
Pregnancy, lactation, menses.
Vitamin and mineral supplements.
Use of drugs that might affect nutrition.

PHYSICAL EXAMINATION

GENERAL	:	Weight as percent of ideal body weight; triceps skin fold ; mid-arm muscle circumference.
SKIN	:	Xerosis, follicularhyperkeratosis, pellagra dermatitis, patechiae, ecchymoses, perifollicular hemorrhages, flaky paint dermatitis, pallor.
HAIR	:	Dyspigmentation, easy pluckability, thinning, staraightening.
HEAD	:	Temporal wasting, parotid enlargement.
EYES	:	Bitot spots, conjunctival and scleral xerosis, keratomalacia, corneal vascularization, angular palpebrites.
MOUTH	:	Cheilosis, angular stomatitis, magenta tongue, atrophic lingual papillae, tongue fissuring, glossitis, spongy gums, dentition.
HEART	:	Cardiomegaly, findings of congestive heart failure.
ABDOMEN	:	Hepatomegaly.
EXTREMITIES	:	Oedema, koilonychia.
NEUROLOGICAL	:	Irritabity, weakness, calf tenderness, loss of deep tendon reflexes.

VII. MILK AND PASTEURISATION OF MILK

Q.2.39. What is milk ?

Milk is an ideal as well as complete food of human being, secreted from the mammary glands of the female individuals after first three days of the birth of the baby.

It is thick in consistency, yellowish in colour and very rich in proteins and salts. It is also the indespensable food of the new borne and the principal food stuff of the growing child.

Q.2.40. What is meant by humanised milk ?

Humanised milk means preparation of cow's milk or goat's milk by adding water, lactose or sugar and cream, and sometimes lime water to form a composition which resembles human milk so far as to its fat, protein and carbohydrate contains and caloric value.

Generally the human milk is richer in lactose, lower in proteins, lower in total salts, poorer in phosphates and chlorides than the milk of cow or a goat. So to form a humanised milk and cow milk is diluted with an equal amount of water and one ounce of sugar and one ounce of ordinary centrifugalised cream (or 50 p.c. codliver oil emulsion) are added to form one pint of milk. (the fats dont mix suddenly, it is done gradually). [* lime water used to prevent the curd from lumping.]

Q.2.41. What are the difference between human milk and cow's milk ?

Cow's milk is commonly used as a substitute of a breast milk for children and used as a good supplementary diet for vegetarian and persons of all age groups particularly children and the aged. Generally cow's milk composition differs from that human milk are as follows :

1. The human milk has much *casein* than cow's milk but total protein content has a higher nutritive value per gram. (Cow's milk contains 3% caseinogen of the total proteins and forms a bigger harder clots in the stomach and is less digestible too.)
2. The concentration and physico-chemical properties of casein in human milk are such that on coagulating, it forms a finer, softer and more uniform curd, which is more easily digested than the former curd formed by cow's milk.

3. The human milk contains more lactose than cow's milk (cow's milk contains 4.5% lactose.)
4. The human milk contains less salts, specially calcium and potassium than cow's milk. Human milk contains about 25-35 mg. calcium and cow's milk about 120 mg. calcium per 100 ml.
5. The buffer effect is less in human than cow's milk.
6. The human milk contains only one tenth the amount of volatile fatty acids like triolein, tripalmitin and tributyrin etc. of cow's milk.

The main difference of the various constituents of human milk and cow's milk are as followes:-

	Human Milk	Cow's Milk
Water%	88.5	87.0
Protein (gm.%)	1.50	3.5
Fat (gm.%)	4.0	3.5
Carbohydrate (gm.%)	6.8	4.8
Salt (gm.%)	0.2	0.7
Vitamins	A,D,B_1,B_2 & C	A,C,B_2, & D
Calcium (mg.%)	.34	1.49
Phosphorus (mg.%)	.12	.96
Iron (mg.%)	-	0.2
Thiamine (mg.)	0.02	0.05
Riboflavin (mg.)	0.02	0.18
Nicotinic acid (mg.)	-	0.1
Vit-C (mg.)	3	2
Caloric value (Kcal.)	65	67

Q.2.42. Why milk is considered as an ideal food for growing infants ? And why it is called complete food for all age groups?

MILK IS AN IDEAL FOOD

Milk is the secretion of mammary glands of the female individuals after the first three days of the birth of the baby.

It is the best and an ideal food for growing infants as it contains all the food factors needed for the growth and maintenance of health. The nutrients exist in the milk in various forms e.g. the protein in colloidal suspension, fats in emulsion, carbohydrates and minerals in solution and the vitamins in solution and fatty emulsion. Quantity of these are also exactly same to the requirements of an infant. So the milk is considered as an ideal food for growing infants.

MILK IS A COMPLETE FOOD

The milk is mainly composed of water and solids:
 i) Water - 88.5%
 ii) Solids - 11.5%

The solids are :

1. Proteins

The milk proteins are casein, lactoalbumin and lactoglobulin. They constitute 3.5 percent of the total weight. Casein which is the chief protein, occurs in combination with calcium as calcium caseinogenate. It is also particularly rich in lysine and methionine.

2. Fats

The fat in milk is composed mainly of (i) the glycerine of butyric, palmitic and oleic acids, (ii) smaller amounts of stearic acid and acids with carbon chain of 4 to 24 carbon atoms; and (iii) phospholipides such as lecithin, cephalin and steroles.

3. Carbohydrates

The carbohydrate of milk is lactose. It is present to the extent of 4 to 5 percent and remains in the dissolved stage in fluid after casein and fat globules have been separated. It is less sweet than cane sugar and can easily be fermented by lactic acid bacilli.

4. Minerals

Milk contains almost all the known minerals needed by the body such as calcium, magnesium, phosphorus, cobalts, copper, iodine and chloride with small quantities of citrate and lactate.

5. Vitamins

Milk is a good source of vitamins A, vit.D thiamine, and riboflavin and niacin. It is a poor source of vit.C and much of its destroy during boiling.

6. Other constitutents

Milk also contain antibodies and certain number of enzymes such as catalase oxidase, reductase etc.

Showing to its composition, it is seen that it has a high nutritive value and contains almost all the proximate principles of well balanced diet required for human body. Generally complete food supplies necessary energy to the body, promotes growth by build up new tissues, repair wear and tear and maintain life by providing necessary nourishment. Like complete food, milk can add the necessary elements to the body and is capable of giving energy to the system for the growth and maintenance of health, so it is called complete food.

Also sugar present in milk supply necessary energy. Proteins present in it, are the first class proteins like lactoalbumin, lactoglobulin, caseinogen etc. are the highest growth promoting substances and will build up tissues and repair losses. The minerals like inorganic salts of potassium, calcium, sodium, phosphates and chloride with small quantities of citrate and lactate etc. help the formation of bone and teeth. The fats like glycerides of oleic, myristic and palmitic acids, and phospholipides such as lecithin, cephalin and sterols, vitamins like vit A, B_1, B_2 etc. and water present in milk help in different metabolic processes and disease prevention. Generally 100 gms. of cow's milk generates 67 calories of heat and it is also easy to digest. So in case of certain disease of human being where nutrition is impair, milk is prescribed as an indespensible food.

So from the above discussion, we easily come to the conclusion that milk is an ideal and complete food for infants as well as adults.

FOOD AND NUTRITION

Q.2.43. "Milk is an ideal food but cannot serve as the only element of our diet"- Explain.

Though milk is an ideal food but it cannot serve as the only element of our diet.

Because :

1) It is poor in iron, nicotinic acid and vitamin C and contains no vitamin E.

2) In order to supply to necessary calories and the nutrients, a large amount of milk has to be taken. But the total supply of milk (both in quantity and quality) is very unsatisfactory in our country and is quite expensive.

3) It is a very good medium for the growth of bacteria and it can also be easily adulterated, so pure clean and fresh milk is difficult to obtain and milk borne disease are largely prevalent.

4) Experimentally it is seen that infants who feed on only milk, usually become anaemic and flabby after 7 to 8 months (milk injury).

Q.2.44. What is meant by milk borne disease ? What are the common sources of contamination ?

Milk borne disease means the disease of man which are spread through the milk.

Generally milk is an efficient vehicle for a great variety of disease agents, due to the fact that it is a very good media for bacterial growth. The common sources for contamination of milk are :

 i) the disease condition of the dairy animals;
 ii) dust from blowing air;
 iii) hands and clothings of milker;
 iv) dirty vessels and utensils;
 v) from impure water which are used for washing cans; and
 vi) during adulteration, storage, transport or distribution of milk.
 vii) sometimes milk is carried in open containers under the cover of hay or leaves of trees to prevent spliting or splashing—a process leading to obvious bacterial contamination.

Q.2.45. What are the common milk borne disease ?

The common milk borne disease are.
1) Bovine tuberculosis prevalent mainly in the west,
2) Strepto and staphylococal infection;
3) Diphtheria and scarlet fever;
4) Brucellosis due to infection with *Brucell abortus* from milk of infected cow;
5) Foot and mouth disease;
6) Enteric infections-typhoid and paratyphiod fevers;
7) Cholera;
8) Diarrhoea and dysentery.

Except tuberculosis and brucellosis all other are extraneous infections contaminating milk. Some of these diseases arise in epidemic form as milk borne infections.

Q.2.46. What are the steps we can take to prevent milk borne disease ?

Various steps to prevent milk borne disease are:-

1. The milk producing animal should be healthy, clean and free from infections. It should be daily groomed and its udder and tail should be cleaned before milking. Common milk borne disease is tuberculosis, so to prevent this, regular veterinary examination of the animals along with tuberculin test at every six months interval are necessary.

2. Milking vessels should be scrupulously clean and kept covered after milking.

3. Milker should be healthy and should not be a carrier of any infection which may have detrimental effect on the health of milk consumers. He should be clean in his personal habits especially while milking. Before milking he must wash his hands and arms.

4. The environment of the milking place should be of a sanitary type, with proper ventilation, water supply and drainage etc.

5. Distribution of milk should be done under hygienic condition.

6. Milk should be preserved by boiling, pasteurisation and sterilisation.

FOOD AND NUTRITION 79

7. Before use milk, it should be boiled.

8. Enforcement of strict legislation and punishment for adulteration is utmost important.

Q.2.47. How we will know that a given sample of milk is pure without the help of chemical and bacteriological examination ?

OR

Is, the specific gravity of milk is only test to ascertain its purity ? If not, Why ?

The purity of milk can be ascertained without the help of bacteriological and chemical examination by finding out the specific gravity of given milk by introducing in it a lactometer. The specific gravity of pure milk varies normally from 1027 to 1034.

The specific gravity test may not be the only test as addition of water lowers the specific gravity after extraction of fat from it. So, if after extraction of fat from milk, water is added proportionately to maintain the specific gravity as a pure milk, then specific gravity test will fail to detect it.

Q.2.48. How we can proceed to check a sample of milk quality and purity ? Or How we can proceed to detect the type of adulteration and comtamination of milk.

A sample of good milk should be opaque, of white colour, without any peculiar taste or smell. Fresh milk is amphoteric due to presence of acid phosphatase of alkalies. It however, soon becomes acid. The acidity amount is 0.4% lactic acid. The specific gravity of milk also varies from 1027 to 1034, with the breed, stage of lactation and the condition of husbandry under which animals are maintained.

But it is a common practice to adulterate milk and the common methods are employed :—

(a) addition of water (b) skimming of milk and (c) skimming and watering. Sometimes milk is also contaminated by various types of bacteria. So for checking a sample of milk to detect quality and purity the common steps are.

1) **For Addition of Water**

   a) Specific gravity test.
   b) Nitrates test.
   c) Freezing point test.

2) **For Skimming Milk**

   a) Lactometer,—Gerber test,—Evaporation.

3) **For skimming and watering followed by addition of cane sugar, gelatin, starch etc.**

   a) Detection of cane sugar.
   b) Detection of starch.
   c) Detection of gelatin.

4) **For Bacteriological Examination**

   a) An estimation of number of living bacteria in milk, and
   b) Detection of pathogenic organisms by the help of microscopes or grows in specific culturemedia.

1. Test of Specific Gravity

The specific gravity of water and of milk are 1000 and 1027 to 1034 (average 1032) respectively, at 15 degree C and can be easily determined by LACTOMETER. The addition of water to milk results lowering of specific gravity.

2. Test of Nitrates

Milk contains no nitrates, but water does. The presence of nitrates in milk indicates adulteration with water, and it can be detected by the following method.

If 5 ml. of suspected milk is taken in a test tube and 1 ml. of acid diphenylamine (1 ml. of diphenylamine with 100 c, c of sulphuric acid) is added slowly, in the side of the tube, a blue colour is seen at the point where acid and milk meet. The proves presence of nitrates i.e. addition of water in milk.

3. Test for Freezing Point

The freezing point of milk is—0.54 to—0.57 degree C and is determined by a CRYOSCOPE. A freezing point nearer to 0 degree C will indicate adulteration with water.

4. Test of Skimming of Milk

If fat is removed from the milk, it can be detected by—*lactometer* (high specific gravity), *Gerbertest* (low fat percentage), and *evaporation* (high percentage of solids but not fat).

5. Detection of Cane Sugar

Taking 5 ml. of milk in a test tube, if 0.1 gm. of resorcin power and a few drops of hydrochloric acid is added and boiled for a few minutes *Blood red colour appears*, indicating the presence of cane sugar in milk.

6. Detection of Starch

Taking 10 ml. of cool boiled milk, if 1 ml. 5 percent of iodine solution is added, blue colour appears, indicate the presence of starch.

7. Detection of Gelatin

Taking 10 ml. of milk in a test tube, if 10 ml. of acid mercuric nitrate is added and after shaking these if 20 ml. water is added and filtered, the filterate will be opalescent ; indicating gelatin. If the filterate is saturated by aqueous solution of picric acid, yellow precipitate or cloudiness appears indicates the presence of gelatin.

8. Bacteriological Test

It is done for two purposes :-
 a) for testing the cleanliness of the milk, and
 b) for determining its safety i.e. freedom from the presence of pathogenic organisms.

a) Test of Measuring Cleanliness

There are many methods but the following are the common :

i) Sedimentation Test:

A pint of milk is filtered through a bottle shaped container over which a cotton pads filled. Dirt sticks to the pad and its colour is compared with standard pads. The test determines the amount of extraneous matter and gross dirt contaminating the milk.

ii) Cellular count :

Under physiological condition milk contains leucocytes on an average about 330,000 per cc. Counts above 1,00,000 per cc. with associated streptococci should be regarded as pathological.

iii) Methylene Blue Reduction test :

Under normal conditions methylene blue is decolourised only by anaerobic conditions. if, however, bacteria are present, methylene blue is reduced even under aerobic conditions. The rate of reduction depends on the number and the metabolic activity on the organisms. It is a *simple and cheap method.*

This test is generally done by the following ways:

10 ml. of sample of milk is taken in a test tube, and added 1 ml. (1 in 3000,000) of a standard solution of methylene blue. Then the test-tube is pluged with a rubber stopper and put it is a waterbath, at 37 degree C. Reduction time of methylene blue are noted and interption is done by the following ways—

Time for reduction of Methylene blue	Quality of the milk
1. 5 hours or more	Good.
2. 2-5 hours	Fair.
3. 20 minutes to 2 hours	Poor.
4. Less than 20 minutes	Very Poor.

iv) Breeding clump counting :

It gives an index of total stainable organisms in milk. It is an *early and rapid method of estimating the number of bacteria in the milk.* It is done by spreading 0.1 ml. of milk over one square centimeter area on a slide and then drying, fixing defating and staining with methylene blue is done. Then the number of bacteria per c.c. is estimated by calculating from the average number of organisms per microscopic field.

Q.2.49. What is meant by pasteurisation of milk ? What are its advantages & disadvantages ?

Pasteurisation is a process of sterilisation and a type of heat treatment which destroys the pathogenic organisms and other bacterial flora of the milk, without altering taste, appearance, flavour, digestibility and nutritive value.

Advantages :

It was first discovered by LOUIS PASTEUR for the prevention of souring of wine or beer. But now this method is used for the preservation of milk, delaying the natural souring of milk about 12 to 14 hours, besides destroying some specific organisms such as, cholera, tuberculosis, typhoid, paratyphoid, staphylococus, scarlet fever and other non-sporing organisms. Generally it consists of heating of milk at various temperature, below boiling point for a variable period of time but sufficiently long enough to kill the most of the organisms without reducing physical and chemical changes in milk. This process neither

FOOD AND NUTRITION

destroys the enzyme (except phosphatase) and nor alters the taste, appearance, flavour and nutritive value of milk. So it is a preventive measure of public health importance and corresponds in all respects to modern principles of safe supply of milk.

Disadvantages :

1. When milk is adequately pasteurised, there is some destruction of enzyme phosphatase and some heat liable vitamins like thiamine, B_{12} & vit. C destroy 20% at 125 degree F.

Q.2.50. What are the various methods of pasteurisation ?

There are two main processes of pasteurisation -, viz.
I. HOLDER PROCESS, and
II. High temperature short time process (H.T.S.T.) or FLASH method.

I. HOLDER'S PROCESS or HOLDING METHOD

In this process milk is heated in a vat. at 61.7 degree C (143 degree F) by holding it for 30 minutes and then cooled at 10 degree C (50 degree F).

The vat is employed in this process, is a double jacket tank, where warm water is drawn out of the bottom of the jacket by a special pump. To obtain through mixing, the milk is agitared by paddles. The milk is then cooled at once in the same vat by passing cold water in its outer jacket. Then the milk is bottled and sealed. In India most of the dairy firm are following this method satisfactorilly.

II. H.T.S.T. PROCESS or FLASHING METHOD

This is an American method and is not considered as a reliable one.

In this process temperature of milk is raised to 71.1 degree C (160 degree F), 15 seconds only, and then rapid cooling is done to not more than 10 degree C (50 degree F).

There are various devices for pasteurisation of milk, by flashmethod, of which plate type is most popular. In plate types a series of thin steel plates are so assembled in a frame, that hot water flows between alternate plates, while the thin sheets of milk flow in the opposite direction. Apart from the plate device there are other methods, e.g. Internal tube heat exchanges and electrical devices etc.

Q.2.51. (a) How we will know that the pasteurisation of milk has been done properly ?

1. BY PHOSPHATASE TEST

Generally when milk is adequtely pasteurised, the enzyme contains of the milk—Phosphatase destroyed adequately in correspondence with the standard timed temperature for pasteurisation. At 60 degree C for 30 minutes phosphatase is completely destroyed, and it is estimated by means of calorimetric method in a *Lovibond Comparator*. Thus the test employed for detection of enzyme phosphatase is the test for checking milk properly (phosphatase test). This test is also widely used to check the efficiency of pasteurisation i.e. it is used to detect inadequate pasteurisation or the addition of raw milk. Here a sample of milk is incubated with buffer disodium phenyl phosphate and the liberated phenol is estimated by calorimetric method after endering it to a blue colour by means of reagent. If the milk is properly pasteurised, the sample of milk should not yield more than 2.3 lovibond unit of phenol.

2. COLIFORM COUNT

Coliform organisms are usually completely destroyed by pasteurisation, and therefore, their presence in pastuerised milk is an indication of improper pasteurisation. The standard in most countries is that coliforms be absent in 1 ml.of milk.

Q.2.51. (b) How long does pasteurised milk keep ?

Pasteurisation destroys much of the bacteria in the milk, but not all. Some bacteria can resist the heat and survive. Milk, naturally, teems with bacteria, a millilitre of good quality milk may contain a million bacteria; and pasteurisation brings this down to about 30,000. As temperature promotes further growth of these bacteria, pasteurised milk is stored below 10 degree C before it is distributed. Once out of the cold storage, pasteurised milk can keep for 9 to 10 hours in our tropical climate.

But the problem is, the milk that we received from the milk booth in the morning might have been taken out of the dairy's cold storage for distribution the previous night and transported in semichilled vans (10 degree C-20 degree C) and badly kept and handled in the milk booths. So by the time it reaches the consumer, it may be already 8 to 9 hours, and the exposure to higher temperature would have caused the bacteria to grow and multiply further. So it needs to be boiled to kill the bacteria after which it may be kept for another 24 hours under refrigeration or any other means of chilling (below 10 degree C). Without refrigeration, boiled milk may keep for another 8 to 10 hours, depending on climatic conditions. Because of all this, there are more complaints about "spoilt milk" even when it is received from the milk booth and heated immediately in the summer months.

High bacterial activity converts the lactose sugar in the milk to lactic acid (which gives the sour smell and taste) and eventually the milk splits, that is, the proteins, mainly casein, and fats, will separate from the water, which may now contain only components which are soluble in water, like traces of lactose etc.

Q.2.52. What are the difference between pasteurised and boiled milk.

Pasteurised milk	Boiled milk
1. All pathogenic organisms are killed and acid forming bacteria are reduced.	1. All pathogenic and spore forming bacillii are destroyed.
2. Calcium is precipetated to the extent of 6%; other minerals are not affected; Iodine is only reduced by 20%.	2. Ca & Mg salts are precipetated and iodine is totally volatilised.
3. Lactose not charred or caramelised;	3. Lactose is caramelised.

Pasteurised milk	Boiled milk
4. No scum is formed ;	4. Ca & Pare taken up by the scum.
5. About 5% Lactoalbumin is coagulated at 158°F.	5. Both lactoalbumin and lactoglobulin are coagulated 158°F and 167°F respectively.
6. Vit C is reduced by 20%.	6. Vit C is destroyed except in brief boiling.
7. Taste, appearance and food values are not altered.	7. Taste is altered and food value affected.
8. Keeping quality of milk improves and souring is delayed.	8. Keeping quality more improved and souring may be prevented for several hours if kept covered after boiling.

Q.2.53. Why breast feeding is better than bottle feeding ?

Breast feeding is better than bottle feeding because :

1. The infant gets the nourishment direct from the mother at a suitable temperature and in an assimilable composition without any exposure to air.

2. Breast milk is free from contamination i.e. clean and pure.

3. It contains protective antibodies, enzymes and vitamins.

But bottle feed babies get their milk exposed to contamination, dusts and other agents from the dairies; enzymes and antibody contents are missing and over and above the phychological satisfaction of the infant derived from breast sucking is absent.

So the breast feeding should be insisted upon unless the breast is dry or the mother is sick.

FOOD AND NUTRITION

VIII. PRESERVATION OF FOOD

Q.2.54. How food can be preserved ?

Food both from animal or vegetable kingdom are likely to decompose in a short time. But the adulteration act of 1954 and rules of 1955, permit the food to be preserved in the following manners as preservatives inhibit, retard or arrest the process of fermentation and decomposition.

Preservation Methods :

1. *Heating and canning*—Heat destroy germs of infection and canning prevents entry of outside germs. But only vit. C is destroyed.
2. *Drying and dehydration*—By this method the germs die, as there is no moisture - examples are dryfish, drymilk powder.
3. *Smoking*—Kills the germs on the surface of meat, fish etc.
4. *Smalting or pickling*—Addition of salt, sugar, spices, oil, vinegar, honey etc. are permitted preservatives.
5. Sulphur di-oxide, benzoic acid, sorbic acids and their salts are also permitted in certain types of food only, and in certain quantity as pecified in the rules. If excess quantity is added, food is considered adulterated.
6. *Cooling and refrigeration*—At a temperature of 0 degree C or even at 10 degree C the pathogenic bacteria cannot multiply. However, the germs do not die. As soon as the temperature is above 10 degree C germs start growing. Fungus grows even at 0 degree C.

Q.2.55. What are the advantages and disadvantages of cooking food?

Advantages :

1. Cooking makes the food more palatable by making it attractive to sight, taste and smell which stimulates gastric secretion and there by digestion.
2. By cooking most of the vegetable dietary articles are made softer, agreeable and easy to masticate. But

they are too hard for mastication and digestion if taken raw.
3. It avoid monotony by the presentation of great variety of food.
4. It helps to delay the putrefaction and decomposition of food than raw food.
5. The food is partly digested by the help of cooking as a result of hydrolysis.
6. The food is sterilised by cooking, as certain microorganisms and the eggs of parasites with which the food may be infected are killed by cooking due to high temperature.

Disadvantages :

1. Some quantity of vitamins is lost.
2. A small part of energy of the food (about 5%) is also lost.

IX. ADULTERATION OF FOOD

Q.2.56. (a) When an article or food should be considered as adulterated ?

Generally an article of food is considered, to be adulterated if.

1. The article is not of the natural one i.e. the quality as demanded by the purchaser is altered viz.:

(a) if cheaper substance has been added, or

(b) the normal constituent has been removed, or

(c) if the article contains an other substance affecting the nature, substance or quality.

2. If the article contains prophibited colour, preservatives or any other poisonous matter.

3. If the article is prepared or kept in any insanitary manner. or the article is decomposed or insect infested.

4. If the article is not the prescribed standard as laid down under rules appendix B.

FOOD AND NUTRITION

Standards of some articles as per Appendix-B under Rule 5:
1. Cow's milk must have 3.5% fat and 8.5% N.F.S.(non-fatty solids).
2. Buffalo's milk must have 6% fat and 9% "
3. Standardised milk must have 4.5% fat and 8.5% "
4. Toned milk must have 3% fat and 8.5% "
5. Double toned milk must have 1.5% fat and 9% "
6. Skimmed milk must have 5% fat and 8.7% "
7. Steparated milk must have Nil fat and 8.7% "

Humanised milk = ½ litre milk + ½ litre water + 15 grams cream + 15 grams milk sugar (Lactose). It is not as per adulteration rules and hence humanised milk cannot be sold.

Q.2.56. (b) What are the various food stuffs commonly adulterad ? How can we prevent them ?

Adulteration of foods are an important social problem. Adulteration of food consists of a large number of practices—mixing, substitution, abstraction, concealment of quality, putting up decomposed foods for sale and addition of poisonous substances. The main object is profiting. Food adulteration practices vary from one part of the country to another and from time to time. Our knowledge about the current practices of food adulteration is meagre. The types of adulteration commonly found in various food stuffs are:

1. *Milk*—By addition of water, removal of fat, addition of starch and skimmed milk powder.
2. *Ghee*—With hydrogenated vegetable oils and fats oil.
3. *Cereals*—Rice and wheat are mixed with stonechips and gravel.
4. *Flours*—Cheap variety of starch, maize flour and saw dust.
5. *Mustard oil*—Argemone oil.
6. *Sugar*—Starch, soap stone.
7. *Tea and coffee*—Tea leaves are adulterated with old tea leaves, leather and saw dust, coffee is adulterated with chicory.
8. *Honey*—Sugar, jaggery, molasses.

PREVENTION OF FOOD ADULTERATION

1. Prevention of Food Adulteration Act

In 1954 the prevention of Food Adulteration Act was enacted by the Indian parliament. The act extends all over

India except in Jammu and Kashmir. In 1955 a few ammendment were made and 'Prevention of Food Adulteration Rules of 1955, was with of 3 parts.

(a) The rules describes the methods of sampling, functions of the public analyst, Food inspectors, conditions of licence, preservatives, colouring agent etc.

(b) Appendix—A Describes the specimen of forms to be issued.

(c) Appendix—B Lays down the standards of articles of food.

But in 1963, again a few ammendments were made in order to make the act more stringent. Under this act standards have been laid down for various foods. The Indian Standard Institute, the Central Committee for food standard, in the Ministry of Health and the Directorate of Marketting and Inspection work in close vision for maintaining food quality in India were made. Act carries severe penalties for infringment and the purpose of the act is to protect the health of the consumer and to assure foods of honest nutritive value.

2. Code of Practice

Every hotel or shop must be registered. A standard code regarding-(i) the measures to limit the infection of food from food handlers, (ii) cleansing of utensils, covering of food and their proper serving etc. (iii) prevention form rodents (iv) provision of minimum requirements of working premises, lighting and ventilation.

3. Health Education

The food handler and food traders should be properly educated about the health hazards of food infection and adulteration.

4. Provision of Public Health Laboratory

This is necessary for investigation off the out break of food poisoning. Such a laboratory may also carry investigations and research on different aspects of food storage etc.

X. POWER OF A FOOD INSPECTOR

A.2.57. What are the power of a food inspector ?

Power of a food Inspector :
1) He can take sample of food when it is being conveyed, sec....10(1).
2) He can enter any place, where food is being manufactured, stored or kept for sale and take sample   sec....10(2).
3. He can break open door, package etc. and take sample ....sec 10(c).
4. He can prohibit the sale of an article of food ....sec 10(1)(c).
5. He pays reasonable cost of the article purchased....sec 10(3).
6. If he thinks that the article is adulterated or misbranded, he can seize and carry away the article, ...sec 10(4).
(After necessary procedure, he produces the article before the magistrate as soon as possible)   .....sec 11(4), 10, 10(a),10(b)
7. He may seize material used for adulteration   ....sec 10(6).
8. He follows the procedure of sampling.
9. He ascertains the address and name of vendor   ....sec 10(8).
10. He may prosecute the vendor or owner or both   ....sec 16(1).
11. He can prosecute the vendor only, for preventing him to take the sample   ...sec 16(1)(6).

XI. FOOD POISONING

Q.2.58. What is meant by food poisoning ?

Food poisoning is an very unsatisfactory term. In public health, for the purpose of notification, the term food poisoning includes the chemical food poisoning and certain bacterial food poisoning. The Ministry of Health, U.K. in the British Medical Journal of 1966 has defined the term food poisoning as:
   i) Presence of *chemical poisons* in food.
   ii) *Bacterial food* poisoning are restricted to.
   a) *Salmonella* types of food poisoning.
   b) *Staphylococcal* type of food poisoning.
   c) *Clostridium botulinus* type of food poisoning.

N.B.

(The infections of food due to cholera, enteric dysentery, helmenthic infections etc. are not included as food poisoning).

Food poisoning is not very serious disease and deaths due to food poisoning are rare. The morbidity is high, but the mortality is low. Generally in food poisoning there is vomiting and diarrhoea and therefore the disease appears to be like cholera. But in food poisoning there is headache, fever, griping and the source of infection is usually obvious. In a house the persons who have eaten motton carry, or dal etc. are the sufferers of gastro—enteritis. This indicate the mutton carry or the dal is containing the thermostable exo-toxin of salmonella of food poisoning type.

In a marriage party of persons who have eaten certain type of milk products are sufferers. Chemical food poisoning are also obvious and point to a certain type of food. Anti-cholera innoculations and other anti-cholera measures are not necessary in obvious case of food poisoning. Contaminated food must be frozen or destroyed. Sample of food, or vomit or stool may be sent for analysis.

However in case of any doubt anti-cholera measures should be taken.

XII. DISEASES FROM FOOD

Q.2.59. Describe the various diseases that originate from food.

A large number of diseases may occur from food. They are generally of following types:

1. Diseases from animal sources.
2. Diseases from vegetable sources.
3. Diseases from chemical sources.
4. Diseases from bacterial sources.
5. Deficiency disease from food, and
6. Allergic diseases.

1. Diseases from animal sources are :

i) *Taenia solium* and *Trichinella spiralis* form *pork*.
ii) *Taenia saginata* and *Tuberculosis* from *beef*.
iii) *Fasciola hepatica* from the liver of *sheep*.
iv) *Diteothreocephalus latus* is from *fish*.
v) *Brucellosis* is from *Goats milk*.

vi) Any meat my give rise to tuberculosis, anthrax and actynomycosis,
vii) Cow's milk may give rise to Bovine tuberculosis, streptococcal infection, Staphylococcal type of food poisoning and brucellosis. Taenia saginata and cowpox are the other diseases from cow.

2. Diseases from vegetable sources are :

i) *Poisonous mushrooms* eaten by mistake will cause food poisonings.
ii) *Ergot* is a fungus, grows on rye, bajra, wheat etc. Gangrene, repeated abortion may occur as his involuntary muscles are in spasm.
iii) *Argemone* in mustard oil cause glaucome, epidemic dropsy, paralysis.
iv) *Lang dal* may cause lathyrism i.e. spastic paralysis of lower limbs.

3. Diseases from chemical sources :

i) It may be accidental poisoning by arsenic, tin, lead, copper, antimony and insecticides.
ii) The inscticides used in agricultural operations are not only harmful to the consumers of food stuff. Poisoning by insecticide may be due to :
   a) Eating food stuff and fruits sprayed with insecticide.
   b) Use of insecticide in beds and clothes, so that there is a prolonged contact with the insecticide.
   c) Using empty containers of insecticides to store grain etc.
   d) Gammexane used as additive and preservative in agricultural products like cereal, pulses etc.
   e) Urethane used to prevent sprouting of stored potatoes. Urethane is carcinogenic.
iii) Use of prohibited preservatives and colouring agents as described under Rules 53 to 57 and 23 to 30 of the P.E.A. Rules.
iv) Adulteration of food stuff by poisonous adulterants. Lubricating oil is commonly used. In 1959, at Morocco over 10,000 persons suffered from

acute food poisoning and paralysis due to adulteration of edible oil with lubricating cantaining T.O.C.P. (a deadly poison). In India hundreds of cases of paralysis have occured due to adulteration of mustard oil with argemone oil.

4. Disease from bacterial sources are :

i) *Salmonella* of the food poisoning type. There are several varieties of salmonella of the food poisoning type. The most common types are salmonella typhimurium and salmonella enteritides found in the urine and the faeces of rats and mice. These bacteria produce an exotoxin which is thermo-stable (i.e. not destroyed by heat). The toxin cause inflammation of stomach and intestine, causing vomiting and diarrhoea, commonly described as gastro-enteritis.

ii) *Staphylococcal* type of food poisoning occur from milk and milk products. A variety of staphylococcus (i.e. staphylococcus aureus) produce a thermostable exo-toxin. This also give rise to actue vomiting and diarrhoea. It is common after marriage parties.

iii) *Botulinus type* of food poisoning occur from canned meat. Due to imperfect sterilzation of meat, the spores of clostridium botulins remain, and the germs multiply, in the canned tin and produce a powerful toxin. The toxin do not produce acute gastro—enteritis. The poison causes paralysis of muscles of the intestine and may cause constipation. Generally the symptoms are of nervous origin. Distorted vision, diplopia, paralysis of muscles and death may follow. However, the tinned meat has an obvious bad smell.

5. Deficiency diseases from food are :

i) Protein deficiency causing marasmus and kwash—iorkor diseases.
ii) Vitamin deficiencies cause—Beri-beri, scurvy, rickets etc.
iii) Mineral deficiency may cause—Anaemia, goitre, dental carries etc.

6. Allergic diseases from proteins :

i) The protein particles from eggs, fish, meat, pollen of flowers, dust of hay particle etc. may produce hypersensitivity. There may occur sneezing urticaria, angeoneurotic oedema, eczema and acute breathing difficulty.

iii) Before innoculating B.C.G. Penicillin, serum etc. sensitivity test is done. A minute dose innoculated intradermally produces reaction and in duration and red areola of skin.

XIII. DIETOTHERAPY

The subject of dietotherapy has developed considerably during the last two decades and varieties of therapeutic diets have been planned, formulated, prepared and tried in various diseases as an adjucent to medicinal theraphy with encouraging results. The importance of food nutrition in preventing a disease, or hastening recovery from a disease has been known to man since ancient days. Hence the question of prescribing a suitable diet for a patient is always uppermost in the mind of the doctor as well as the patient in time of any sickness.

Most of the common diseases occuring in man lead to depletion of nutrient reserves of the body, by increasing their metabolic requirements of the tissues and also by depressing the appetite and thereby lowering the net absorption of nutrients. Under nutrition, thus produced, lowers the body resistance, and prolongs the convalescence period. In this way, a vicious cycle is set up.

The *purpose of dietotherapy* in diseases is to break this vicious cycle by :
   i) maintaining good nutritional standard,
   ii) correcting deficiencies that might have occured
   iii) affording rest to the affected organs, and
   iv) fulfilling metabolic needs of the body.

While planning any therapeutic diet for any disease conditions, the normal diet is generally used as the basis, and the necessary modifications are brought about, keeping in view the ailments of the patient and his over all nutritional requirements.

For example, a normal diet can be modified to:
  i) provide changes in consistency as in fluid and soft diets,
  ii) increase or decrease other energy values,
  iii) include greater or lesser amounts of one or more nutrients e.g. a high protein diet or a low-sodium diet,
  iv) increase or decrease of the bulk, and
  v) include or exclude some specific foods.

RECOMMENDED DIETS IN DIFFERENT DISEASES

1. Diabetes Mellitus

The object of dietotherapy in this disease is to adjust the carbohydrate intake, with or without insulin with in body's colerana. The calories should be sufficient to maintain normal weight, over-nutrition being avoided, carbohydrates should be restricted and amount of fat should be enough to meet caloric needs.

RECOMMENDED DIET

Items	Quality and Quantity
1. Milk	— 1 cup milk or ½ cup evaporate milk.
2A. Vegetable	— Unlimited amount of cabbage, palak, lettuce, celery, greencucumber, cauliflour, brinjal, ladiesfinger.
2B. Vegetable	— ½ ent beets, carrots, onions or peas.
3. Fruits	— 1 orange, 1 small apple, ½ banana, 12 grapes, ¼ muskmelon, 2 dates, 2 fresh figs, ½ medium papaya.
4. Bread	— Flour 2½ table spoons, 1 slice bread, 1 small potato, 2 graham crackers, ½ cup cooked rice.
5. Meat	— 1 oz. meat, 1 egg, 1 oz. cheese, 1 oz. fish.
6. Fat	— 1 teaspoon margarine or butter, 6 small nuts.

2. Gout

The diet should be resistricted in calories with a low protein content. The amount of carbohydrate should be high with quantity of fat with in caloric limits. Milk, egg, bread, potato and fruits are advised while meat, fish coffee, cocoa, alcohol and rich highly seasoned foods are to be avoided.

FOOD AND NUTRITION

3. Peptic Ulcer

Diet of during pain of the peptic ulcer (vegetarian)

On Rising : Milk 1 glass
8-00 A.M.—Orange juice 3/4 cup, milk with sugar 3/4 cup.
10-00 A.M.—Cream-or butter 1 tablespoon with bread.
12-00 noon—Cheese, potato, bread with butter, banana.
2-00 P.M.—Curd 3/4 cup.
4-00 P.M.—Milk 1 cup.
6-00 P.M.—Custard or curd 1 cup.
8-00 P.M..—Curd 1 cup, boiled potato, bread with butter or chapatis-2.
Before Retiring—milk 1 glass.
**Chillies and fried and spicey food, sauces, pickles, tea, coffee, alcohol and fruits should be better avoided.

4. Cirrhosis of Liver

Total calories—2000
Proteins—110 gms.
Fat—50 gms.
Carbohydrates—290 gms.
Breakfast—Coffee or tea 1 cup,
Porriadge with 3/4 cup milk with sugar 1 teaspoon, 2 toasts or 4 khakhra, butter 2 teaspoons, orange or banana.
Midmorning—Skimmedmilk—1 cup.
Lunch—Beetroot salad, curd, prepared form skimmed milk 1 cup, rice 2 tablespoons, dal—1 cup, 2 bread or chappati, 4 cooked brinjals 3/4 cup.
4-00 P.M.—Tea with bread and butter, groundnuts 20.
Dinner—Skimmed milk curd 1—cup; boiled potato—1, cooked spinach—½ cup, 2 slices bread or chapatis, 4.
Before Retiring—Skimmed milk—1 cup.

5. Acute Nephritis

Total calories—1,700.
Proteins—30 gm.
Carbohydrates—250 gm.
Fats—60 gm.
Morning—Tea or coffee 1 cup.
Breakfast—Toast or bread—2 slices with butter—2 teaspoon, jam 2 teaspoon, banana—2, tea or coffee—2 cup.
Lunch—Mashed potato, lettuce and cucumber salad, cooked cauliflour, rice—4 tablespoons, with tomato soup—½ cup, biscuits 2-3.
4-00 P.M.—Tea—1 cup, biscuits 2-3.
Dinner—2 chappati with butter, baked apple with sugar and cream (1 tablespoon).
** No salt in cooking or at the table.

6. Obesity.

Vagetarian

Morning—Tea 1 cup with skimmed milk 2 tablespoon or sugar 1 teaspoon.

Breakfast

Lunch—skimmed milk 1 cup, 1 slice bread, mixed vegetable 1 cup, thin dal 3/4 cup, cooked pumkin, bread-1 slice, chappati-1.

4-P.M.—Tea with 2 tablespoon of skimmed milk and 1 teaspoon of sugar.

6-P.M.—1 banana or orange.

Dinner—Tomato soup...1 cup, thin dal 3/4 cup, bread slices or chappati 2, cooked carrots.

CHAPTER-III

AIR, LIGHT, SUNSHINE IN RELATION TO HEALTH

DISCUSSION FOR LEARNING

I. Air and it's importance.
II. Composition of air.
III. How air becomes impured due to man's activities.
IV. What are the effects of the changes of air on man.
V. Over-crowding and its bad effects.
VI. How air is purified in nature.
VII. Ventilation—Natural and Artificial.
VIII. Lighting and its importance.
IX. Sunshine and its importance.

AIR IN RELATION TO HEALTH

I. AIR AND IT'S IMPORTANCE

Q. 3.1. Why air is necessary for life?

Of the two most essential elements that sustain life, air is of greater importance than water, as life cannot be sustain without air (oxygen) for more than three minutes, but one can survive for a few days without water. For maintenance of healthy life pure air of clean atmosphere is necessary as:

  i) it purifies the blood by inter change of O_2 with CO_2, in the lungs.
 ii) regulated body temperature.
iii) promotes digestion and assimilation.
 iv) strengthen the body and nerves.
  v) improves metabolism, and
 vi) increase resistance against disease.

II. COMPOSITION OF AIR

Q. 3.2. What are the composition of air ?

Air is mixture of gases and not a chemical compound. It has the following compositions :

Oxygen—20.96%
Nitrogen—79.00%
Carbon di-oxide 0.04% (.03-.04%),

Argon, Neon, Krypton, Xenon, Helium and other inert gases in trace and varying proportion of water vapour. In addition there are present traces of ammonia, ozone, salts of sodium, methane, sulphur di-oxide, nitrous and nitric acids and other gases resulting from decomposition, combustion and manufacturing processes, and in cities and industrial towns smoke, dust, aldehydes, gases and effuvia from sewers, industries and offensive trades, pathogenic and non-pathogenic bacteria, pollens, vegetable fibres, spores of fungi, moulds, starch etc.

Q. 3.3. What are the factors responsible for maintaining constant composition of air?

The various factors which are mostly responsible for maintaining constant composition of air in the open are :
  i) its enormous amount,
  ii) mizing action of winds,
  iii) diffusion and convection current,
  iv) absorption of CO_2 emanated from animal respiration by plants in exchange of O_2, and
  v) solution of gases etc. in water.

III. HOW AIR BECOMES IMPURE DUE TO HUMAN ACTIVITIES

Q. 3.4. What are the changes occur in the composition of air due to human activities ? Or How air becomes impure ?

The changes in the composition of air due to human activities are (or the air becomes impure by) :
1. Breathing of men and animals,
2. Combustion of coal, gas, oil etc.,
3. Human occupancy in ill ventilated room,
4. Decomposition of organic matters, and
5. Trade, traffic and many factory process.

1. Breathing of man : The O_2 becomes less and CO_2, temperature, humidity and organic impurities are increased. A man usually respires 18 times a minutes and each time expires about 500 ml. of air. The expired air contains about 4.5 percent less oxygen and about the same quantity of increased CO_2. The expired air is warmer and saturated with moisture and also contains bacteria and small amount of organic matter. So changes due to breathing *or the composition of inspired and expired air are* :

	Inspired Air	Expired Air	Change
Oxygen	20.96%	16.40%	O_2 is less by 4.56%
Carbon dioxide	.04%	4.44%	CO_2 is use by 4.40%
Nitrogen	79.00%	79.00%	No change
Water vapour	As in air (varies)	Saturated	Increased
Temperature	As in air (varies)	Body temperature	Increased
Organic matters	As in air	Increased	Increased
Other gases	In traces	Remains same	No change

2. Combustion : (i.e.burning)—By combustion, O_2 becomes less and CO_2, Co, soot, So_2 etc. are given out. Temperature becomes more.

a) *Burning coal*—For burning 500 grams of coal, 350 cu.ft. of air is required. It gives out 1% unburnt carbon particles as soot. CO_2, Co, Cs_2, H_2S, So, O_2, NH_3, and water vapour are also given out.

b) *Production of coal gas*—It is produced by destructive distillation of coal i.e. by heating coal without oxygen, the gas has 4.6% H_2, 37%, marsh gas, 7% Co and a few other gas.

c) *Burning oil*—Kerosene, vegetable oil and paraffin are burnt for lighting purpose. An ordinary sperm candle on complete combustion yields 0.4 cu. ft of CO_2 and about the same amount of water, 1 oz. of paraffin oils gives of 3.2 cu.ft. of CO_2 and about 2.25 cu.ft. of water. Kerosene gives off considerable quantity of soot during burning. An ordinary gas burner gives about 3 cu.ft. of CO_2 per hour. Thus fuel combustion more or less vitiates the air raising the temperature of the room, increase the moisture, Co and CO_2, compounds of NH_2, and soot to the air.

3. Occupancy : Generally the following *main changes occur due to human occupancy in a room :*

  i) the oxygen contents is reduced.
  ii) the amount of CO_2 present is increased.
  iii) organic matter and odours are given off from the skin, clothing, and mouths of the occupants.
  iv) humidity is increased by the moisture, and
  v) the temperature of the room is increased.

N.B.—A person breathing for one hour gives out O.6 cu.ft. of CO_2. If the movement of the air is 10 times per hour, then O.6. cu.ft. of CO_2, will become 0.4% (i.e. in normal air). Besides these—household wastes—

(*Decomposable organic matters*) added CO_2, NH_3, H_2S etc. to the air during their decomposition. In industrial and trading area the air is not only received heat and soot, but also vapour, fumes and industrial dusts and becomes impure.

IV. WHAT ARE THE EFFECTS OF THE CHANGES OF AIR ON MAN

Q. 3.5. Describe the effects of the changes of air on man ?

1. OXYGEN : In the air oxygen never becomes less than 20%. So due to human occupation there is no physiological effect on human health. In mines the oxygen is 18%. If oxygen becomes 10% or less then a person may become unconscious.

2. CARBON DI-OXIDE : If in the air CO_2, becomes 0.7% no ill effect occurs. Normally, CO_2, can never be more than 0.09% in the air. In the more worst ventilated place CO_2 may be 0.1%. But this has no physiological bad effect.

3. WATER-VAPOUR : Normally by breathing, a person gives out 10 oz. water in the form of water vapour per day, and 20 oz. of water is excreted by perspiration. But if the air warm and the humidity in air is more, evaporation of perspiration become less. Then the body heat is not lost but this creats a feeling of suffocation. This will be more, if there is *lack* of movement of the air.

4. TEMPERATURE : Heat is lost from the body by conduction, convection, radiation and evaporation. Evaporation is the most important to remove heat produced in our body. If temperature becomes high discomfort is felt.

5. ORGANIC MATTER : The increase of the organic matter due to breathing has no physiological effect. Specific germs like tuberculosis, virus etc. may cause the specific disease, but the normal organic matters thrown out during expiration has no harmful effect on our body.

V. OVER CROWDING AND ITS BAD EFFECTS

Q. 3.6. What is meant by overcrowding ?

The overcrowding is expressed in various ways but the following are most important :

1. Persons per room :

The degree of overcrowding expressed as the number of persons per room i.e. number of persons present in excess against the general standards in a dwelling room. General standards in this respect are :

1 Room for	—	2 persons.
2 Rooms	—	3 persons.
3 Rooms	—	5 persons.
4 Rooms	—	7½ persons.
5 or more	—	10 persons.

****Additional 2 for each further one room is necessary.

2. Standard floor space per person :

110 sq.ft. or more	—	2 persons.
90-100 sq.ft.	—	1½ person.
70-90 sq.ft.	—	1 person.
under 50 sq.ft.	—	½ person.

**A baby under 12 months is not counted while children between 1 to 10 years old should be counted as half a unit.

3. Sex separation :

Overcrowding is considered to exist if 2 persons, with over 9 years of aged children, is not husband and wife.

Q. 3.7. What are the disadvantages (or bad effects) of over-crowding in bad ventilated or poorly ventilated class-room or cinema hall?

Overcrowding is an evil and has bad effects on physical as well as social aspects. Generally overcrowding cause— increase of temperature, humidity and stagnation of air i.e. increase CO_2% and decrease O_2 in a room. Generally these factors lower the vitality of the students or people and they are easily prone to infection.

The *acute bad* effects of over crowding are—lassitude, headache, vertigo, etc. The *Chronic bad effects* are— anaemia, debility, digestive disturbance, lower vitality and diminishes resistance to infection. Besides these:

a) if some persons in the crowd are suffering from contagious disease; like scabies and ringworm, or respiratory diseases like influenza, and tuberculosis, small pox, chicken pox, measles then there is great risk to other people contracting these infections. Even louse brone typhus is also associated with overcrowding.

b) Excess of CO_2 produces ill effects on the health such as headache, inability to concentrate mind, drowsiness, lassitude etc. It may even cause death especially in a closed room where coal is burning.

c) In humid atmosphere due to overcrowding the lungs and the skin are unable to get rid of the moisture and thus a feeling of oppression and stuffiness is experienced.

d) *Apart from its association on disease, overcrowding has a bad social effect specially when persons of opposite sexes occupy the same sleeping room. The lack of privacy preforce an adverse and degrading influence specially on children and adolescents.*

AIR, LIGHT, SUNSHINE IN RELATION TO HEALTH

Q. 3.8. What measures would be taken to prevent the bad effect of overcrowding of a class room?

OR

How we can maintain the proper ventilation of a class-room?

Minimum 100 cu.ft. space is necessary per head for proper ventilation of a class room. Generally the proper ventilation of a class room can be done by planning school building. In planning building the windows and doors should be so arranged that they can easily provide a crossed draught. The perflation action of the wind can be effectively utilised by opening windows facing the wind. This action is considerably enhanced when windows and doors on the opposite side of the rooms are also kept open. The rooms are there—by rapidly and continuously flushed with fresh air and it becomes feasible to renew the air of a room at the rate of 100 times an hour.

The ventilation of the class room also can be maintained by adopting admistrative measures, viz-no lesson should be continued for more than an hour at a stretch and an interval of at least 10 to 15 minutes should be maintained between two consecutive lessons. During this period class room should be kept empty. The out going teacher should be taken responsible for ascertaining that all windows and doors of the class room are flung open as soon as it is vacated. The incoming teacher may close as many windows of the class room as he considers necessary, depending upon prevailing weather, conditions and temperature. This gives the room a flush of pure air for about 10-15 minutes. Sometimes artificial ventilation are also done by the help of different types of fans.

VI. HOW AIR IS PURIFIED IN NATURE

Q. 3.9. Describe how air is purified in nature?

Air is purified in nature by :
1. *Action of the wind*—It dilutes the impurities.
2. *Rain washes out impurities of air*—i.e. dust, soot, gases.

3. Sunlight due to its heat kills the insects and germs, and ultraviolet rays of sunlight is protoplasmic poison to the germs.
4. Oxygen and ozone in air oxidise and kill the germ.
5. During photosynthesis plant takes up CO_2, from the air, breaks up CO_2 to carbon and oxygen. O_2 is given out in air and hence air contain more oxygen and less CO_2.
6. Diffusion of gases dilutes the impurities in the air.

$$Diffusion\ of\ gas = \frac{1}{\sqrt{density\ of\ gas}}\ as\ per\ Grahm's\ Law.$$

Q. 3.10. How air can be disinfected ?

Air can be disinfected by :
1) U.V. rays,
2) Triethylene Glycol,
3. Chloramine T mist, or
4) Mist of Sodium Hypochlorite (Aerosol).

VII. VENTILATION—NATURAL AND ARTIFICIAL

Q. 3.11. What is meant by ventilation ?

Ventilation is the science of maintaining atmospheric conditions which are comfortable and helpful to the human body.

It also means the constant replacement of foul air by fresh air through inlets and outlets or the control of the quality of incoming air with regards to its temperature, humidity and purity.

Q. 3.12. What are its main objects ?

The main objects of ventilation are:
i) supply of pure air from out side which is comfortable and free from risk of infection with a proper temperature and humidity.
ii) prevents chilling and drying of the body as well as stagnation of the body heat.

AIR, LIGHT, SUNSHINE IN RELATION TO HEALTH

iii) removes gases, odours, bacteria, dust etc. which contaminate the air and also it removes the impurities produced inside the room through vitiating process.

Q. 3.13. What is meant by internal ventilation and external ventilation ? How these can be ensured ?

Generally *Ventilation* is divided into two forms : (i) *Internal* and (ii) *External*.

i) *Internal Ventilation* means the removal or dilution of the atmosphere of a place which has become stagnent, warm and moist through the vitiating process by air, which is comparatively drier, cooler and in motion.

ii) *External Ventilation* means admission of fresh air into a house, from the surrounding air spaces such as streets, garden etc. This is generally done by making the streets broad, building houses moderately high and not very close to one another etc. It is also ensured :

    a) by preventing impurities from entering the air,
    b) by watering the streets to lay the dust down,
    c) by careful inspection of all drains and sewers,
    d) by transporting all offensive trades and occupations to special quarters,
    e) by the speedy removal of street and other refuse,
    f) by such regulations which will prevent nuisance from smoke, and
    g) by keeping plants in open spaces and parks.

Q. 3.14. What is the principal object of ventilation ?

The principal object of ventilation is the *stimulating effects of moving air upon the skin*, which depends largely upon the evaporative power of the air.

Q. 3.15. What are the amount of air required for proper ventilation ?

The amount of air required for proper ventilation depends on several factors namely, the size of the room, the number of persons occupying it, type of lights burning, other sources in the room which may vitiate the air and the existing arrangement for natural or artificial ventilation. The amount of fresh air required for a healthy living in a room is calculated by the formula $e/_p = d$, where

e = CoDiffusion of gas = emitted per hour per head (av. 0.6 cu.ft.);

p = limit of respiratory CO_2 cu.ft. of air (0.02 cu.ft. per 100 cu.ft.);

and d= amount of fresh air require per cu.ft. per head per hour.

So it comes to $\dfrac{0.6}{0.002}$ = 3000 cu.ft.

Based on this standard an average adult requires 3000 cu.ft. of air per hour and a child about 200 cu.ft per head per hour.

Residential house 500 cu.ft.,

General hospital (teaching) 1,800 cu.ft., and

Sick person in a room 3,000-5,200 cu.ft.

Q. 3.16. When the air of a place or room would be considered as poorly ventilated or ill-ventilated ?

Generally a man entering a room from the open air should not perceive any smell or stuffiness. But when the CO_2, of the air of a room exceeded the percentage in the out side air by more than 0.02 percent, the feeling of stuffiness become perceptable to the sense. So by the sense of smell and stuffiness one can detect the impurity of air in a room or places. Also estimation of temperature, humidity can give a better indication of proper ventilation.

i) For temperature of the air use thermometer.
ii) For humidity use any type of Hygrometer or Dry and Wet Buble Thermometer.
iii) For find out the cooling power of air use Kata-Thermometer.

Q. 3.17. What are the various systems of ventilation ?

What method are used to achieve good ventilation in a house/room?

There are two systems of ventilation depending upon the motive power, viz.
1. *Natural* and 2. *Artificial*

1. VENTILATION OF A HOUSE OR ROOM

In any system of ventilation the size and shape of the room are important. Generally the minimum space of about one-third the quantity of air required per hour i.e. 700 to 1000 cu.ft. per person is required. But the space by itself has a little value unless the air is replaced by free circulation of fresh air. Actually in any case the room will be a large enough to allow the air to be replaced two or three times an hour without any perceptable draught.

Generally good ventilation of a house or room can be achieved by 2 ways—(a) *Naturally* and (b) *Artificially.*

A. NATURAL VENTILATION

Natural ventilation is generally achieved by building houses having *sufficient open space and by having a large number of window opening direct into the open air.* Fresh air enters the room though windows and doors and replaces the foul air. This is due to (i) *perflation and aspiration*, (ii) *temperature difference* and (iii) *diffusion of gases.*

Generally when the doors and windows are open, the wind naturally blows through the room (perflation) causing the surrounding air to move towards it by aspiration.

Perflation action: Wind going in the room through doors, windows, ventilators etc. The normal blowing of the wind from one direction to other, air enters the room, and changes the air of the room by perflation action.

Aspiration action of the wind : When air current is blowing outside the wall of a building or over the chimney, the inside air is sucked out of the room, and from some other openings air enters the room to fill up the space.

For such natural ventilation there must be an inlet or exit for the air, so that the air may move in and out in every possible direction and *diffusion* can take place inversely as the square root of their densities. The rate of flow can be measured with an *Anemometer* or with the aid of Katathermometer and the cross-sectional area of the inlet will give the total amount of air entering the room in a given time. In the tropics the usual practice is to have cross ventilation, the windows and doors being placed opposite each other, for which at least one-fifth of the floor space should be used.

Difference of temperature is another factor which also helps natural ventilation. If the air of the room is heated by fire, as in the cold countries, or by the respiration of men or animals it expands and rises up to escape through openings. This causes the outer colder air to enter into the room until the temperature of the inside air becomes equal to that of the outside air.

Besides, natural ventilation, ventilation of a room also can be maintained naturally by inlet and outlet ventilators. Inlet ventilators throw the air in the room and outlet ventilators throws out the air from the room.

(a) The common inlet ventilators are :
   1. Double sash window.
   2. Hopper inlet ventilator.
   3. Coppers ventilator.
   4. Sheringham valves.
   5. Ellisons bricks.
   6. Tobin tube.
   7. Louver's ventilator.

(b) Outlet ventuators are :
   1. Macknnels ventilator,
   2. Ridge ventilator, and
   3. Chimney flonacts as outlet ventilator.

But where a number of people are congregated for a considerably long period and where climate conditions do not permit free use of open windows and doors, and inlet and outlet ventilators are not able to produce satisfactory results i.e. in *cinema hall, theater hall, examination halls, schools, hotels, factories* etc., proper ventilation is done by various mechanical means such as exhaust fan, extraction fans and propulsion fans etc. and these are known as *Mechanical ventilation methods* or *Artificial system of ventilation.*

B. ARTIFICIAL SYSTEM OF VENTILATION

Q. 3.18. What is meant by artificial ventilation ? Describe the various mechanical methods for improving ventilation.

Artificial ventilation is a process of moving the air by a mechanical device, like various inlets and outlets with the electric fans.

Various Mechanical Methods :

Where a number of people are congugated for a considerably long period and where climate conditions do not permit free use of open windows and doors or the inlets and outlets ventilators are not able to maintain proper ventilation, various mechanical means are used to facilitate the removal of air and are known as mechanical system of ventilation. These methods are generally adopted in cinema hall, theater hall, examination hall, hotels, schools, factories etc. Mechanical methods of ventilation are of 4 types namely

1) *Vaccum system,*
2) *Plenum system,*
3) *Combined system,* and
4) *Air conditioning.*

1. VACCUM SYSTEM

Here exhaust fans are used to expel out the air from a room, such as cinema hall, factories, kitchen room of an eating house etc.

A two feet diameter fan with 600 revolutions per minute can throw out 6000 cubic feet of air.

2. PLENUM SYSTEM

Here propulsion fans are used to throw fresh air from outside in a hall room. They are mainly used in factories. The air is carried by a duct in the factory premisses and the ducts have openings where the workers are working. The outside fresh air is thus uniformly distributed amongst the workers.

3. COMBINED SYSTEM OR BALANCED SYSTEM

This is a combination of the extraction and plenum system of ventilation. Here air under controlled conditions of temperature and humidity is driven into by means of ducts by the plenum method and extraction is done by means of a fan of a furnace; it is essential that there should be no leakage through windows or doors. This is specially for ventilation of large halls and factories and also used in air conditioning.

4. AIR CONDITIONING

Air conditioning is process by which the air is simultaneously purified, cooled or heated and the moisture content regulated. Thus this is a combination of ventilation, heating or cooling to the desired humidity or temperature.

Mechanism :

The air drawn from outside and in combination with the recirculated air is passed through a set of filters and dried and then cooled by mechanical refrigerator, ice or cold water in cooling coils and then passed through a humidifier to take up a predetermined amount of water vapour. This *humidification* takes place in a chamber containing nozzles which project water into it in the form of fine sprays. In the next stage the eliminator plates remove dirts and droplets and air current is pushed into the room by electric fan.

AIR CONDITIONING PLANT :

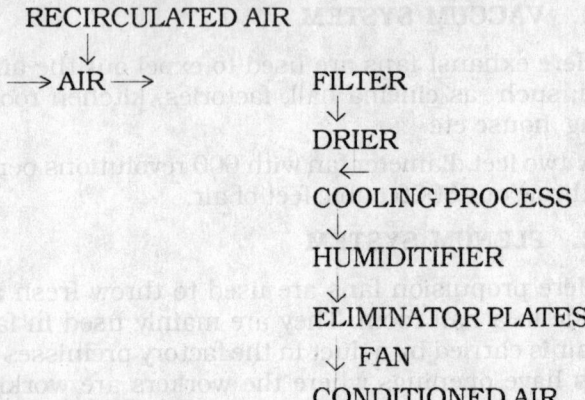

```
        RECIRCULATED AIR
                ↓
    → AIR →     FILTER
                ↓
                DRIER
                ←
                COOLING PROCESS
                ↓
                HUMIDITIFIER
                ↓
                ELIMINATOR PLATES
                ↓ FAN
                CONDITIONED AIR
```

AIR, LIGHT, SUNSHINE IN RELATION TO HEALTH

N.B. a) So in air conditioning, the air is conditioned regarding the temperature and humidity.
b) The dust is filtered.
c) The temperature is increased or decreased by the heating or cooling process.
d) The humidity is increased or decreased by adding moisture or cooling so that the humidity gets saturated and then the necessary amount of water is removed, in form of water drops. This water is then drained away, and there by the humidity is adjusted as desired.

In India, air condition means only filtering the air of dust and cooling the temperature to desired level. In the cooling process, whatever quantity of moisture falls out as water drop is only removed.

N.B. I. COMFORTABLE AIR

The amount of humidity and temperature required to give comfort varies from person to person. Some may like temp. of 70 degree F. with relative humidity as 60%. Other may not like this. On an average, a room is considered comfortable if :

1. Temperature is 75 degree F.
2. Relative humidity is 70%.
3. There is no dust.
4. D.K. (Dry Kata)- reading is 5 to 6.
5. W.K. (Wet Kata)- reading is 15 to 20.
6. There is movement of air of the room 10 times per hour.

2. COMFORT-ZONES

Comfort-zones may be defined as the range of effective temperature over which the majority of adults feel comfortable. There is no unanimous decision on a single zone of comfort for all people because comfort is quite a complex subjective experience which depends not only on physical, physiological factors, but also on phychological factors which are difficult to determine.

Considering only the environmental factors in India, the comfortable thermal condition are as follow, under which a person can maintain normal balance between production of heat and loss of heat i.e. maintain normal body temperature without sweating.

Effective Temperature -O degree F.

1. Pleasant and cool — 69
2. Comfortable and cool — 69-78
3. Comfortable — 77-80
4. Hot and uncomfortable — 81-82
5. Extremely hot — 83+
6. Intolerably hot — 86+

Predicted four hour sweat rate (P_4 SR)

1. Comfortzone — 1-3 litres.
2. Just tolerable — 3-4.5 litres.
3. Intolerable — 4.5 litres.

P_4SR-Maximum allowable sweat rate compatible with physiological normal reaction of acclimatized, healthy young man for repeated exposures to heat.

VIII. LIGHT AND ITS IMPORTANCE

Q. 3.19. What are the importance of lighting ?

Good illumination is necessary for performing work. Inadequate or defective illumination causes eye strain and fatigue, poor performance and accidents. The illumination of any surface is measured in *foot-scandles* which is the illumination of a white surface placed at right angles to the rays one foot away from a standard scandle. It is conveniently measured by photo-electric light metres.

In the tropics, during the day the intensity of illumination from sky (not direct sunlight) is very high almost all the year around. Sufficient illumination is obtained inside the premises by having enough openings in the walls (or even in the roofs), so that a good deal of the sky is visible from inside. A convenient rule is that the area of the opening (windows etc.) should be at least one fifth of the floor area for adequate illumination inside a room. For working in evenings or at nights or in working in larges factories of such construction which do not allow a sufficiency of illumination in all portions of the factory as well as in a countries geographically so, situated and with such climates that clear daylight is available only for short periods, artificial illumination is necessary. For rough tasks a level of illumination of about 6 foot candle is sufficient, where as for continued work demanding high degree of visual acuity and precision, the levels of illumination required for proper performance of the task may be upto 50 foot candles. But the illumination should be such as to prevent the formation of excessively dark shadows, the other principal requirement is that these should not be bright light sources or very brightly illuminated surface in the visual field of workers. These constitute glare and interfere with vision by interfering with the convergence accommodation reflex.

Very poor illumination, as usually obtains inside the dark depths of the coal mines, may result in the development of Nystagmus in miners who have spent long years in underground work.

IX. SUNSHINE (SUNLIGHT) AND ITS IMPORTANCE

Q. 3.20. What are the effects of sunlight in our body or Why sunshine are more important for us?

The importance of sunshine (sunlight) for physical development and preservation is not duly appreciated. Women and children, as well as men, in order to be healthy, and well developed, should spend a portion of each day where the solar rays can reach them directly, this being particularly necessary when there is a tendency to tuberculosis.

The value of sunshine recognised for the preservation of health has been recommended, as we see in case of putting an infants to a bask under the sunshine after anointing the body with musterd oil. But with the advancement of modern civilisation, this practice is being given up, at least cities, with the result that the children are ill-developed, rickets and grow with poor physique.

Generally the sunshine helps by its ultraviolet rays to synthesis vitamin-D from ergosterol and helps and calcium metabolism, forming bones, preventing disease like rickets and osteomalacia of a baby or children. It is also seen that children and adults who live almost entirely dark room or houses or kitchen, dingly alleys, badly lighted workshops, are pale cheeked and feeble. Houses are only fit to be occupied at night when, they have been purified by the solar rays of the day. It is also evident that during the prevalance of certain epidemic diseases, the inhabitants who occupy houses on the side of the street upon which the sunshines directly fall, are less subjected to the prevailing disease than those who live on the shaded side. So it is proved that the sunshine is more effective to destroy infectious agents which are present in dust, smoke and other organic matter of atmosphere by its ultravioletrays.

"HEALTH IS BEAUTY AND BEAUTY IS HEALTH"

CHAPTER-IV

EFFECT OF CLIMATE

(HUMIDITY, TEMPERATURE AND PRESSURE)

I. Climate.
II. Humidity and its effect on health.
III. Temperature and its effects on health.
IV. Pressure and its changes effecting health.

I. CLIMATE

Introduction

The general experience is that climate and wheather have marked effects on health and diseases. For intance, gastro-intestinal disorders occur with a greater frequency in the weather conditions obtaining in the summer and rainy seasons than at other times. Respiratory infections, in general, tend to be high during the colder months and in the colder climates.

But there is no clear cut answers how the weather and climate affect the health of a man. Most of the effects are considered to be indirect. But in any case we can not deni the relationship of climate and weather on health and disease, though the underlying mechanisms are obscure due to the fluctuating patterns of incidences of many diseases as mentioned above. So in public health, we are naturally concerned with the characteristics of the weather or the climate which are usually important in the natural history of many disease.

Major climatic factors are :
1) Temperature.
2) Moisture content of air (pressure & humidity).
3) Air velocity and direction.
4) Latitude and distance from the sea.
5) Nearness of mountains and hills.

6) Sunshine (Radiant heat).
7) Rainfall.

N.B. Of these according to D.H.M.S. and B.H.M.S. syllabus—temperature, moisture content of air (humidity & pressure) should be studied.

Q. 4.1. What is meant by climate ?

Climate—It is the average conditions of the atmosphere and the character of the earth's surface of a particular place or region for a long time and is also the some-total of all the meteorological conditions in relation to animal and vegetable life.

Q. 4.2. What is meant by meteorology ?

Meteorology is the science which deals with atmospheric phenomena in relation to weather *and climate, i.e. atmospheric pressure, air temperature, humidity, direction and speed of wind, rainfall, proximity of mountain and sea, height above the sea level etc. It also includes the interpretation of the sum-total effect of all these factors.

*Weather—it denotes a single occurance or event in the series of conditions which make up climate.

II. HUMIDITY AND ITS EFFECTS ON HEALTH

Q. 4.3. What is meant by humidity ?

Humidity—denotes the amount of moisture in the air. The amount of water vapour necessary to cause saturation of the air varies directly with the temperature. The higher the temperature the more water vapour can it hold, before saturation point is reached. The following two terms also related to humidity—absolute humidity and relative humidity.

Absolute humidity—is the exact amount of water vapour actually present in the air, and expressed as number of water in each cubic metre of air.

Relative humidity—can be expressed as the percentage of the amount of water vapour actually present in the air,

EFFECT OF CLIMATE 119

at a given temperature in relation to the amount that would have been present, had the air been saturated with water vapour at the same temperature.

Q. 4.4. What are the effects of humidity on health?

According to the moisture contents (i.e. the degree of humidity), the climates are classified into moist and dry but always a certain amount of moisture is present in the air. We have seen that the sensation of freshness or sultiness depends upon the rate of cooling of the body temperature which is turn depends upon the rate of air movement and the percentage of relative humidity. *Halden* has also seen that the maximum temperature which can be borne for some hours without the development of heat stroke, depends mostly upon the amount of moisture present in the air.

Generally excessive humidity retards evaporation from the lungs and skin and as it has a very little drying effects or no effects the perspiration do not take place and the normal functions of the lungs become impaired. So the person fells uneassy and oppression. Most climates are also less healthy than dry ones, as it favours the growth and development of micro organisms and hastens putrefactive changes. For good health, generally 75 percent of humidity is best.

N.B. : [GENERALLY HUMIDITY IS DETERMINED BY WET AND DRYBULB THERMOMETERS.

III. EFFECT OF TEMPERATURE ON HUMAN HEALTH

1. EFFECT OF HIGH TEMPERATURE

Q. 4.5. What are the effects of high temperature on man's health.

Generally variations in the external temperature set in motion on physiological corrective mechanisms which act both on the production of heat and on its loss by the body.

In the cells, important chemical reactions are continually taking place. this activity is acompanied by liberation of energy, and part of this appears as heat. It is a common place that physical exercise is a source of heat production, but this applies to all types of cellular activity. Even at rest, the human body loses about, 2,000 calories every twenty four hours. This is the 'central heating' which enables man to maintain a body temperature generally above that of his surroundings. The loss of heat, except that lost in respiration (expired air is warmer than inspired air and is saturated with water vapour), occurs form the skin by *radiation, by convection, or through the evaporation of water.*

In case of excessive use in temperature, man, the homoeothermic subject reduces the production of heat as much as possible (which is relatively little), and increase heat loss by a cutaneous vasodilation and especially, if the surrounding temperature is raised, through perspiration. As seen a man weighing 70 kg. can thus lose from 1 to 3 litres of perspiration in one hour, and the evaparation of this represents the loss of several thousand calories—a considerable amount. Thus in case of high rise of temperature heavy perspiration occurs and heavy perspiration corresponds to complex interchanges of water between blood, the intertitial spaces, and the tissues. If it is prolonged, it leads to a real dehydration. As we seen in the desert in summer a man can lose 10 to 12 litres of water a day. Such losses must be made good by the drinking of at least the same quantity of water with salts.

But experiences shows that even in dry climates the organisms can endure very high external temperatures only for very short periods. If the body's defences are overwhlemed by a high temperature and the internal temperature increase, "*heat disorders*" syndromes like heat stroke, heat exhaustion, heat crams etc. occur. The margins of internal temperature variations is a very narrow i.e. 44° C to 45° C (110° F to 113° F) represents the upper extreme temperature compatible with life. So the effect of excessive rise of temperature on the human health are.

EFFECT OF CLIMATE

1. **Directly**—It causes heat disorder syndromes like heat cram, heat exhaustion and heat stroke (sunstroke) or fever due to interferance or suspended some of the important and natural functions of the body.

   a) *Heat cramp*—This occurs in men who are doing heavy muscular work and sweating profusely in high external temperature. It is characterised by painful cramps of the skeletal muscles. Body temperature may be normal or sligtly increased. (cramps may be treated by administration of salt). It is generally occurs due to loss of sodium chlorides from the blood.

   b) *Heat exhaustion*—It is a mild form of heat collapse caused by continued exposure to heat, high relative humidity and insufficient ventilation as these upset the heat regulation mechanism of the body.

   Signs and symptoms—are dizziness, headache, fatigue, cold and clammy skin. Complete collapse due to circulatory failure or unconsciousness. The body temperature may be normal or as low as 96 degree F. The underlying cause is gradual loss of water and chlorides from the body which upsets the normal chemical balances of the body. (This condition may be treated by rest, suitable clothings, by intake of salt, administration of cardiac stimulants and by reducing muscular exertion).

   c) *Heat stroke*—It is the most clinical condition and often flows heat exhaustion.

   Body temperature may be high as 110 degree F associated with cessation of sweating and dry skin. There may be headache, stupor and delirium. (Treatment is the lowering of body temperature by ice water bath, ice packs and ice enemate).

2. **Indirectly**, high rise of temperature produces heat syncopes, changes in metabolism and congestive disorder affecting the liver and bowels. Stimulation of the nervous system followed by depression is the rule in tropical climates.

2. EFFECT OF LOW TEMPERATURE

Q.4.6. What are the effects of low temperature on human health with reference to the surgical importance?

A man exposed to cold reduces his heat loss (cutaneous vaso-constriction) and increase heat production. The cellular combustion is raised through the influence of nervous and endrocrine regulatory mechanisms and through muscular exercise. However, the efficiency of these mechanisms has its limits. In a person exposed to very low temperatures certain parts of the body become vulnerable; for instances, the feet and hands. Cold leads to localized vasodilator reactions of which chilblains are a first indication. If the action of cold is too intense, serious circulatory troubles will follows and will lead to gangrene. The internal temperature is safe guarded for the time being, but the most exposed parts of the body are sacrificed. Clothing plays the part of an insulator. It can be adapted to the temperatures expected and, if necessary, heated, as in fly suits. These give protection to the wearer even at temperatures of -40° C to 52° C.

But when a man is exposed to lower temperatures without sufficient protection, his thermo-regulatory system runs the risk of breaking down. The struggle against cold is lost and the internal temperature beings to fall, this is called hypothermy. The main functions of the body are progressively slow down. Below 30 degree C (86 degree F) consciousness is lost. Then the circulation shows down, while the respiratory movements diminish in amplitude. If no help is forthcoming, death supervens, usually between 25° C and 20° C (72° F & 68° F). Death from cold involves, infact, a general 'bogging down', of all the main functions of the body. Experiences show that in worm blooded animals that have been cooled to 20 degree C (68 degree F), all the tissues are in a state of 'slow motion'. the celluler activity is reduced and failure of nervous action dominates the picture, leading to failure of the important functions, particularly respiration.

On the basis of these findings, it is possible to-day to use 'controlled hypothermy' during surgical operations, such as those on the heart, which entail prolonged arrest of circulation. This arrest is well supported at low temperatures. While at normal temperatures an arrest of the cerebral circulation for three or four minutes causes grave secondary damage, such an arrest can be continued for thirty five to forty minutes at a temperature of 16° C to 18° C (60.8° F to 64.4° F).

The study of hypothermy, its effects and the way in which disturbances are produced has thus enable us to use low temperature techniques in connection with surgery. In medical therapy, chilling, under the debatable name of hibernation involves a drop of temperature of only 2° C or 3° C, this is generally brought about by the use of various chemical products which reduce the activity of the normal thermo-regulatory mechanisms.

SUMMARY

EFFECTS OF HIGH AND LOW TEMPERATURE

High Temperature :

Common effects of high temperature are heat crams from loss of sodium chloride in the sweat; if saline drinks are taken, the crams can be prevented. In heat stroke, sweating suddenly ceases and the body temperatures may rise as high as 108° F (42° C). If this state is unrelieved, coma and death may ensure. *Heat exhaustion* occurs during excessively hot weather in workers not acclimatized to heat. Sweating is profuse and body temperature are normal. It is caused by dilatation of the peripheral blood vessels. Recovery is rapid after rest. High temperatures generally occur in a verity of occupations such as mining, refining and casting, brick making, construction work in the tropics, and work in engine rooms abords ships. Other than summer (season), heat syncope is also a common bad effect of high temperature. In its milder form, the person standing in the sun become pale, his blood pressure falls and he collapses suddenly. There is particularly no rise in body temperature. The condition results from pooling of blood in lower limbs due to dilatation of blood vessels, with the result that the amount of blood returning to the heat is reduced, which in turn is responsible for lowering of blood pressure, and lack of blood supply to the brain. This condition is quite common among soldiers when they are standing long time for parades in the summer.

Treatment is quite simple. The patient should be made to lie in the shade with the head slightly down, recovery usually comes with in 5 to 10 minutes.

Low Temperature:

Exposure to low temperature i.e. cold occurs among workers in artificially cooled or naturally cold environments. Such persons include building workers, commercial fishermen, food storage attendants, and dry ice makers. Generally the effects are *chilblains, frost-bite* and *immersion foot or trench foot*. These conditions may prevented by protective clothing or by using water at 44 degree C. Warming should be last for 20 minutes at a time. In take of hot fluids also promotes general rewarming. But the common injury due to cold may be general or local. In general cold injury (hypo-thermia), the individual is said to be suffering from exposure to cold. This is characterised by numbness, loss of sensation, muscular weakness, desire for sleep, coma and death.

Local cold injury may occur at temperature above freezing (wet cold conditions) as in *immersion* or *trench foot*. At temperatures below freezing (dry cold conditions) frostbite occurs ; and also the tissues freeze and ice crystals form in between the cells.

IV. EFFECTS OF THE CHANGES OF PRESSURE ON HUMAN'S HEALTH

1. EFFECTS OF LOW PRESSURE—Chemical Effects

Q. 4.7. What are the chemical effects of pressure on man when he ascends from normal atmospheric pressure to high altitudes ?

EFFECT OF CLIMATE

Man is accustomed to living under a pressure of 760 mm of mercury. He takes his respiratory requirements from the air, which consists of approximately 80 percent nitrogen and 20 percent oxygen. When the barometric pressure falls, as happens at high altitudes, the partial pressure of the oxygen falls in proportion. The respiratory exchanges in the lungs are determined by the differences between the pressure of the air in the alveoli and that in the venous, blood, and so the exchanges are reduced. Thus the blood no longer becomes sufficiently oxygeneted during its passage through the lung and there arises a state of hypoxia (i.e. deep breathing, quick pulse, nausea, fainting with bleeding from nose and ears, and impaired vision), which is known as the *chemical effect of the falls of pressure or mountain sickness.*

Observation at the hight of 2,500 to 3,000 meters (8,000 to 9,500 ft.) seen that tissues of a young person in good health begin to suffer from lack of oxygen. In older people, and even more in those with pulmonary or cardiac trouble, this threshold is lower. At about 3,000 m. (10,000 ft.) a phase of cortical hyper excitability occurs. But more than this height i.e. at higher altitudes errors of judgement become more and more frequent. It becomes impossible to make mental calculations and the reaction time becomes longer. At about 7,000 to 8,000 m. (22,000 to 25,000 ft.) loss of consciousness may supervene. The effect is dramatic. The individual loses all contact with external world, but regains it at once, if oxygen is administered. He will remember absolutely nothing of the period of anoxic faint. So inorder to protect the organism against the chemical effects of lowering of the barometric pressure e.g. in an aeroplane, it is necessary, to inhale oxygen above 3,000 meters i.e. 10,000 ft.

2. PHYSICAL EFFECTS OF LOW PRESSURE

Q. 4.8. What are the physical effects of pressure on man during ascending and descending from normal atmosphere.

Due to lowering of barometric pressure, some of the physical effects are relatively harmless. But due to expansion of gases (when the pressure is lowered) the main problems are generally associated with the ears.

Pain and sensation of deafness may occur, which are quickly relieved by a simple swallowing movement or by yawing widely in order to open the Eustachian tubes and so equalise the pressure on each side of ear-drums. If there is a complete blockage of the communication between the middle ear and the nasopharynx, a rapid descent may lead to rupture of the ear-drums, but this seldom occurs.

Generally this mishaps, resulting from too swift a descent are also well known to drivers and aqualung fisherman. Each descent of 10 m. (approximately 32 ft.) below the surface of the sea corresponds to an increase of pressure by one atmosphere. Equilibrium of the pressures on each side of the ear-drums must therefore be re-established both during the descent and on the return to the surface.

But much more serious accidents may befall a man at high altitudes, or a diver returning quickly to the surface. If the human organism is subjected to an abrupt decompression, i.e. reduction of atmospheric pressure, gas will come out of solution. Nitrogen, an inert gas, is the most important in this respect and at atmospheric pressure at sea level a man weighing 70 kg. will contain 1,000 cu.ft. of nitrogen in solution. When the pressure is rapidly reduced, this gas tends to come out of solution and the free gas may appear as bubbles in many different parts of the body. The disturbances which result from this, caused by physical changes, may take different forms, according to where the gas is. Among the most frequent minor forms are *pains in the joints or on the course of the nerves and sensations of itching with cutaneous reddening.* Unfortunately, *when central nervous system, the pulmonary circulation, or the coronary arteries are affected, these disturbances are more serious and prove fatal.* Such a release of gas from solution may occur at a height of 8,000 to 9,000 m. (25,000 to 28,000 ft.).

EFFECT OF CLIMATE

B. EFFECT OF HIGH PRESSURE

The human body can endure, pressures of several atmosphere, but the higher the pressure, the more gas will be dissolved. Even oxygen itself can then become harmful in excess. Mental disturbances with hallucinations have been occured under pressure of 8-10 atmospheres. But once again, it is nitrogen which is the most important, it dissolves in the body an average at about, 1,000 c.c. for each atmosphere. After fairly prolonged stay at high pressure the quantities of nitrogen dissolve may be considerable and produced cassion's disease. When the driver returns to the surface, thus undergoing the decompression, there is considerable risk of air embolisms being produced.

Q. 4.9. Why the works of deep sea drivers and of tunnal workers and flyers are vigorously regulated ?

The physical mechanisms and the physiological and pathological aspects are the same for a man adapted to normal pressure who ascends in the air to regions of lower pressure, as for a man adapted to high pressure who returns to regions of normal pressure. Each time the pressure is reduced rapidly by half, whether it be from 6 to 3 atmosphere, or from 4 to 2, or from 2 to 1 or from 1 to 1/2 or from 1/2 to 1/4, the risk of air embolism is present.

We can thus understand why, on the basis of these data the work of deep sea drivers and of tunnel workers is vigorously regulated. The compression must be sufficiently slow for the removal through the lungs of the excess of nitrogen which has been dissolved, calculated from the pressures experienced and the duration of the stay at a depth. This determines the different levels at which stops are made during the return to the surface, which can amount to several hours, if the excess of pressure has been considerable and fairly prolonged. There are also tables which lay down precisely the length of time to be spent at each level during to ascent.

It is important to understand that from the biological point of view the studies concerning flyers and astronants are exactly similar to those based on observations concerning drivers and tunnel workers. The problems set by the decompression of the flyer who rises above sea level are the same as those of the driver who rises to it from the depths, they obey the same physical laws and give rise to the same type of accidents.

SUMMARY

Effects of high and low pressure :

Exposures to high or low atmospheric pressures can cause *decompression sickness*. It occurs, for example, when workers in compressed air, as in constructing tunnels under rivers, are too rapidly returned to ordinary air pressures or when airman ascends too rapidly to high altitudes. The symptoms include pains in the joints and bones, difficulty in breathing, or even asphyxia, and staggers, dizziness and vomiting. All these symptoms are caused by the release of nitrogen from solution in the blood and tissues and then formation of nitrogen bubbles.

CHAPTER-V

PERSONAL HYGIENE

DISCUSSION FOR LEARNING

I. Personal hygiene and its main objects.
II. Various health care for the maintenance of personal hygiene.
III. Health care and avoidable habits of children.
IV. Health care of a house wife for maintaining her personal hygiene.

I. PERSONAL HYGIENE AND ITS MAIN OBJECTS

Q. 5.1. What is meant by personal hygiene? What are its main objects?

Def: The science that deals with the various aspects of the health of a person, and help through his own efforts to attain the highest possible standard of health is known as personal hygiene.

It consists of two words—Personal and Hygiene which means laws of health and sanitation to be practised by the individual at personal level.

Personal hygiene includs *Physical personal* and *Mental personal hygiene*. Physical personal hygiene is also divided into :

A. *Hygiene of body parts*, and
B. *Hygiene for maintenance of physiological functions.*

A. *Hygiene of the body parts care about* :

1) Mouth and teeth
2) Eyes
3) Ears
4) Nose and throat
5) Skin
6) Hair
7) Nails and hands
8) Bowel care
9) Exercise
10) Bath and cleanliness

B. *Hygiene for maintenance of physiological functions* are :

1) Clothing
2) Shoes and boots
3) Food habits
4) Control of weight
5) Hunger and mid-day lunch
6) Idiosyncrasy
7) Sleep and rest
8) Sex hygiene

Main objects :

1) Its main objects are the maintenance of promotion of individual health both mental and physical, and involves him into certain practices which enables him to lead a healthy and blissful life and serve himself and the society with satisfaction.

2) From the personal hygiene man also recognised the limitations of the human machine, and he has to regulate his activities according to his physical and mental make up and guards against the adverse effect which the environment in which he lives may bring to bear upon him.

II. VARIOUS CARE FOR THE MAINTENANCE OF PERSONAL HEALTH AND HYGIENE.

Q. 5.2. What should be followed to maintain personal hygiene ?

"*Health is wealth*" and "Health is beauty and beauty is health" expresses an eternal truth. A person with good health makes an impressive personality. This is largely achieved through care of personal hygiene. Certain habits and practices Pertaining to personal health are prevalent in India. Some of which have scientific background but perhaps wrongly practiced and some have been steeped more in superstition than in their hygienic value and some still have the practice value.

The practice of personal hygiene is as old as the origin or mainkind and is the oldest form of preventive medicine. In *Vedas* the practice of personal hygiene has been greatly streassed in daily morning and evening prayers. In the same manner at all our sacred and religious occasions, its principles have preached and practised. Similar accounts are available in the holy books of Buddhism, Jainism and Sikhism, and also in the practice of all other religious. Practice of personal hygiene is also common to us and our children generally learn it sub-consciously from their parents at home or from the teachers at school etc., just as they adopt language, religion, values of life and other habits from parents. But the role of mother is supreme.

Generally cleanliness is the first step of healthful living.

CLEANLINESS

"Cleanliness is next to godliness." There cannot be any truth than this epithat. This truth was realized by the Hindu long long ago and from the vedic age bathing was prescribed before any religious work or function. This cleanliness covers almost all aspects of our living, namely, body, parts of the body, air, water, food, drink, clothing, beds and beddings, utensils, house, and so on.

1st step of cleanliness is bathing :

Bathing : Regular bathing throughout the year is a healthy practice. During the cold season, it is necessary not only for cleanliness but also for the beneficient action on the skin the internal organs. This can be taken in ponds, rivers, lakes, tanks, swimming pool, shower in house, water tap or by pouring water on the body. Full immersion methods is the best of all types of bathing.

Sick people are cleansed with spongs instead of a bath. Tepid bath, cold bath, warm bath, hot bath, milk and curd bath etc. are also used in various times for various purposes. It is the best practice to massage with mustard and olive oil before bathing, and for privacy and to avoid unnecessary exposure baths in house should be taken in covered enclosure or room. For the cleanliness of the body bath preferably with soap is useful, because soap dissolves the oily matters on the body and the pores of the skin are opened up.

Besides regular bathing cleanliness must be extended to skin, mouth and teeth, eyes, ears, nose and throat, hairs, hands and nails etc. which are as follows :

1. SKIN

Skin is also cleaned by bathing. Regular bathing with or without soap and massaging the body with oil are good hygienic measures to keep the skin healthy, addition of balanced diet containing unsaturated fats and vitamin A & D is useful.

Use of soap with towel will open up the pores of the skin and there by skin diseases are avoided. Cutaneous circulation is also improved.

2. MOUTH AND TEETH

Teeth should be brushed twice daily in the morning and before going to bed, besides the washing of mouth and teeth after every meals.

The use of tooth powder and a heard brush is desirable. After use, the brush should be cleaned, rinsed and dried. Many people use sticks made out of branches of certain trees like neem, mulberry varanda, mango etc., particularly for its cheapness and also for some medicinal value but it is not very suitable process. It should be always used after washing stick well. Cleaning of tongue is also practised to remove foul ordour, particularly by the mouth breathers and smokers.

3. EYES

Eyes should be regularly washed and cleaned with cold and clean water in the morning, during bathing and at anytime following exposure to dust, smoke and heat etc. Goggles are useful to protect from glaring heat and dust etc.

4. NOSE AND THROAT

Washing of nose and throat should be a daily routine as muchas of others parts of the body. To avoid obstruction

PERSONAL HYGIENE

of breathing and those are susceptable to attacks of cold and tonsillitis cleanliness accompanied by judicious dieting and clothing is helpful. Proper disposal of nasal secretion and phlegm is of extreme importance in preventing the spread of respiratory infections and public health hazards that are entailed in their indiscriminate throwing. Use of handkerchief for blowing the nose and during sneezing and coughing is helpful in protecting others against droplet infection. It hands are used these should be properly washed subsequently. For any obstruction of passage by polypus, adenoids etc. a competent doctor should be consulted.

5. EARS

Ears should be properly cleansed. If wax accumulated, it should be removed carefully. External ears are needed protection in extreme cold climate by ear muffs to prevent earach. Special precaution should also be taken to cover the ear during swimming and diving. Competent doctor should be consulted on slightest suspicion of deafness in a child.

6. HAIRS

Cleanliness of hair is essential to keep away the dirts, louse infestation and fungal infections. Daily bathing keeps the hair supple, and shining. Persons having long hair should, in addition have head bath once or twice a week. Regular cutting of hairs short at intervals and shaving of beard are helpful in maintaining cleanliness. All precaution should be taken by the barber in keeping his instruments clean after each shave to protect customers against infections of strepto and staphylococci, syphilis, scabies fungal diseases etc. Hair should be regularly brushed and combed. Razor and blades should be separate for every individuals.

7. HANDS AND NAILS

Hand should be washed with soap and water before taking meals, or after every ablution. Nail should be timmed otherwise dirt will collect in the nails and ultimately enter into our body through food. The dirt from the nails enter the eyes, or scratching it may enter the skin producing various disease. Long nails and habits of nail biting are unhygienic, so nail brushing and use of soap for removing dirts from the nail essential. Certain other rules of health for cleanliness must also be performed namely use of clean clothing, use of clean utensils for keeping cooked food and for eating, clean food and drinks, clean house and surrounding etc.

Q. 5.3. (a) What is meant by cleanliness ? Describe it in brief.

B. After cleanliness the 2nd thing for maintaining personal hygiene is temperance i.e. Be moderate and avoid extreme.

1. **CLOTHING** : So the choice of clothing should be cotton.

i) Porous and permeable to air, should be light and tight fittings. Underwears should be absorbant.

ii) Wollen and silk clothes are bad conductors, hence they are useful to retain the body heat in cold climate.

iii) Garters and string elastic belts should be avoided as these may hamper circulation.

iv) For health point of view in the tropics synthetic fabrics, nylon, orlon, polyester etc. are not suitable. It is rather uncomfortable in the summer and rainy season and may cause allergy, irritation and even toxic symptoms.

v) Socks and stocking are generally made of cotton fibres, silk and nylon. In the tropics these should be worn with boots and shoes during the winter months. In the summer it is not suitable due to sweat and odour. They must be washed and exposed to sun daily, if used.

vi) Foot wears are hygienic and protective. The types of shoes varies with the nature of activity of the person and season. Generally airy, light and open type shoe i.e. slipper are desirable during hot seasons and more close and protective type in the winter; for sking, skating, playing, hiking,

PERSONAL HYGIENE

hunting, mountainering, walking on snow etc. special types of shoes are used.

On the whole, footwears should be comfortable, neither loose nor tight, and fitting with conformation and arch of the foot.

Q. 5.3. (b) What are the principal objectives of clothing ?

The principal objective of clothings are :
1) to protect the body from external effects of weather, temperature, external injuries, bites of insects and also of animals,
2) to maintain body temperature, and
3) for personal decoration.

Next to cleanliness and moderate clothing, food habit is the essential part for maintaining personal hygiene and the foods should also be moderate in quantity and quality.

2. FOOD AND FOOD HABITS

Food is the prime necessity of life. Although several aspects of food should always by kept in mind viz. adequacy, balancing of constituents, digestion, assimilation and safety (food hygiene), the basic things of foods and food habits are:-

1. Food is to be taken with a good appetite at regular intervals, to be taken at regular hours each day.
2. Food should be well masticated.
3. Food should be clean, prepared in clean utensils in a clean premises and kept covered and better still in a refrigerator.
4. Salads (fresh vegetables), fruits and green vegetables should from a part of each food meal.
5. Milk, as far as practicable, should also form a part of the meal.
6. It should be preferable to take fluid either before or sometime after the principal meals to help digestion and also in between meals.

7. Food rich in carbohydrates and fats are harmful.
8. Quantity should be adjusted according to age, sex and other necessities, eating too much is as bed as too little.
9. Fasting or light dieting at fortnightly or weekly interval helps to maintain good health.
10. The following foods should be avoided : Under-ripe and over- ripe fruits, food contaminated with dust, flies, dirt, overspiced and highly irritant food frequent drinks of tea of coffee, alcoholic drink etc. and narcotic substances like opium, cocaine, dhatura, bhang, charas, heavy smoking, tobacco and pan-chewing etc. are definitely harmful to health and demoralizing and should be strictly avoided.
11. Night meal should be lighter and person should not go to sleep with a heavy loaded stomach.
12. Certain types of food do not suit some people as they cause allergic symptoms e.g. eggs, prawns, shell-fish, certain fruits like oranges and certain vegetables like ladies fingers, so these should be differentiated from mere fancy as seen in some children.

Q. 5.3 (c) What should be our food and food habits to maintain personal health ?

After taken up foods for maintaining hygiene of the body parts and physiological functions-

***Bowel care** i.e. regular evacuation habit is boon to health.

3. BOWEL CARE

All foods taken cannot be completely transformed into forms which can be assimilated in the body and hence a good part of them is excreted out. As food intake at regular intervals is necessary, excretion should be also be equally regulated to keep the body in fit and healthy condition. Accumulation of these excretory material inside the bowels is definitely harmful for the body by producing fermentation, gas and even toxic material. It may create congestion of

PERSONAL HYGIENE

liver and may cause headache, lassitude, disturbed sleep and lowering of the capacity for mental work. Hence every body should cultivate the habit of evacuating the bowels at regular hours. The practice should start from childhood and the parents must train their children to create this regular habit. Those who are constipated relief to constipation by purgatives is often avoidable.

In order to develop regular normal bowel reflex, one must attend to latrine in the morning regularly whether one suceeds initially in complete evacuation or not. Every person can develop his own norm. Regular exercise; morning or evening taking a tumbler of water or a cup of tea a first thing in the morning before attending can be tried. Yogic exercises are sometimes helpful.

4. SLEEP AND REST

Sound sleep is very essential to sound health and to increase longevity. It is a natural process to remove the fatigue and recouperate the energy and vigour spent during working hours. Normally the prescribed hours of sleep are :

For—		
0-1 years	18-20	hours
1-2 years	14-15	hours
upto 8 years	11-13	hours
9-12 years	9-11	hours
13-15 years	8-10	hours
Young adults	8	hours
Adults	7	hours
After middle age	6	hours
Aged persons	6	hours
Ill and convalescents	More rest and sleep are needed for recovery.	

For enjoying good sleep and maximum benefit to the health the following should be maintained :

Principles for good sleep :

1. Avoid mental work or excitement before going to bed.

2. Always go to bed at fixed time (develop sleep reflex).
3. Avoid going to bed with full or empty stomach.
4. In cold countries a warm bath before going to bed is helpful.
5. Bed should be comfortable with soft pillow and not too hard bedding.
6. Dress should be light and loose.
7. It is good to have pleasant thoughts supplemented by prayers to God before sleeping.

Additional care :

(i) Mind is to be trained to be at rest when one intends to go to bed.
(ii) Sensitive persons must avoid tea or coffee in the evening and at night.
(iii) A tumbler of milk, as per one's taste followed by thorough rinsing of mouth at bed time or a warm bath may help in many cases.
(iv) Indigestion or any kind of bowel upset, fermentation and gas formation is to be avoided and thoroughly treated.
(v) Any constitutional disease like high blood pressure, heart disease, asthma, brain complaints or nervous disorders etc. should be adequately treated.
(vi) Regular practice of taking sleeping pill or draught should be avoided.
(vii) One must keep lying in bed quietly with eyes closed to enable himself to get some amount of physical rest.

Q. 5.3.(d) What are the basic principles for sleep and rest ?

5. EXERCISE

For maintaining personal hygiene exercise is the basic and is essential for growth and development, particularly during childhood and early manhood. It is certainly better if a habit of exercise in the form of walking, playing games and even instrumental or free hand exercise of Yoga is maintained till ripe old age.

Exercise keep the body fit signifying the old proverb :

"A healthy mind is in a healthy body."

Exercise is useful for the following purposes :

1. It tones up all organs of the body cutaneous, respiratory, circulatory, muscular and nervous system, digestion and evacuation and also other excretions.
2. It promotes oxygenation, utilization of food and repair of tissues, and help physical development of weakling.
3. It can relieve certain conditions of debility, obesity and deformity (during young age).
4. It has a restorative value during convalescene and healing after injury.
5. It counteracts the baneful effect of heavy mental work and prevents metabolic disease like, gout, rheumatism, diabetes, degenerative arterial diseases.
6. It has a very good effect as an educational measure for the mentally deficient.
7. It prevents aged persons from lapsing into habits of inactivity and indolence.

Rules of exercises :

1. Exercise should be strictly regulated. Generally exercise should be followed by rest for sometime, 15 minutes to 1 hour, and then the body should be washed or sponged or better a bath taken to clean the sweat, salt and other excretions resulting from the exercise. Persons always feel fresh both mentally and physically after the above procedures. Excessive exercise may cause nervous and muscular fatigue.

2. Beginners or sedentary persons and convalescent should start with graduated exercise till a physical optimum is reached.
3. It should be taken in open air as far as possible, repeated daily at about the same hour and not immediately after or before a meal.
4. It should be regular and systematic involving every part of the body in the process.
5. The amount of exercise should be regulated according to the age and physical capacity of the person.
6. Maintain proper posture of the body during exercise.

Type of exercise :

For *children*—Playing, running, swimming, skipping, dancing etc.

For *school boys*—Playing, drill, running, swimming, skipping, sliding, gymnastics, free hand physical, instrumental, sport and junior cadet corps excercise.

For *adolescents*—All kinds of outdoor and indoor games, regulatedphysical with or without instruments, National Cadet Corps exercises, skipping and dancing for girls.

For *adults*—Regulated exercise for half to one hour daily with or without instruments, outdoor or indoor games, gymnastics upto the middle age, breathing exercises, dancing, massage of body with mustard oil before bathing.

For *older people*—Continuation of regulated exercises as for as practicable. Playing of certain games according to choice—tennis, cricket, badminton etc., free hand exercise, breathing exercises and best of all walking (morning and evening).

Q. 5.3. (e) Why exercise is necessary for health ? What are the basic rules of exercise ?

After cleanliness and temperance the main points are to be observed in personal hygiene is prevention of diseases :

Prevention of Diseases of Infections

(1) Early rising from the bed, having a walk or exercise and a bath, moderate dieting and early going to bed at night is the basic principle for maintain health and preventing diseases.

(2) For prevention of disease avoid places where infection exists. As far as possible one should not go to the places where there are cases of smallpox cholera etc. Avoid cinemas and swimming pools if there is an epidemic of influenza or meningo-coccal meningitis.

(3) Get yourself vaccinated as per the schedule of immunization.

(4) Do not eat food exposed to flies and dirt. Do not eat over ripe or rotten fruits, such food may cause cholera, enteric diarrhoea, dysentery etc.

(5) Do not drink ice, water or cold drinks with ice. Ice does not kill germs. It is bacteriostatic. Germ in ice will cause the disease by ingestion.

(6) Cook the food properly so as to avoid infection from vegetables and meat.

(7) Fruit and vegetables that are to be eaten raw should be dipped in solution of potassium permanganent and then properly washed. Taken form $KMnO_4$ kills the germ.

(8) Boiled milk and water to be used for drinking.

(9) Water receptable should have a tap at the bottom. If glasses are dipped by hand in water, water receives the germ from the hand as well as the dust on the glass.

Finally, added to these are sex education, good hobbies, good friend's circle, picnics, and educational or pleasure trip which will make the mind of a person cheerful and are the factors contributing to "Positive health".

Q. 5.3.(f) What steps to be taken to prevent health from diseases.

For maintaining personal hygiene care to be taken :

(1) Cleanliness ⟶
(2) Clothing
(3) Food habits
(4) Bowel care
(5) Sleeps and rests
(6) Exercise
(7) Prevention of infection.

(a) Bathing
(b) Skin
(c) Mouth and teeth
(d) Eyes
(e) Nose
(f) Ears
(g) Hair
(h) Hands nails

Above and all 'habit' is regarded as the second nature of man so maintaining personal hygiene habit should be healthy. With good food, housing, sanitation, economic security, suitable working facilities i.e. proper environmental, biological and social conditions.

III. HEALTH CARE AND AVOIDABLE HABITS OF CHILDREN

Q. 5.4. What should be the care of a children to maintain personal hygiene ?

OR

Instruction to a mother to taking care about the personal hygiene of her son aged 14 years.

All children and adolescents are to be taught all aspects of personal hygiene by their parents and teachers at school, though the role of mother is unique. Generally mother should teach the principles of hygiene as mentioned earlier for maintaining personal hygiene.

(A) **HEALTH PRACTICES**
1. Going to bed early and sleeping long hours with windows open and rising before sunrise.

2. Brushing the teeth atleast twice a day, after each meal, if possible.
3. Habits of regular eating, sleeping, going to toilet and taking out-door exercise etc.
4. A full bath daily after massaging the body with mustard oil.
5. Wearing of clean garments.
6. Drinking milk as much as possible but no tea or coffee.
7. Drinking at least 4 glasses of water.
8. Eating some fresh fruits and green vegetables.
9. Habits of personal cleanliness, especially that of washing hands before meals.
10. Habits of being cheerful.
11. Keeping objects out of mouth (fingers, pencils, books etc).
12. Having a clean handkerchief and using it properly to prevent droplet infection.
13. Maintaining good posture in standing, sitting and working.
14. Reading books in good light but avoiding direct sunlight on books.
15. Urinating and defaceating should be followed by cleaning of hands preferably with soap and water.

(B) **OBJECTIONABLE HABITS WHICH SHOULD BE AVOIDED**

1. Answering the call of nature in the open field should be avoided.
2. Indiscriminate spitting, blowing nose and throwing nasal secretion should be stopped, they should be taught to use wash basins and handkerchiefs.
3. Cleaning of slate with saliva and putting the pencil or pen in the mouth should be stoped.
4. Both nail biting and finger sucking are bad habits and should be stopped.

5. Attending school bare-footed which exposes them to many risks should be discouraged.
6. School should not be attended in empty stomach, because hunger, pain and discomfort are deterimental to his studies.
7. Buying of eatables and infant foods from hawkers during recess period should be strongly discouraged as it may lead to infection and gastric upset. Instead, midday meals should be arranged.
8. Taking meals in a great hurry should be avoided as leads to indigestion, if diarrhoea, abdominal discomfort and pain.
9. Going to bed in full stomach at night leads to indigestion and disturb sleep.
10. Studing while dying down causes eye strain. Defective light and posture are to be corrected.
11. Stealing, abusing, fighting and quarrelling are bad practices and should be corrected.
12. Running after vehicles is dangerous and must be avoided.
13. Practice of keeping pet like dogs, cats, etc. may give rise to many kind of diseases from animals and birds. Strict vigilance and watch should be kept for proper cleanliness. Dogs may be immunised against rabies and dewormed for hydatidosis.

IV. HEALTH CARE OF A HOUSE WIFE

Q. 5.5. What are the measures to be followed by a house wife to maintain her personal hygiene and family hygiene.

A great deal of hygienic measures in the household depends on house wife as a cook, server of food and bearer of children. Most of the gastro-intestinal disease would be greatly minimised if the house wife sees to it that food is prepared, preserved and served hygienically. So she must follow certain principles of hygiene apart from her own personal hygiene discussed earlier. They are cleanliness,

PERSONAL HYGIENE

clothing, food habits, sleep and rest, bowel care, exercise etc. for maintaining her personal and family hygiene.

1. Use soap and water for washing hands, after going to lavatory, attending a child, handling excreta, refuse and garbage.
2. Use clean utensils and clean water for cooking and serving food.
3. Keep the nails well trimmed and wear clean clothes and aprons.
4. Cook food in a sanitary kitchen built separate from other rooms, arrange smokeless chulah is such a manner that she can cook on standing or high sitting posture for her own safety. Keep the kitchen tidy and cover all cooked foods and eatables to protect from flies, rates, cats, dogs, cockroaches and ants etc.
5. Collect all kitchen garbage and refuse in drums for proper disposal.
6. Handle all eatables after cooking by spoon or ladle and not by bare hands.
7. Keep the cooked foods in a village kitchen in a built-in-safe.
8. Teach all children to use latrine and have a soap and water wash afterwards, to have mouth and dental by hygiene and to practise other personal hygiene.
9. Have knowledge on applied nutrition so that she can improve nutrition of children and all other members in the family within her economic means.
10. Store drinking water and all food materials in clean containers.

PART II

ENVIRONMENTAL SANITATION

"HEALTH IS WEALTH"

CHAPTER-VI
ENVIRONMENTAL SANITATION

DEFINATION AND ITS IMPORTANCE

Q. 6.1. What is meant by environmental sanitation ?

Environmental Sanitation is that branch of Preventive and Social Medicine which seeks to control all the factors of the physical environment, which exercise or may exercise a deleterious effect on man's physical, mental and social well-being. Generally this control are :-

I. the water he drinks,
II. the food he eats,
III. the light he sees,
IV. the house he live in,
V. the disposal of body wastes and other wastes attendant upon his community living,
VI. the atmosphere,
VII. the insect and parasitic enemies of man,
VIII. his working place, and conditions of work,
IX. recreational areas.

It is also a specialised field in which engineering principles and techniques are employed to control various noxious agents of the environment to which a man is exposed and are of his own made. So it deals with those essential measures which are found disirable for promoting optimum conditions for man's health and well-being and for survival.

Q. 6.2. Why environmental sanitations are needed ?

Like all other living creatures men are constantly exposed to te influence of the action of the various agents in the enviornments. *In most of our villages*-the sources of water like rivers, tanks and wells are constantly polluted. The soil is polluted, our houses having no latrines, mosquitoes and flies swarm about and rats abound in the huts. *Most of our towns*—which have grown up haphazardly without plan also prevailing this conditions. It is estimated that 75% of the people living in urban areas lack protected water supply, while over 85% lack the amenities of sewerage system. In the villages, only 4% of the population have protected sources of water their water from unprotected sources mostly from *wells*, as also from tanks, ponds, lakes, river, springs etc.

More than 95% of the 'houses have no latrine. Naturally, we suffer most from the diseases carried by filth due to our poor enviornmental sanitation. Many of such diseases are endemic in our country and some also assume epidemic properties. Gastro-intestinal diseases like cholera, dysentery, diarrhoea, enteric group of fevers, helminthic infestations, insect borne diseases like malaria, filaria, plague and others continue to remain as our problem diseases. So *environmental sanitation is basically needed* :

(i) to reduce the incidence of these disease which are commonly acquired or transmitted through excreta, or conveyed to man by contaminated water supplies, food or drink, or transmitted by vectors, of diseases, environmental sanitation is needed.

(ii) Environmental Sanitation is also needed to improve the other hygienic conditions of Environmental—Social and Economic to influences the attitude of the people in the pattern of their living and is conductive to social development.

*** But the *Government view* is to the general improvement of environment which led to economic gain and improve the way of living by controlling morbidity and to releating trained person to carry out sanitation and reducing expenses on treatment of illness.

Q. 6.3. What is meant by sanitation and what are the various sanitary measures ?

The word *sanitation* comes from a French word '*sanita*' which means *cleanliness*. So *Sanitation* is a procedure involving measures to keep the environment or whole ecology of man clean and free from waste and decaying matters, animal and human excreta, putrefactive agents, gases,

ENVIRONMENTAL SANITATION

poisons, smoke, infective and obnoxious materials dangerous to life, insects and other agents associated with human diseases, and to provide safe and sufficient air, water and food etc.

Basic Sanitary measures are :
1. Safe water supply.
2. Housing.
3. Disposal of refuse and garbage.
4. Disposal of human and animal excreta.
5. Prevention of air pollution.
6. Food sanitation.
7. Vector control.
8. Control of diseases of animals : communicable to men.
9. Control of occupational hazards. (WHO).

Q. 6.4. What is meant by environment ?

Environment has been defined as the *"aggregate of all external conditions and influences affecting the life and development of an organism, human, behaviour, society."* Generally it comprises of four major elements-*Physical, Biological, Social and Economical. Physical environments* are climate, season, weather, geography and geological structures. It included air, food water, house, occupation, travels andrecreation in which a man always comes in contact. *Biological environments* are the animals, insects, parasites and other organisms of biological forms. *Social environment* includes the persons of a family and community other than himself and *Economicl environments* are his way of livng and opportunities of life influenced by economical circumstances.

CHAPTER-VII

ATMOSPHERIC POLLUTION AND ITS PREVENTION

DISCUSSION FOR LEARNING

I. Atmospheric pollution—Definition.
II. Various pollutants and their sources.
III. Effects of pollution on health.
IV. Prevention of air pollution.
V. Airborne diseases and their control.

I. ATMOSPHERIC POLLUTION

Q. 7.1. What is meant by atmospheric pollution ?

Atmospheric pollution means an excessive concentration of foreign matter in the outdoor atmosphere which is harmful to man or his environment.

Generally air contains many substances some of which are essential for life at a certain level of concentration. But the air may be said to be polluted when substances in it, are present at higher concentrations than their normal ambient levels to produce a measurable effect on human health. These substances may be natural or man made, chemcial elements or compounds, capable of being air born. These substances may exist in the atmosphere as gases, liquid drops or solid particles.

II. POLLUTANTS AND THEIR SOURCES

Q. 7.2. What are the pollutants generally occur in our modern age ?

The type of pollutants in our modern age varies according to their nature of sources. But the variety of born matter is so large it is difficult to put them in a precise classification.

Generally we place them in two categories.

1) Primary *pollutants*—those directly from sources

2) *Secondary pollutants*—those formed in the atmosphere by chemical intractions among primary pollutants and normal atmospheric constituents.

Besides these, pollutants can also be listed on the basis of materials as under :
1. *Sulphur containing compounds* i.e. SO_2, SO_4, etc.
2. Nitrogen *containting compounds* i.e NH_3, Oxides of nitrogen.
3. *Carbon containing campounds* i.e. CO, CO_2 etc.
4. *Halogen compounds* e.g. chlorine.
5. *Organic compounds like* aldehydes, acetones and polycyclic hydrocarbons.
6. *Carcinogenic particles* like radioactive isotopes, benzepyrine etc.
7. *Allergic pollens.*
8. *Particulate matters.*

The particulate matter consists of fine *solids*, or *liquid droplets* suspended in air. The large size particles are *grit fly ash*, dust, and *soot* ; and smaller sizes are *smoke, mist* and *aerosoles*.

N.B.— The different types of particulates have definite means which are as follows:
a) *grit*—solid particles suspended in air with a diameter of over 500 µm;
b) *dust*—solid particles suspended in air with a diameter between 0.25 to 500 µm;
c) *smoke*—gas born solids with particles usually less then 2 µm in diameter;
d) *fumes*—suspended solids in air less them 1.0 µm in diameters normally released from chemical or metallurgical processes;
e) *mist*—liquid droplets suspended in air with a diameter of less than 2.0 µm; and
f) *aerosol*—solid or liquid particles in suspension in air, or some other gas, with diameter of les than 1.0 µm.

Q. 7.3. What are the sources of air pollutants ?

The naturally occuring pollutants of air are dust from organic and inorganic sources, bacteria, forest fires, decomposing plants and animals. But these are transient and of minor importance. From hygienic point of view, air pollution due to the presence of foreign substances in the natrual air through man's activities are mostly considered. So the various sources which contribute the pollution of the atmosphere particularly, in the cities and towns are :

1) *Industries*—gaseous wastes in industries result, from burning of fuels of various types, coal being the most common. Crude oils like naptha are also burnt in many industrial furnaces in place of coal.

2) *Plants*—for generating coal gas and electricity for power supply and lighting. Generally coal is used as fuel in these plants.

3) *Steam locomotives*—as are used in railways, steamers, launches etc.

4) *Motor transport and internal combustion engines*—burning large quantities of petrol diesel, kerosine, naptha and other fuel oils.

5) *Incinerators of large municipalities*—a large quantity of gaseous effluents is emitted from these incinerators.

6) *Domestic kitchens*—using coal, coal gas, kerosene, cowdung cakes etc.

7) *Lighting in houses*—by burning vegetable oils, paraffin, kerosene, coal gas, water gas etc. producing by products of combustion not conductive of heat.

8) *Sewers and house drains*—The various contents of sewer & house drains in the cities and towns are products of decomposition of night soil, domestic refuse, industrial and trade wastes oils, grease, e.g. acids from engineering works, carbide, resin, alkali, ammoniacal liquids, phenol and tar products, paraffin, petrol, diesel oil from garages, and animal wastes etc. So a large number of gases emitted from the sewers due to interaction of the above products. These are generally coalgas, methane, acetylene, benzene. H_2S, HCN, besides CO_2, NH_3, chlorine, phosphagene, nitrous fumes, SO_2, CS_2, CO etc.

9) *Offensive trades*—give off disagreeable organic vapours bad odours and certain pyroligeneous matters which are injurious to health.

10) *Street dust & house dust*—The street dust is composed of both organic and inorganic matters, bacteria, scales of epithelium, allergic pollens, fibres of cotton, linen and wool, particles of hair, dried sputum and excreta, soot, silica, and other minerals, decaying leaves, etc which enters into the rooms and contaminate food exposed for sale or consumption.

11) *Atmosphere*—The effect of atmospheric conditions and of sun-rays also accentuate the air pollution by forming new toxic products from the less harmful substances. Organic compounds and oxides of nitrogen together with vaperised fuel under go chemcial changes in the air especialy in strong sunlight and toxic compunds like ozone and other oxidants are formed.

12) *Radioactive substance*—Increase manufacture of ratio-active substance for the use of medical and power generating purpose add the radioactive pollutants in the atmosphere which are harmful to man.

III. EFFECT OF POLLUTANTS

Q. 7.4. What are the effects of pollutants on atmosphere and human health ?

Usually contaminants or pollutants which are present in small concentration in the atmosphere exert no toxic effect on human beings, but there are evidences that continous exposure to such an atmosphere has resulted in increase of chronic pulmonary ailments including cancer. It is possible that the effects observed are due to synergism of many pollutants acting together over some years. Generally the effects are as follows :

1. Effect on Atmospehre

(a) The high concentration of pollutants in the atmosphere over large urban and industrial areas can produce a number of general effects. Smoke and fumes increase the atmosphere turbidity and reduce the amount of solar radiation. Particulates absorbe and reflect incoming solar radiation to the ground and causes 15-20% decrease in large cities compared to "cleaner rural areas."

(b) *In urban area*—solid particulates take part in increase water vapour emission resulting upto 20% increased cloud and upto 10% more wetdays, mist, fog and smog.

2. Effects on Human Health

Air pollutant effects on human health are of two types :
  A. Immediate effects.
  B. Delayed effects.

A. IMMEDIATE EFFECTS

Epidemological studies have shown that a sudden increase in air polluation has been associated with immediate increase in the mortality and morbidity. The symptoms are usually referable to the *respiratory system* as seen in Bhopal (1984).

B. DELAYED EFFECTS

Generally the delayed effects of air pollutants are various types of diseases, but the more significant diseases are chronic bronchitis, emphysema and allergic disorder which are significant between urban and rural air pollution.

Generally the delayed effects are :

1. Effects of Smoke and Smog

(i) Both petrol fumes and diesel exhaust contain carcinogenic agents and harmful to human health.

(ii) Smoke causes serious damage to properties, building, clothings and furnitures, and is irritating to the respiratory passages and increases pulmonary disease.

(iii) In the winter smoke creats—SMOG (smoke+fog), causing high cardio-respiratory morbidity and excess of death among the two extremes of age. Generally smog contain a large amount of SO_2 compunds. Dur to SO_2, people commonly suffered from different respiratory symptoms, such as naso-pharingitis, coughing, and shortness of breath. Urban dewellers are also subjected to smoke and smog, so they suffer respiratory disease like bronchitis, asthma and emphysema.

ATMOSPHERIC POLLUTION AND ITS PREVENTION

(iv) Effect of smoke on the mental health :

1. The depressing effects of gloom and smoky atmosphere on mental health of the population is known to every body. The house wife suffers from feelings of frustation and depression when she would see that their efforts at promoting cleanliness of the house, mosquito curtains, soft furnishing and carpets grow quickly shabby, windows can never kept open to receive fresh air from outside. So smoke is a heavy taxation on the house wife time and temper and eventually affects the physical and emotional health of the family rendering many of the member irritable and neurotic.

2. Effects of Particulates or Dusts

Particulates—includes house dust, mineral dusts, fibres and a range of manufactured chemical compounds. Dust is a normal and important constituents of air. Ordinary dust is not harmful to health. But house dust is more injurous than dust of the outside air as it contains pathogenic organigms like tubercle bacilli, staphylococci, pneumococci, diphtheria bacilli and dried small pox scabes etc. Generally these pass into the dust during coughing, sneezing and talking as droplets and from pus, wounds, sputum and excreta thrown on the ground or floor. Still more dangerious are teanus, anthrax, and gas gangrene spores which by contaminating wounds cause tetanus, maliganant boils, and gangrene. Other pathological conditions due to dust are asthma and allergic disorders, conjunctivitis and trachoma.

Industrial dust—Jute mill, cotton mill, flour mill, paper mill etc. produces harmful effects on health of the workers and the diseases produces are bronchitis, tuberculosis, asthma etc.

Mineral dust—of coal, stone fire-clay, mica, china clay, graphite fibres including asbestors, and glass and rock work which are used in insulation purposes causes deposits over lungs for a long period of time. Scaning or fibrosis of the lung lining, if silicosis, asbestosis and other such dust diseases are well known as industrial pollution diseases. prolonged exposure to asbestors, and possibly glass fibres over a period of 20 years or longer is known to cause mesothelioma, or cancer of the lining of abdomen.

3. Effects of Most Important Gaseous Pollutants :

(i) *Carbon monoxide* (CO) — This colourless, odourless gas is produced by the incomplete combustion of fossil fuels, the refinings of petroleum, wood pulp processing, and iron and steel smelting process. The average global concentration in the atmosphere is 0.1 - 0.2 ppm and little produced from natural biological process. This pollutant is a cumulative toxin and an acute concentration of 1000 ppm or more is invariably fatal.

Increase cencentration over 100 ppm causes headache, dizziness, lassitude, nausea, vomiting, palpitation, breathing defficulty, muscular weakness, convulsion and unconciousness.

(ii) *Sulphur compounds*—They are the most common and harmful pollutants of our life. The most common sulphur compounds are sulphur dioxide and sulphur trioxide besides hydrogen sulphides. The sources of sulphur compounds are combustion of fossil fuels, decomposition and combusion of organic matter etc. The main effects of these pollutants are respiratory diseases like bronchitis, asthma and emphysema.

(iii) *Ozone* (O_3)—It is formed in the atmospheric air by the production of nitrogen oxides particularly nitric oxide and nitrogen dioxide by road vehicles.

Ozone at high concentration between 1.5 to 200 ppm can cause temporary effects within 2 hours, producing irritation of eyes, throat and lungs, retarded mental growth. People pron to asthma attack and can be adversely affected by conc. low as 0.25 ppm. There is uncertanity about long term effects of this. Apart from aggravating respiratory complaints, it may act as a tumour acclator.

(iv) *Nitrogen compounds*—main symptoms are pulmonary fibrosis and emphysema of the lungs.

4. Effect of Radio Active Substance

Radio active pollution of atmosphere has been defined as "any increase in the natural background radiation arising out of human activities involving the use of naturally occuring or artifically produced radioactive substance." Such a pollution creates hazards not only for those who are engaged in radiation work but also for general public. This causes long term effects on life, inducing genetic aberation like cancer, mental retardation and physically handicapped etc. Already there have been several accidental pollutions of atmosphere as recently reported of throwing away the radium needles by a cancer patient in a calcutta hospital.

IV. PREVENTION OF AIR POLLUTION

Q. 7.5. What steps would be taken to prevent and control atmospheric pollution in our modern age ?

Present atmospheric pollution originates from two main sources, namely,

(i) the inefficient combustion of primary energy sources, and
(ii) the emission of waste, industrial and domestic products into the air.

So there are broadly three possible changes that could reduce the level of pollution :

a) first, if the uses of coal, oil and gas are to be reduced :
b) secondly, if the process of combustion becomes more efficient, and
c) thirdly, if less waste products are discharged into the atmosphere.

A number of measures have been suggested for control had prevention of air pollution in general, but atmosphere tends to purify itself by dilution, dispertion, and chemical degradation of the pollutants, which are under the general heading of :

Self Purification or Natural Purification of Air.

VARIOUS MEASURES

Generally proposed measures for control and prevention for atmospheric pollution are :

1. DOMESTIC MEASURES

a) Public education and publicity regarding harmful effects of smoke, and its methods of control and value of fresh air is first and foremost steps of measure to prevent air pollution.

    b) Careful planning and selecting sites for factories and dwelling houses are important. The factories should be in the outskrits of the town.

    c) Increased use of electricity and natural gas at home and in the industry lower the pollution ratio.

    d) Domestic smoke problem can be solved by using smokeless fuels or coal.

2. TRANSPORT

Enforcement of laws relating to smoke nuisance and improvement in the vehicles and traffic management can reduce pollution from automobile vehicles. Reduction of smoke and fumes by efficient engine maintenance, avoidance of over rich mixture and idling in traffic james cause less pollution.

3. INDUSTRIES

Industrial smoke can be considerably prevented by adopting the following methods :

    a) Use of smokeless fuels e.g coke in boiler and furnaces,

    b) Use of mechanical stokes or employment of skilled labour for careful stoking of furnaces.

    c) Provision of efficient furnace plant with accurately maintained draughts.

    d) Zoning of industries away from residential districts.

    e) Installing of offensive trades far away from human localities and maintenance of strict sanitary supervision,

    f) Recently various filtering devices are used to absorb, absorb or chemically alter the pollutants gas into other products which can be collected. Particulate matters are widely present as dirt and dust which may contain a wide range of materials both inorganic and organic. The particulates are generally soot, soil, lint etc. and their removal can be achieved by three types of devices, namely- *dry filters, viscous filter and electrostatic precipitators.*

g) For the protection of industrial—workers from pollution—Susceptable persons should remain in a well warmed room and uses of mask is compulsory as it keeps him out of polluted droplets.

4. **SPECIAL MEASURES** (Proposed measures for control) :

   a) Dust in the streets and houses can be disposed of by regular sweeping and washing and efficient screening and ventilation of the rooms. The rooms may be sprayed with triethylene glycocol vapour to a concentration of 1 in 400,000 or 0.0025 mg. per litre, chloramine T, Catechol and sodium hypochlorite (1% solution) may be used for spraying hospitals, schools and other confined spaces. Ultra violet rays may be used for sterilising the children's ward.

   b) Establishment of certain standards of air quality by the present state of our knowledge.

   c) Establishment of air-monitaring agencies to issue warning when the pollution goes beyond the set standards and approximate action under those conditions to reduce the domestic and industrial gaseous effluents.

   d) Researches on pre-treatment of industrial and automobile exhaust for reduction of their pollutional load before discharging into the atmosphere.

   e) As in this atomic era atmosphere pollution by dispers of ionizing radiation in air is assuming a great importance. No concentration can be ignored as its effect is cummulative have lasting on life. So legislative devices such as, Environments Pollution Act, TLV (Threshold Limit Values) for substance etc. should be adopted.

Conclusion :

As modern atmospheric pollution is essentially a product of industrial revolution which attracts and collects the populance in towns and cities, so establishment of *green belts* between industrial areas and residential houses are utmost important to prevent and reduce air pollution by plants.

V. AIR BORN DISEASES AND THEIR CONTROL

Q. 7.6. What is mean by air born disease ?

The term *air born* diseases have been applied loosely to acute respiratory and exanthematous diseases although these are known to spread in many instances by contact. A more precise definition of air-born diseases can be given as under :

"The air born diseases are those in which the primary pathology lies in the respiratory tract or the portal entry of the agent is through the respiratory tract."

Q. 7.7. What are the air borne diseases ?

The various diseases which can be included in list of air borne diseases are :

1. *Viral diseases* like influenza, caused by influenza or other newer respiratory viruses which involves with the respiratory epithelium.

2. *The exanthematous or so-called acute contagious diseases of childhood,* e.g. smallpox, chickenpox, measles, rubella etc. which are also caused by viruses.

3. *Acute bacterial infective diseases* like diphtheriae, whooping-cough, meningitis etc. are caused by a specific bacteria.

4. *Various other diseases* in which the portal of entry is respiratory tract, e.g. mumps tuberculosis, pneumonia plague, Q-fever etc.

5. *Fungal diseases* caused by monilialies, coccidioiodmycosis, histoplasmosis, blastomycosis, candida albicans etc. infection.

VI. GENERAL METHODS OF CONTROL OF AIR BORNE DISEASES

Q. 7.8. How we can control air borne diseases ?

Microbial contamination of the air may be controlled by four general methods :
1) *Ventilation*
2) *Ultraviolet radiation*
3) *Use of disinfectants vapours*
4) *Dust suppression.*

1. *Ventilation* : The simplest of all measures for removing contaminates from enclosed spaces, is natural ventilation or ventilation from open windows or by the helps of mechanical ventilation.

2. *Ultraviolet radiation* : The disinfectant action of ultraviolet light has long been known and have been accurately quantitated. Wave lengths in the rang of 2500^0 A are most bactericidal. Low pressure mercury vapour lamp, which emits its maximum radiation in the wave length 2531^0 A has been a reasonable economical device.

3. *Disinfectant vapours* : Many chemicals have been shown to have marked bactericidal action when dispersed in air. These include the halogens, hypochlorites, lactic acid, hexylresorcinols and the glycols. Of these glycols, particularle triethylene glycol, appears to be the most practical because of their high bactericidal potency, reasonable cost, freedom from odours, toxicity and corrosiveness.

4. *Dust suppression* : Dust particles carrying disease organisms can be suppressed by using light paraffin which makes sticky. Floors treated with paraffin makes them greasy and restrict the movements of dust, blankets, beddings and clothes can also be oil-treated in a similar way while laundering.

CHAPTER-VIII

WATER

(IN RELATION TO HEALTH AND DISEASES)
DISCUSSION FOR LEARNING

I. Properties of water.
II. Biological importance of water.
III. Uses of water.
IV. Quantity of water required.
V. Quality of water.
VI. Sources of water.
VII. Water supply of rural areas.
VIII. Water supplies of cities. (Calcutta water supply constant, intermittent and dual water supply).
IX. Impurities of water—Natural and artificial.
X. Effects of impurities of water on health.
XI. Water borne diseases.
XII. Purification water (various methods.)
XIII. Purification of water in Inidan villages.
XIV. Purification of water in the cities like Calcutta and Delhi.
XV. Filteration of water—Slow Sand Filter and Rapid Sand Filter.
XVI. Hardness of water.
XVII. Removal of hardness of water.
XVIII. Hydrological cycle.

Water is the most important fluid in earth. Without it life, as we know it on this planet, would be impossible. Not only would all living things dry up, the earth itself would be subject to such extreme temperature fluctuations as to make it inhabitable. According to the Hindu scriptures one of the synonyms of water is 'Jivana' i.e. life, as because without it life cannot be sustained.

WATER

Let us examine a few of the important characteristics of this remarkable fluid.

I. PROPERTIES OF WATER

Q. 8.1. What are the properties of water?

In the *first place*, water is abundant. If we take the crust of the earth to be about 2 kilometers deep, we have a shell of 2,540 million cubic kilometers of which about 1,500 million, or more than half, are water. *Second*, water has an unusual *molecular structure*. A water molecule consists of one atom of *Oxygen* and two atoms of *Hydrogen* (H_2O). There is a strong bond between these three atoms, which results in a molecule, that, unlike most other molecules is asymmetric and electrically charged. Because in most minerals that occur in nature the atoms are held together by electrical attraction, the water molecule with its positive and negative charges can easily squaree between atoms in other molecules. This ability is the cause of the enormous dissolving power of water. No other fluid can match it. It also explains in part, the action of water upon the earth's surface, known as erosion. Mountains are continously dissolved and over the cons, washed into the sea.

The *irregular* shape of the water molecule has other consequences of great importance to our lives. When water becomes a solid (freezes), the molecules becomes arranged in open, crystal like structures. Ice is therefore less dense than water and floats on the water's surface. If ice melts, that is, goes from solid to the liquid phases, the molecules move around more freely, filling up the holes, and the water gets denser. The densest point is reached at 4°C with rising temperatures the molecules begin to move faster and faster, occuring more and more liquid until at 100°C, the water boils, that is, goes from the liquid to the gaseous phase. However, because of the strong molecular attraction, it takes enoromous energy to bring water into the gaseous stage.

The opposite is also true, when water condenses. This happens in the summer in our cumulus clouds, which is only an hour or so many build up into a thunderstorm. One average thunderstorm has the same energy as is created by the burning of 6,000 metric tons of coal.

Water—H_2O.

Boiling point $100°C$ *Freezing point $0°C$.*

Specific gravity — 1.

Latent heat fusion—80 Cal.   *Latent heat of evaporation— 539 Kcal.*

II. BIOLOGICAL IMPORTANCE OF WATER

Q. 8.2. Why water is essential ?

It is fairly certain the first living things on earth were formed in watery surroundings and the inheritance of this origin is still with us. There are only a few living things that contain less than 10% of their weight is water, for examples plants, seeds and spores of bacteria and fungus. Most of the vegetable matter that we use for food, such as tomatoes, potatoes, lettuce and carrots, contains at the time of harvest 85 to 90% water by weight. Even such derived food and bread contain more than 30% water.

Plants use large quantities of water, but only small part is used for building plant material. The rest is transpired into the air via stomata. But man himself is extremely watery. This author weighs 50 kg. about 70% of this or more than 35 kg is water and he must continously strive to keep this ratio as is or he will die of dehydration, long before the water is completely evaporated out of his body. This fact suggests the necessity of water, though the amount of water man needs varies in the circumstances in which he lives and works. Also the physiological functions suggest the necessity of water.

Water is necessary for the performance of the physiological functions in all living beings in the world. It enters into the system either as a circulating fluid or as a vehicle of nourishment or for the supply of dissolved oxygen necessary to convert food into vital energy and for removing the waste products. The supply of pure water performs a major role in the health recovery and well being of all concerned. Despite the marvels of modern science no suitable substitute of water has yet been discovered.

Generally water is essential for the regulation of body temperature, excretion of waste products, maintains fludity of blood and lymph and balancing the body loss resulting from breathings, sweatings and excretion of urine and faeces. It is also essential for maintaining personal body hygiene and freedom from disease.

III. USES OF WATER

Q. 8.3. What are the uses of water ?

PERSONAL USE :

Water is a basic natural resource required by human beings, and by the modern technological society in which they live. Man requires a minimum body intake of water that varies from 2.8 to 13 liters per head per day depending upon the climate and the temperature. Water is normally taken into the body in food and drink, and the intake must balance the body loss resulting from sweating and the excretion of urine and faces. If there is no intake of water into the body, death will be inevitable within 10 days.

Water is also essential to man for maintaing personal body hygiene and freedom from disease.

Water intake in ml. per day	Water output in ml. per day
Water intake as such = 1100 Water intake in diet = 900 Water produced during metabolism = 200	Water excreted in urine = 1000 Water excreted in stools = 200 Water lost through— skin & lungs = 1000
Total intake = 2200	Total out put = 2200

In addition to personal use, water is required for many other purposes of which our chief concern in Preventive and Social Medicine is with the consumption of water by human being for :

a) **Domestic or household purposes** : generally *two-thirds* portion of supplies are used by *domestic or household's* for drinking, cooking, dishwashing, general cleaning, laundrings, personal washing and bathing, lavatory flushing, car washing, garden watering, maintenance of parks and fountains.

The other *one-third* is used by *industry* and *commercial* and *trade premises*.

b) **Industrial process** : require large quantities of water for coaling purposes, steam raising, material processing and the disposal of waste. Water is also used as a fluid carrier for processing materials such as paper fibres, or crushed etc.

c) **Agricultural industry** : used comparatively small quantities of water for dairy processing, animal hygiene, stock watering and land irrigation. The horticultural industry uses water for land irrigation, glass house watering and washing marketable vegetable crops.

d) **Other purposes** : water is also required for *amenity* and *amusment* or *relaxational purpose*. This category differs from previous three types because water is not abstracted from the hydrological cycle. The so-called water space includes streams, rivers, reservoirs, cannals and coastal water. It is used for all types of water sports such as swimming, fishing, boating, sailing, skeing and as a means of transportation for pleasure or commercial purposes. The presence areas of water also adds to the amenity value of the country side and enjoyment of the general public.

IV. QUANTITY OF WATER REQUIRED

Q. 8.4. State the quantity of water required per head per day.

The *Indian standard code of water supply, drainage* and *sanitation* recommends a minimum 30 *gallons* (136.34 litres) of *water per capita per day for residences* provided with water carriage system of sanitation. Although a minimum of 15 to 20 *gallons* may be considered adequate for domestic requirements which would vary according to the habits and standard of life of a population, the season and climate of the country and other civil and sanitary amenities of the places.

Recommended Standard of Environmental Hygiene Committee

Sl. No.	Communities with the Population range	Gallons per Capita per day
1.	1,000—5,000	15
2.	5,000—10,000	20
3.	10,000—50,000	25
4.	50,000—200,000	40
5.	200,000—and above	45 *
6.	Calcutta Metropolitan District	50
7.	Calcutta and Howrah Corporation	60

(*Add 5 gallons per capita per day where sewage is contemplated).

In the *rural community* the minimum rate are above 5 gallons per capita per day. According to *Parkes and Kenword* daily requirement of water per persons per day for all purposes are the following :

1. **Household/Domestic Purpose :**

Fluid as drink	—0.35 gallons.
Cooking	—0.65 gallons.
Bathing and ablution	—8.00 gallons.
Utensils and house washing	—3.00 gallons.
Laundry	—3.00 gallons.
Water closet	—5.00 gallons.

2. **Trade and Manufacturing :** —5.00 gallons.
3. **Municipal :**
   (for watering streets, public   —5.00 gallons.
   baths, fountains, flushing sewers
   and fire extinguishing etc.)

   Total —30.00 gallons

IN HOSPITAL — 40 to 50 gallons per head must be required daily.

IN CULCUTTA — The daily requirement is 45.7 gallons filtered water and atleast 5.00 gallons unfilterd river water for flushing water closets, drains etc.

V. QUALITY OF WATER

Q. 8.5. What are the chief qualities of drinking water or good water or potable water?

Or

What are the requirement of a wholesome drinking water?

1. Drinking water should be soft i.e. neither corrosive nor scale forming. Generally more than 20 per 100,000 hardness is unsuitable.

2. It should be free from taste, colour, smell, suspended and dissolved impurities which produce undesirable physiological action.

3. It should contain some amount of dissolved oxygen and also CO_2 and trace elements like iodine and fluorine.

4. It should be free from pathogenic organisms, nitrogenous organic matter and poisonous substance like aresenic, lead and iron. So from the above points the drinking water should be absolutely free from impurities, *physically and chemically, but practically impurities* to a certain extent in water is inevitable.

So the following permissive and excessive standards for physical, chemical, toxic and radioactive as well as bacteriological quality of drinking water are recommended in the Manual & Code of Practice, Ministry of Health and WHO (1971).

Recommended Standards of Quality of Drinking Water Per Litre

Character and Content	Permissive (mg)	Maximum allowable limit in mg. or PPM (mg)
A. Physical		
Total dissolved solids	500	1500
Turbidity (units)	5	25
Taste and Odour	Nothing	disagreeable
Temperature	—	50° F
B. Chemical		
pH	7.85	6.5 to 9.2
Sulphates (SO_4)	250	1000
Chlorides (Cl)	250	500
Nitrates (NO_3)	20	50
Nitrites (NO_2)	even trade is not	permitted
Fluorides (F)	1.0	2.0
Hardness ($CaCO_3$)	300	600
Calcium (Ca)	75	200
Magnesium (Mg)	20	150
Iron (Fe)	0.3	10
Copper (Cu)	10	30
Zinc (Zn)	5.0	15.0
Poenolic substances	0.001	0.002
Maganese (Mn)	0.1	0.5
C. Toxic		
Arsenic (As)		0.2
Chromium (Cr)		
Cyanides (CN)	0.01	0.01
Selenium (Se)		0.01
Lead (Pb)		0.05
D. Radio-activity		
Alfa-emitters		10 µc/ml
Beta-emitters		20 µc/ml

E. Standards of Bacteriological Quality

(i) **Treated water**—The MPN (most probable number) index of coliform bacteria should be zero or less than 1.0 per 100 ml. and no sample exceed 10 per 100 ml.

(ii) **Untreated water**—The MPN index of colifrom should normally be less than 10 per 10 ml. None of the sample should show an MPN greater than 20.

Q. 8.6. (a) What is pure water in the sanitary sense?

The clean or pure water in the sanitary sense is one which is free from contamination and safe for human consumption as determined by chemical, bacteriological examination of the sample water.

Q. 8.6. (b) What will be the standards of a Potable Water?

Standards of Potable Water

A. Physical :
1) Turbidity—Limit 10 units (By Platinum Rod Method).
2) Colour—Limit 5 (By Colorimeter).
3) Taste—Pleasant.
4) Odour—Nil.
5) Total solids 5500 PPM.

B. Chemical :
1) Hardness upto $20°$.
2) Lead upto 0.1 PPM.
3) Iron—0.3 PPM.
4) Nitrites—Nil.
5) Nitrates—10 PPM.
6) Free NH_3—0.06 PPM.
7) Albuminoid NH_3—0.1 PPM.

C. Bacteriological—Water is unfit for consumption if it has more than 10 B. coli per 100 c.c of water.

D. Microscopic—It should not show presence of tissue cells.

N.B. : (1) Yellow colouration of water suggests faecal contamination. (2) Presence of Nitrites and free NH_3 suggest recent faecal contamination. (3) Presence of Nitrates, and Albuminoid ammonia suggest past faecal contamination. (4) More than 10 B. coli in 100 ml suggest faecal contamination. (5) Presence of tissue cells seen under microscope suggest faecal contamination, (6) High chloride suggests faecal contamination (Except nearer to the sea).

VI. SOURCES OF WATER

Q. 8.7. Name the different sources of water.

The primary source of all water on land surface of the earth is the condensed water in the air evaporated from the ocean at the rate of 700 gallons per square mile per minute, which comes down as rain, snow, dew, mist and hail. On reaching the hills and earth's surface it is collected in the hills as snow and in the plains as lakes, tanks, ponds etc or passes as rivers in the direction of the natural fall towards the sea, being forced by the melted snow from the hills. A part of the rains percolate into the earth and form the *subsoil* and *ground* water or resurges out as spring. Thus three sources of water are available for various human requirements namely :

I. **RAIN WATER**

II. **SURFACE WATER**
   (a) Upland surface water i.e. Impounding Reservoirs
   (b) Low land surface water
      (i) Tanks and ponds
      (ii) Rivers and streams

III. **GROUND WATER**
   (a) Springs
   (b) Wells-shallow and Deep.
   (c) Tube wells.

Q.8.8. What are the different (natural) sources of drinking water? Describe their advantages and isadvantages.

Different sources of drinking water are:

I. RAIN WATER	II. SURFACE WATER	III. GROUND WATER
	1) Upland surface water	a) Springs
	2) Low land surface water	b) Wells.
	a) TANKS, PONDS and LAKES.	
	b) RIVERS AND STREAMS.	

ADVANTAGES AND DISADVANTAGES

RAIN WATER	II. SURFACE WATER		III. GROUND WATER
	1. Upland surface water (Impounding Reserviors).	2. Lowland surface water A. Tanks, Ponds and Lakes B. River and Streams.	(Springs, Deep and shallow wells)
Advantages : Rain water is purest water in nature. Physically clear, bright and sparkling. Chemically, it is a very soft, containing only	**Advantages :** 1. The water is clear, and palatable and poure, next to rain water, but if the surrounding	**Advantages :** Tanks, ponds and lakes water undergoes self purification. Generally self purification occurs due to	**Advantages :** Selt purification or natural purification occurs by dilution, sedimentation, aeration, oxidation, sunlight etc.	**Advantages :** 1. It is free from pathogenic organism. 2. It is usually requires no treatment. 3. The supply of water is constant

traces of dissolved solids.
4. Bacteriologically, it is free from pathogenic organisms.

Disadvantages:

1. It contains suspended impurities of the atmosphere, such as dust soot and micro organisms & gases like CO_2 nitrogen, oxygen & ammonia but they are generally negligible.
2. It becomes impure when it passes through the atmosphere.
3. As it is soft in nature it has a corrosive action.

hills are covered with peat, the water becomes brownish colour.
2. Usually it is soft and free from pathogenic organisms.

Disadvantages:

1. It becomes impure by human excreta and animal waste products, if the catchment are is contaminated by wild animal or human habitation.
2. Storage of water for long times causes growth of algae & other micro-organisms which im-

storage oxidation and by other agencies.

Disadvantages:

Although these water under so self purification, but not sufficient to render safe water. Because they are recipients of all sorts of contamination as they are always used for washing of clothes, cattle, cooking pots, children use them for swimming and there may be a regular defection around the edges which washed into the

Disadvantages:

1. River water is turbid during rainy season although may be clear in other seasons, but clearity is no guarantee
2. It contains dissolved and suspened impurities of all kinds which derived from surface washing, sewage and sullage water, industrial and trade wastes and drainage from agricultural areas.
 The customs and habits of the people like bath-

even during dry season.
4. Generally the water of these sources are sparklingly clear, cool and palatable being charged with CO_2 gas. Sometimes it contains dissolved minerals and is hard. Hot springs are used for therapeutic purposes particularly for rheumatic patients.

Disadvantages:

The water of the shallow wells become polluted either from contamination of

Comments :
For human consumption the steps of purification are same as those of surface water. In the Sundarban area of West Bengal, the river water being saline, rain water collected in tanks and from the roof are the source of water for drinking and cooking.

part bad tastes and odours.

Comments :
To keep it pure, it is necessary to keep the catchment are free from human or animal intrusion.

tank or ponds by rain. Old tanks or ponds as full of aquatic vegetation and old leaves of trees of the sides undergoes decay and added impurities like H_2S gases etc.

Comments :
Generally purification is done by boiling Filteration, chemically by Hallogen tablet, potassium chlorate and Bleaching powder etc.

ing, animal washing & disposal of dead body added, more pollution.
3. The bacterial count including human intestinal organisms are very high.

Comments :
For human consumption it should be disinfected and supplied through pipes.

subsoil like latrines, urinales, drains cesspoles etc. and usually goes dry in summer.

Comments :
It requires pumping or some arrangement to lift the water.
Springs are natural sources of drinking water and these water are safe for human consumption.

Q. 8.9. What is well ? What are the different types of well ? What is meant by ideal or sanitary well ?

Def : A *well* is an artificial pit or hole sunk into the earth to reach the water level into which the subsoil water percolates.

There are four types of wells :
1) **Shallow well or Dug well.**
2) **Deep well.**
3) **Norton's Abyssinial tube well.**
4) **Artesian well.**

The *shallow* or *dugwell* tap the ground water above the first imprevious layer of the soil and hence may be subjected to surface contamination. *Deep wells* or driven wells (tube wells) yield safer water as they pass through one or more imprevious layers of the soil. The yield is also larger. An *Artesian* well is a deep well yielding water under pressure between the imprevious strata. When this level is taped, water flows by itself. Deep tube wells are in reality a type of artesian well.

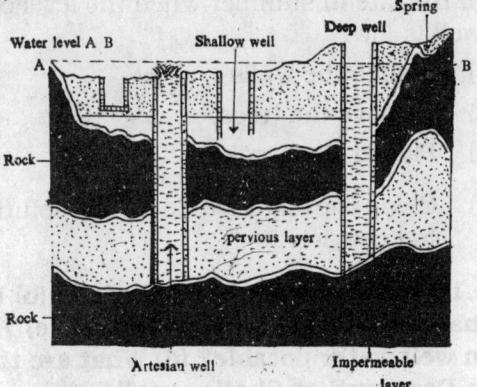

Fig. 1. Different types of wells

Wells are main sources of water supply in Indian villages and towns. Those *well have the following characteristics, they are ideal or sanitary well.*

Ideal or Sanitary Well
(1) It is a deep well.
(2) It is dug in good soil.

(3) It is at least 200 feet from any cesspool or drain.
(4) It has a paraper 3' high all around.
(5) Surrounding 6' is made imprevious and a circular half channel drain, leads the water away.
(6) The wall of the well should have a puddle 12" thick and over this, the bricks, stones or masonary are fixed. This layer should go down at least a foot or more, below the first impervious layer of the soil.
(7) It should have a bucket and a rope for drawing out water. An ideal well should preferably be completely covered, and a hand pump should be fitted to draw out water.
(8) No washing of utensils, clothes, animals etc is allowed on the 6' paved space around the well.
(9) Cut away trees, and fill up rat holes and ditches around the well.
(10) Provide iron hooks for going down in the well for cleaning etc,
(11) Clean the well once every year. This is generally done at the late in summer when the level of water in the well is low.
  (i) Scmbs the walls,
  (ii) Remove the trees,
  (iii) Plaster the cracks,
  (iv) Clean the sides with a strong solution of bleaching powder.

Q. 8.10. (a) How wells are polluted? (b) How will you know that well's water are polluted? (c) How can you make an well water potable? (d) What are the difference between Deep well or Shallow well.

(a) Generally the wells are polluted by :
  (i) *surface washings,*
  (ii) *cracks and fissures,*
  (iii) *drains and cesspools* or *dug well latrine close by,*
  (iv) trees near the edge polluted the well through bird and dead leaves,

(v) vessels or ropes used for pulling water,
(vi) rise of subsoil water during the rains, and
(vii) over flow by flood water.

(b) Detection of Pollution

Whether well water polluted or not is detected by introducing a solution of fluorescine and caustic soda (1% each) or common salts; paraffin oil or culture of *Bacillus-prodigiosus, yeast* or any other non pathogenic micro organism, and by examining the water at different intervals of time by the testing material. Fluorescine can be detected at a dilution of 1 and 200,000.

(c) How we can Make an Well Water Potable

Well water can be made potable by periodical purification and by proper construction and maintenance of the wells :

PURIFICATION

Purification of a well water is generally done by dewatering and periodically cleansing at least once a year, and disinfecting at least once a week.

(a) *Dewatering and purification :*

The dewatering and cleansing is done at the hot season, when the water is at the lowest level. The water of a well which has neither been used nor cleansed for sometimes contains large amounts of organic matter. Purification is done by scarping the sides and removing all muds specially at the bottom of the well. The sides and the bottom of the well should be then treated with a solution of one part of freshly made slaked lime to 4 parts of water or strong solution of bleaching powder. Usually bleaching powder with 25% or more chlorine or 1/3 rd gr. per gallon is used.

(b) *Disinfection :*

Principles : For disinfection of a well the amount of water is first determined by the formula $D^2 \times W \times 5$ gallons (D = diameter and W = depth of water in feet). Then the calculated quantity of bleaching powder 1/3 rd per gallon) is mixed in a bucket so as to get an even solution of chlorine. This is then lowered into the well 2 feet below the water level and mixing it by giving rotatory movement to the rope tied to the bucket and by down the water surface. After half an hour the residual chlorine is tested by the *orthotoluidine test*.

(c) Proper construction and maintenance is also the main factor to make the well's water potable.

(d) **Difference between shallow well and deep well :**

No.	Items	Shallow well	Deep well
1.	Depth	12'-25'	25'-50
2.	Supply	Temporary	Permanent all-the year, Must pass-through at least one impervious layer.
3.	Layers	Passes through previous layer	
4.	Cone of filtration	Nil	Present
5.	Water tapped	Subsoil or ground water.	Deep water between 2 impervious layers.
6.	Casing	Need not be of impervious.	Must be of impervious material.
7.	Impurities		
	(a) Inorganic	Less	More
	(b) Organic	More	Nil
8.	Character of water.	Soft	Hard due to the pre-presence of $CaCO_3$.
9.	In maintence	Both surface & sub-soil contaminations to be prevented.	Only surface conta-minations to be pre-vented.
10.	Domestic purpose	Better served due to softness.	Not so
11.	Hand pumping	Harmful	Allowable depending on critical velocity of water at the depth.

N.B. DIS-INFECTION IN PRACTICE

WATER

Q. 8.11. How will you disinfect the water of a well? Discuss with examples?

Examples : (How disinfection is done in case of cholera or typhoid epidemic or when an animal has fallen in the well and has died).

The *methods of disinfection of well is as follows :*

1) Find out the volume of water in the well to be disinfected. If diameter of the well is 10' and hight of water is 24' then the volume of water in the well is $10^2 \times 24 \times 5 = 12,000$ gallons.

[Diameter^2 of well in ft x Hight of water in ft x 5 = gallon of water on the well.]

2. Find out by Horrocks test the chlorine demand of the water. Horrock's set has a black cup with a mark, and 6 white cups with marks. There is a bottle of starch solution and another bottle with solution of cadmium iodide. There is a stirrer, a chopper and a spoon which holds 2 gms of $CaOCl_2$ (Bleaching powder).

Given water to be tested and the Bleaching Powder to be used.

i) Put 1 spoon of $CaOCl_2$ in Black cup and add H_2O up to the mark.

ii) 6 white cups contain water to be tested up to the mark.

iii) Put one drop of liquid from the black cup to the white cup No. 1, Two drops in white cup No. 2, and so on i.e. 6 drops in white cup No. 6.

iv) Wait for 30 minutes.

v) Then put 1 drop of starch-solution in every white cup, and 1 drop of cadmium Iodide in each cup. If 4th cup shows blue colour (i.e. 4th, 5th show blue colour) $CaOCl_2$ required = $4 \times 2 = 8$ grams for 100 gallons of water.

Hence for 12,000 gallons of water 960 gms of Bleaching powder is required.

N.B. : If one spoon of $CaOCl_2$ does not show the blue colour, then put 2 spoons, or 3 spoons etc.

Suppose :

If two spoons are put and 3rd cups shows blue colour, then $CaOCl_2$ required = 2x2x3=12 grms 100 gallons. If 4 spoons of $CaOCl_2$ is put and 6th cup shows blue colour. $CaOCl_2$ required = 2x4x6=48 grms for 100 gallons.

*** [Instead of cadmium Iodide and starch solution, Orthotoluidine solution can be put (one drop for 5cc).

If 2 PPM chlorine is present there is yellow colour. If more than. 2 PPM chlorine is present then the colour becomes brown by orrhotoluidine test).

POT-CHLORINATION

This is the best method for continous chlorination of well water.

Wells are the sources of water supply for 75% population. Hence all wells should be chlorinated by pot chlorination.

The method of "pot chlorination" of wells are as follows :

i) A pot of 12 litres capacity is taken.

1.5 kg of $CaOCl_2$+3 kgs of sand are mixed.

If well has about 10,000 litres of water and draw is about 1000 litres daily, then this will be sufficient for 7 days. The pot has holes at the sides of .6 cm in diameter. The mouth is covered by plastic paper and the pot is kept dipped in the water (about a meter below).

Water enters through the holes and chlorinated water comes out through the same hole. The chlorination will be .2 PPM and will be sufficient for 7 days.

* **Bleaching powder** is the disinfectant of choice. If pH of water is more than 7, then "ocl" is liberated. It is less efficient as germicide. If pH is less, then "Hocl" is liberated. It is powerful germicide.

** **Potassium Permanganate** ($KMnO_4$) is used to kill germs in water.

It is costly and unplasant taste remains for a long time.

WATER

In fairs, fruits and vegetables are washed with $KMnO_4$. It oxidises the germs as long as the water is pink in colour.

One ounce of $KMnO_4$, will disinfect 1500 gallons of water.

VII. WATER SUPPLY OF RURAL AREAS

Q. 8.11. (a) What are the main sources of drinking water in a village of the plain ? (b) Which of them would you suggest more suitable for drinking purpose and why ?

(a) Sources of Drinking Water

In the *village* the sources of drinking water are :

1. *Tanks and ponds.*
2. *Dugwells*—Shallow of Deep.
3. *Tube well* and
4. *Sometimes river.*

To become good sources of drinking water the sources of water must fullfil the following two criteria—

i) The quality of water must be acceptable, and

ii) The quantity must be sufficient to meet the present and future requirement.

Now come to the different sources of drinking water in the Indian village of the plain.

1. TANKS AND PONDS : These are the easily available sources of water of our village nearer to our dwelling house. Its water generally used for drinking and cooking purpose when these water are free from pollution i.e adequetly protected and well stored.

But tanks and ponds are commonly used for washing and bathing purposes. The washing of clothes and utensils and bathings of man, cattle and domestic animals directly pollute the water by the passage of excrement direct into the

Why tanks and ponds water are not suitable for drinking, without Purification. water. Jute steeping direct is a common practice in the ponds of the village which makes the water very foul and offensive. Even surface drains are allowed to empty into most of the ponds in village and in the hot weather from putrifactive changes tanks water deteriorates. Growth of algae and the accumulation of the decayed aquatic plants gradually from a layer of very offensive mud at the bottom and putrifactive changes makes water unpleasent to taste and give off H_2S.

So the tanks and ponds water of the our village are not ideal for drinking purpose without purification, although the water undergoes natural purification.

2. DUGWELLS : Dugwells are of two types :

a) *Shallow well* and b) *Deep well*.

a) **Shallow well and deep well** : Shallow well tap the ground water above the first impervious layer of the soil and can be used for drinking purpose. It is generally useful in a village for isolated houses, camps, melas and fair etc. But the water of the shallow wells are easily polluted by flooding the surrounding uplands and from the contamination of the subsoil water by crackes and fissures which exists in the soil or subsoil, or percolating impurities of the soil through the porous soil or open drain close to the wells or the rate holes of the soil. The individual bucket the rope also add contamination.

Merits and demerits of shallow well and deep well.

In the summer the water level of the shallow well drop remarkably. So for the above reasons shallow well of the traditional type is looseing ground. The shallow well is being increasingly converted into protected deep well by covering it with a removeable heavy cement concreate lid and fitted with a hand pump.

So *Deep wells* are the best sources of drinking water as the tap water contained in an area between first and second or more impervious strata. The water of the deep wells are free from organic impurities but inorganic impurities are more common. They contain an excess of lime and common salt and become hard. They are however exposed to contamination from surface washing and other sources as in the cases of shallow well. But this is a much more permanent supply than shallow well.

WATER

3. TUBE WELLS : Tube wells sunk through one or more impervious strata to an underlying water bearing formation depending upon the depth of soil strata from which the water is tapped, they are 100 ft or more long with a diameter of 1 to 1½ inches or 9 inches and are the best sources of drinking water in Indian villages.

Because the water obtained from the tube well is free from organic materials and bacteria as the water travel a long distance through the soil after falling on the earth. Chemically, it contains greater quantity of minerals and inorganic salts than surface water i.e. tanks and ponds or rivers. It contains sodium chloride in variable quantity, traces of iron and other minerals which are essential for life. The water is hard for the presence of calcium carbonate ($CaCO_3$) but hard up to 25 degree are not harmful for drinking purposes, even hard water are more palatable than soft water.

Why tubewell is the best for supply drinking water ?

Recent experience has seen that a tube well with a hand pump can be installed at a reasonable cost and thirty families can meet their requirement of water from such a tube well. Even in congested village with heavy contamination of ground surface, the location of the tube well is not so important as design and construction are specific.

4. RIVER : Sometimes the villager who lives nearer to the river use its water for drinking purpose. But without purification it is dangerous to drink. The river water is fairly pure and unpolluted at its source but during its course through town and villages it often takes up impurities derived from sweage and industrial effluents, particularly near the bank. In our country most of the places for pilgrimage are situated on the banks of rivers and popular customs of bathing in the rivers make the water polluted. Most of the rivers are very muddy and contain much suspended matters and organic matter and also polluted by human and animal excreta accidently or purposefully. The customs of burning dead bodies in of the rivers is also a source of pollution as the infected materials like beddings, clothings and even half burnt dead bodies are thrown into the water.

So for these reason water of the river are not suitable for drinking purposes.

From the above discussion, we come to the conclusion that *Tube well* water is the best suitable for drinking purpose.

Q. 8.11. (c) How disinfection of tube well water is done ?

The idea of disinfection of tube well water is not disinfection of the subsoil water, but only disinfection of the tube. Never use bleaching powder, as it will corrode the tube. The pump is opened up and strong solution of $KMnO_4$ is used to fillup the tube. Do not draw water for 24 hours.

Q. 8.12. Describe the different steps by which you can make tank and pond water suitable for drinking purpose.

In rural areas tanks and ponds are the sources of water supply. For drinking and cooking purposes only water from the reserved tanks should be used. The following steps are to be taken for building a reserved tank from which water can be drawn for *drinking purpose* :

1. *Ponds and tanks* should be excavated in good and appropriate soil avoiding sandy and 'made soil'.

2. It should be deep and large.

3. The banks should be sloping and covered with grass and protected by a fence. No water from outside should enter into the tank.

4. Bathing by men and animals and all kinds of washing should be prohibited.

5. Water should be drawn from a platfrom or jetty or by means of a hand punp.

6. No trees should be allowed to grow on the banks except at a safe distance to prevent soiling of the tank by bird and droppings leaves.

7. The tank should be free from growth of algae, water hyacinth and pistia or any other vegetations.

N.B. : For purfication see *Q. No. 8.22.*

VIII. CALCUTTA WATER SUPPLY

Q. 8.13. Describe briefly the sources of water and water supply of the city Calcutta.

The question of supplying pure water to Calcutta is of great importance and requires careful consideration about *collection, storage and distribution of water.*

1. COLLECTION AND STORAGE

For Calcutta water supply water is collected from the river *Hoogly. Palta 18* miles from Calcutta is the main power house for receiving water from the river Hoogly and 85 million gallons of water is received by means of 5 big pipes. Generally from *Palta* pumping station water goes to the *Pre-settling tank* from which again it goes to the *Settling tanks* by gravity, then by *Slow Sand Filter* and *Rapid Sand Filter* to a well where all the water from Rapid and Slow Sand Filter are collected. From this chlorinated water of about 80 to 81 million gallons are send to *Tala Tank* at Calcutta by three pipes.

In the Palta station 12 Rapid Sand Filter in addition to 59 Slow Sand Filter are functioning since 1940. Generally in the settling tank the water is allowed to remain at least 24 to 48 hours and at that time natural purification takes place. The solid matter in suspension falls to the bottom by gravity, coagulation and precipitation of colloid colouring matter occurs, thus colour disappears.

In the rainy season as the water becomes more turbid process of sedimentation hastened by the Alum Coagulants Chamber. Laboratory examination at palta is done after the filter water is received in the well. From Tala Tank water is distributed to different place in Calcutta but before distribution chlorination is again done by chlorine gas at Tala.

2. DISTRIBUTION OF WATER

The distribution system of water includes the system of pipes connecting the water supply reservoir or the pumping station with the individual service pipes and taps of the

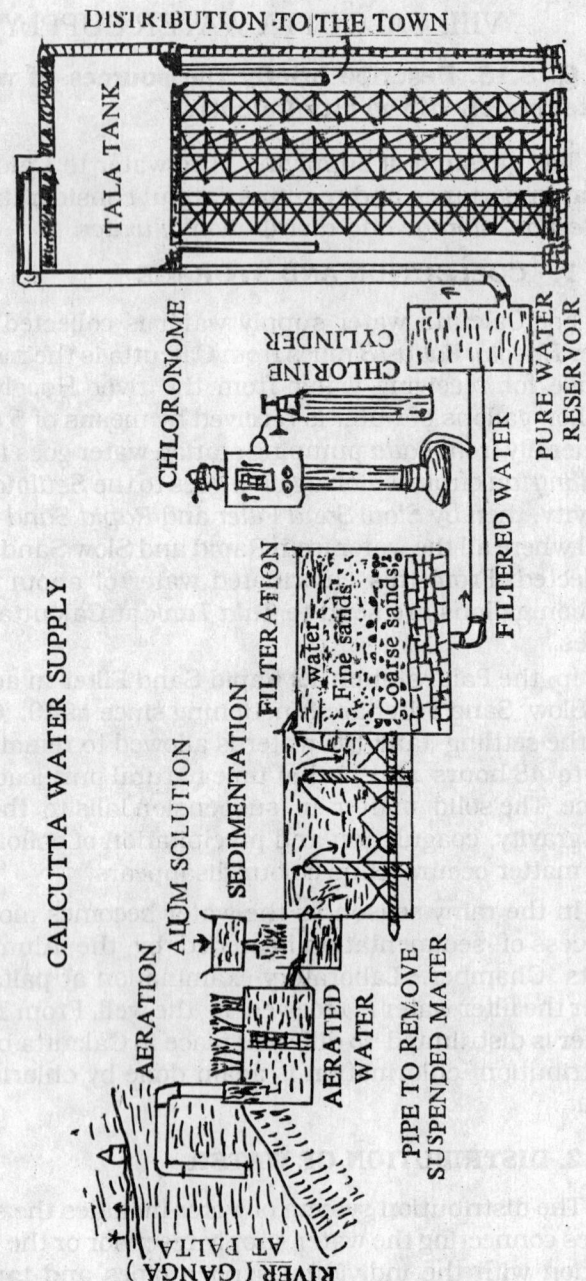

houses. This is a very complex one, as the size and characteristics of this varies from place to place. In Calcutta distribution is carried on by steel pipes of 3/4 inch thickness having a diameter of 5 feet to 6 feet and coated with a special asphalt preparation. The whole network of water supply is divided into :

(a) *Trunk mains*, and (b) *Service main types* and are usually laid in the public streets.

The main criteria of design is to see; the service mains are able to provide at any time a rate of flow which will meet the combined demand of the various services, which have to be supplied with water.

The water supply of Calcutta is of two types :

(i) *Constant* and

(ii) *Intermittent*.

(i) Constant Water Supply

*** [What is meant by dual water supply ?]

Generally constant supply of water in Calcutta is considered as a dual water supply. Due to increased demands and inadequate availability of pipe water, Calcutta has Dual water distribution. i.e. (a) Impured unfiltered water is now chlorinated and supplied for flushing sewers and closets, or watering streets, extingushing fires and for manufacturing or trade purpose and (b) The pure water is supplied for drinking, bathing and cooking purpose only.

In Calcutta the minimum amount of water supply is only 45 gallons per head per day for all purposes, of which 30 gallons are filtered and 15 gallons are unfiltered.

Tube wells are also supply additional water in some parts of the city.

ii) Intermittent Water Supply

*** [What do you meant by intermittent water supply.]

For the sake of economy, the water is also supplied for only a few hours of a day which is known as intermittent supply. In Calcutta the intermittent supply is also done at various pressure-which are as follows :

Pressure	Time
100 ft	5 to 9.30 a.m. and 3.30 to 5.30 p.m.
60 ft.	12.30 to 1.30 p.m.
20 ft.	rest of the day.

Q. 8.14. What are the advantages and disadvantages of : (a) Dual water supply, (b) Intermittent water supply and (c) Constant water supply ?

(a) Advantages and disadvantages of dual water supply :

Advantages :

The Dual supply of water is economically beneficial, because :

i) Less cost in incured to supply unfiltered water and also.

ii) Continues supply of unfiltered water is of much helpful for extinguishing fires, flushing sewers and closets or watering streets etc.

Disadvantages :

1. Amount of pure water supplies being less, with the dual supply of water there is a possibility of using unfiltered water for drinking purpose which can spread water-borne diseases easily.

2. *Dual supply* involves a second system of mains and *supply pipes* being costly to set up, there is also a possibility of cross connection between the supplies due to leakage in distribution pipes.

(B) Merits and Demerits or Advantages and Disadvantages of Intermittent Water Supply

Advantages :

1. The advantages of intermittent water supply that less number of attendants are required for operation.

2. The repair and pipe connection from the mains can be done easily during non-pumping hours without interfering with the period supply.

Disadvantages :

1. The serious disadvantage of the said method is that no water is available for fire fighting during non-pumping hours.

2. Underground or overhead storage tanks are essential at consumer, place to meet the demand during non-pumping hours. So there is additional expenses of transmission cost and feeding for storage tanks.

3. The size of the distribution main should be larger so that the total quantity of water to be delivered within a shorter period will necessitate the use of bigger diameter mains and therefore larger capital investment in pipe lines.

4. Emptying of mains during non-pumping hours tends to create vacuum in certain portion of the main where there is likelihood of polluting sub-soil water to enter through undetected leaks and thereby likely to contaminate the water supply.

(C) Advantages and disadvantages or Merits and demerits of Constant Water Supply

Advantages :

1. Constant supplies of water is of much helpful for extinguishing fires and other emergencies.

2. No water is required to be stored for the house consumers.

3. There is no chance of contamination and pollution by the sucking of gas.

Disadvantages :

1. In constant supply due to non availability of large storage tank at consumer's house the water is often wasted. Even imperfect joints or any kind of defect or leakage of the pipes cause water to be wasted.

IX. IMPURITIES OF WATER

Q. 8.15. What are the impurities of water ?

OR

What different kinds of chemical, mineral and biological impurities are found in water ?

Quality water should be cool and clear, pleasant to taste, free from pathogenic organisms, should neither be corrosive nor scale forming. It should also be free from excessive concentration of minerals which would produce undesirable physiological effects on human health. But no water which occurs in nature is so pure as to satisfy all these qualities as because all natural water are impure to a greater or lesser extent. Being an universal solvent, it dissolves something of everything it touches. Mainly the nature of impurities that water picks up depends on the nature of the materials it encounters during its formation and flow over the land. Generally natural impurities derived from atmosphere, catchment area and the soil, but artificial impurities are derived from our activities for mordernisation i.e. urbanisation and industrialization.

1. Natural Impurities

The following are the list of impurities which water contains both in dissolved and suspended forms :

Natural Impurities of Water

```
                          Impurities
          ┌──────────────────┼──────────────────┐
        Organic           Microbes           Inorganic
                       Algae, Bacteria
 ┌──────────┬──────────┐   Larve of parasites.
Dissolved Colloidal  Suspended  Animal cules.
          Albumin.   Animal matter  Living plants.
          Organic waste. Vegetable matter
 ┌────┬────────┬─────────┐              ┌─────
Gases  Acids      Poison              Salts
CO₂, H₂S  Humic Acid  Soluble, Organic  Alumina
Methane. and others.   matter.        Chloride nitric.
          Dissolved                 Colloidal      Suspended
                                    Alumina       clay, soil, wast,
                                    Iron oxide,   minarals.
 ┌─────┬─────────┬────────┬────── Mica, Silica Fireclay.
Gases  Acids    Poisons   Salts
CO₂,   Nitric   Sb, As,   Alumina,
O₂,    Nitrous, Pb, Cu,   Carbonates, Bicarbonates,
H.     Sulphuric. Hg, CN, Chlorides, Nitrates, Sulphates,
               Tn, Zn.    Phosphates, Silicate, Iron.
```

2. Artificial Impurities

In our modern age impurities like detergent cyanids, heavy metals, bleaching agents, pigments, sulfides, various toxic and biocidal organic compounds produced due to our day to day activities for urbanisation and industrialization of our country are some of the forms of artificial impurities. Water also contains decomposable organic matter and pathogenic agents from sewage. It also contains toxic agents ranging from metal salts to complex synthetic organic chemical from industrial and trade water. Various agricultural pollutants like fertilizers and pesticides are also the chief impurities of water. Basically physical pollutants viz. heat (thermal pollutants) and radio-active substances are the main impurities of water in our atomic era.

X. EFFECTS OF IMPURITIES OF WATER

Q. 8.16. What are the effects of impurities of water on water itself and on human health ?

A. EFFECTS OF IMPURITIES ON WATER

Water of a particular quality at its source gets changed in its composition and behaviour during the interval between the time it is procured and the time it reaches the consumer due to impurities :

1. Generally all suspended matter makes the water *turbid.*
2. Due to presence of organic matter from extracted decaying vegetation the *colouring of water* occurs which is objectionable from aesthetic point of view.
3. *Taste and odour of water are changed* due to the decomposition of organic materials or due to volatile essential oils liberated from the bodies of algae or due to the presence of free gases like H_2S and NH_3, phenolic compound and chlorine.
4. Mineral content makes the *water hard.*
5. Organic impurities and atmospheric dirt favour development of biological organisms, changes the quality of water considerably becoming *turbid.*

B. EFFECTS OF IMPURITIES ON HEALTH

1. Effects of dissolved inorganic materials :

Generally inorganic materials are included metals and salts of lead, Copper, Zinc, Aluminium, Iron, Calcium, Magnesium, Bicarbonates, Sulphates, Chloride and Phosphates. Their effect are :

i) *Lead* (Pb)   The use of water containing 1/100 grs. lead per gallon gives rise to symptoms of lead poisoning i.e. plumbism. Chief symptoms are anemia, constipation, colic, wrist drop, and other symptoms are of peripheral nurities as well as depression, renal disease and finally death.

ii) *Iron and zinc* etc. causes constipation and dyspepsia.

iii) *Calcium and magnesium* — bicarbonates, sulphates, chlorides and nitrates causes hardness of water producing diarrhoea and dyspepsia of man.

iv) *Sodium* salts like sulphates and chlorides in excess causes purging and vomiting.

v) Excessive *mica* causes diarrhoea in hilly regions.

vi) Excesses of *nitrates* are responsible for poisoning of infants.

vii) Excess of *fluorine* causes dental distrophy (fluorosis).

viii) Lack of *iodine* causes goitre.

2. Effects of suspended inorganic impurities :

Suspended inorganic impurities are particles of sand, clay, slit, mud and other insoluble minerals which cause diarrhoea by mechanical irritation of the intestines.

3. Effects of dissolved and suspended organic impurities :

Generally the organic impurities are bacteria— both pathogenic and nonpathogenic, algae, iron and sulphur bacteria and host of other organic growths, suspended solids from sewage and industrial waste etc.

WATER

Their main effects are :

i) Vegetable and cellulos—cause diarrhoea and intestinal troubles.

ii) Organic impurities from soil, sewage and seepage change the quality of water to cause constipation and diarrhoea.

iii) Faecal contamination and by other specific organisms like vibrio cholerae, bacillus typhosa, B.Coli, Entamoeba histolytica, Ascaris lumbricoides, Guinea worm, etc. causes Cholera, Typhoid, B. coli, Dysentery, Roundworm, Threadworm etc. diseases. Even virus of polimyelitis and infective hepatitis cause the respective diseases.

4. Effects of various impurities other than natural impurities i.e. artificial impurities :

The artificial impurities are various industrial and trade wastes, agricultural pollutants and physical pollutants like radioactive substance etc.

Generally the chemical impurities affect man's health directly by producing diarrhoea, constipation etc. but modern chemical impurities of water are not so much related to their acute toxic effects on human health, their effects have long term effect which are difficult to detect immediately but shows genetical aberration in the long run, causing tumours, cancer etc.

XI. WATER BORNE DISEASE

Q. 8.17. What do you mean by water borne disease ?

Water contains various organic and inorganic impurities. The organic impurities are mainly from human sources like urine and excreta and his activities for industrialization and urbanisation of his country. Generally the germs which are present in impure water can live and multiply in water and communicate the diseases to the people. So the water acts as a vehicle in carrying germs, and the diseases arise from the contaminated water are known as *water borne diseases.*

Q. 8.18. What are the diseases commonly spreaded or transmitted by water ?

The following are the diseases which are spreaded by water :

1. Water borne diseases due to the presence of biological agents :

Group — A

1. Bacteria

    (a) Cholera.

    (b) Dysentery—Bacillary (Shigellosis).

    (c) Leptospirosis (Weil's disease).

    (d) Typhoid (Enteric fever).

    (e) Paratyphoid.

2. Protozoa — Amoebiasis (Amoebic dysentery).

3. Virus

    (a) Infective hepatitis, poliomyelitis.

    (b) Pleurodynia.

Group — B

Entozoai Diseases

    a) *Diacontiatis* (guinea worm disease).

    b) *Echinococciasis* (Hydatodosis).

    c) *Schistosomiasis* (Bilbarziasis).

    d) *Ascaris lumbricoides* (Round worm).

II. *Disease due to presence of chemical agent* :

Gastro-enteric diseases like—Diarrhoea, constipation, dyspepsia, purging and vomiting are the common water borne diseases, but these are a group of illness having the main symptoms of diarrhoea. Generally they constitute a major health problem in many countries of the world but all of them are not etiologically defined.

III. *Diseases due to presence of agricultural, industrial and trade wastes and physical agents like radioactive wastes :*

The chemical agents affect man's health directly by producing diarrhoea, constipation etc. But the modern chemical agents of water production no such acute toxic effect on human health. Generally their effects are long terms effects which are expressed by genetically aberrated disease like tumours and cancer etc.

Q. 8.19. What steps will you take to prevent water-borne disease ?

The occurrence of infection through water is extensive; since water is used raw, unlike foods which are mostly cooked. In most cases the water is infected directly by various pollutent and the tanks, wells and river water are largely responsible for the water borne disease.

So to prevent water borne disease every effort should be made to avoid water pollution at their sources and to supply purified water for consumption.

These can be achieved by the following ways :

1. Prevention of Water Pollution at Sources

(A) *Tanks, ponds* and *wells* are chief sources of drinking water in Indian villages.

i) So they should be excavated in good soil and at a fair distance from sources of pollution like cess-pool, drain etc.

ii) They should be carefully examined and thoroughly cleansed at regular interval of the seasons, especially after a time of drought and before the approach of winter, otherwise they should be periodically disinfected.

iii) The water should be drawn by pump, or by using a separate bucket.

iv) Bathing and washing of clothes, untensils etc. are to be totally forbidden.

(B) *River water* is mainly polluted by bathing, washing, trade effluents and the discharge of sewage etc.

　i) So these types of willful pollution should be guarded by making "The River Pollution Act" or preventive act" as has been done in other country.

　ii) By taking river water 20-30 ft. away from the bank by using hand pump with a pipe or from above the spot where sewage and other impurities are discharged into the river, the contamination of water can be checked to some extent.

(C) *In town* where supply is intermittent and the pipes are occasionally left empty, sewage may be drawn the empty pipes through leaky joints and cracks, so to avoid the pollution it is necessary to lay water mains at a distance from gas pipes, drains, sewers etc. or on a solid so as to prevent by cracks occurring from subsidence.

(D) In many places water is distributed by *Bhistis* i.e. through a special leather bag but it is very much difficult to keep these bags clean so as far as possible this system should be avoided or stopped.

2. Purification of Water

(A) *In villages* where drinking water is obtained from tanks, wells, river etc. should be purified by boiling, or disinfected by chemicals like potassium permanganate. Bleaching powder, or tablets like Hallogen etc. or by using domestic filters before drinking.

(B) *In town* water should be supplied after proper disinfection and filtration. Also in the town where the water is supplied in large scale, all employees should be examined medically with bacteriological examination of their stool, nose and throat swabs etc. for preventing water pollution. Also there should be arrangement for water analysis. Above all during an epidemic water should be taken always after boiling.

Q. 8.20. How does the water become impure ?

In the chemical sense the water is never pure. It contains various natural impurities both dissolved and suspended forms. Dissolved impurities are various dissolved gases like H_2S, CO_2, NH_3 etc., and dissolved minerals like salts of calcium, magnesium etc. and suspended impurities are clay, slit, sand, mud and microscopic plant and animals.

Generally water becomes impure at its :
1) *sources,*
2) *during transit from sources to the reserviors,*
3) *at the storage, and*
4) *during distribution.*

So these are the following ways in which water becomes impure :

(1) At the Sources

All natural sources of water are impure to a greater or lesser extent, because it is an universal solvent and dissolves something of everything it touches.

Rain water is the purest water when occurs in the nature, but its purity, however, does not remain as it receives impurities from air or from the surface where it falls. It absorbs gases and take up dirt from the lower regions of the atmosphere. Thus it contains nitrogens, oxygen and carbonic acid, and near the sea contain salt, suspended matter and also microb.

Surface water includes upland water, impounding reserviors, lakes, tanks or ponds, river and streams etc. Generally the character of water depends upon the geological structure through which it travels. In case of *upland surface water* it is seen that if the hills are covered with peat, the water becomes brownish, yellowish, or when the rock contains soluble minerals, then the water will dissolve those minerals. Thus a upland surface water contains salts of magnesia, nitrate, common salt or calcium carbonate derived from lime stone rocks.

Tanks and ponds water are commonly impure by being used for washing or bathing purposes by the passage of excrement direct into the water or by the rotten leaves. Cattle and domestic animal are often bathed and washed in the tanks and surface drains are allowed to empty into most them. Growth of algae make the water unpleasant to taste. Jute steeping or the dieing of the aquatic plants gives of H_2S and makes the water very foul and and offensive.

Ground water i.e. springs and wells are free from organic impurities but inorganic impurities are sometimes common which renders water unfit for domestic purpose. It may also contain excess of lime and common salt. The water of the wells often gets polluted either from surface water or from contamination of the subsoil water.

(2) During Transit from Sources to Reservior

Upland surface water is the water which is stored in the form of natural lakes or artificially constructed impounding reserviors in hilly districts at the head of rivulets or streams. The surrounding areas from which the water is collected is called the catchment area. Depending upon the characteristic of the catchment are the impurities of the upland surface water are various dissolved organic impurities and decayed vegetable matter.

The river water is fairly pure and unpolluted at its source but during its course, it becomes more or less polluted, as most riyers and streams form and natural drainage channels of regions they pass through. As a rule river water contains a large amount of organic matter, industrial effluents, sewage, waste, human excreta etc. The custom of burning dead bodies on the banks of rivers add impurities by the infected materials like bedding, clothing and even unburnt or half burnt bodies which are thrown in the river.

(3) At the Storage :

Generally water taken from different sources are stored in gharas (earthen pots) or metal vessels for drinking purpose. When water kept in metal vessels and protected by a cover for a long time, the water partly loses its aerated character. If the water are stored in masonary tanks or wooden tubs for a long time the water often deteriorated by contamination from dust, dirt, cockroaches etc. or by losing its sparkling character gradually becomes flat and insipid. If stored in earthen pot it may be contaminated due to the porous character of the pot.

(4) During Distribution

When the supply of water is intermittent and the pipes are occasionally left empty, outside impurities may be drawn into the empty pipes through leaky joints or cracks. If soft water passed through lead pipes, lead is dissolved.

In many places water is distributed, by special water carriers—*Bhistees* who use bhitis (leather bags) for carrying water, contaminate the water as it is not possible to keep these bags clean. Moreover these bhistees also live in a very insanitary environment so all sorts of contamination occurs.

From the above discussion we come to know that natural impurities are derived from the atmosphere, catchment area and from the soil. But in our modern age the main impurities are our own activities for urbanization and industrialization of our country.

Several types of decomposable organic matters, pathogenic agents, industrial and trade wastes, fertilizer and pesticides etc. are also the impurities of water which make the water of rivers impure.

XII. PURIFICATION OF WATER

Q. 8.21. What are the different methods of purification of water ?

Generally the impurities of water are grouped into five categories, namely :

1. Floating and suspended solids of visible size;
2. Small suspended and colloidal solids, causes turbidity;
3. Micro organisms;

4. Dissolved solids producing hardness and acidity, and
5. Dissolved gases, such as O_2, CO_2, H_2S etc.

Water purification aims to remove most of these impurities, and methods used are related to the particle size and chemical composition. The type of surface water treatment for purification is not standarized. It varies according to the raw quantity and the extent of water purification that is required.

Nature often helps to purify water by various means which are included under the heading of *Natural methods of purification*. But purification by nature is not dependable, so the natural supplies are required purification by artificial methods which are included under the heading of *Artificial methods of purification*.

Generally the different methods of purification are of the following types :

METHODS OF PURIFICATION OF WATER

Natural
1. Evaporation and condensation
2. Storage and settlement
3. Aeration, oxidation, sunlight
4. Filtration through earth
5. Self-purification of rivers and streams
6. Biological purification

N.B.:—Various—*artificial* methods of treatment may also classified according to their purposes rather then their made of action are—

Artificial
1. *Physical* :
   a) Boiling
   b) Distillation
   c) Aeration
   d) Sedimentation

2. *Chemical* :
   a) Coagulation (precipitation)
   b) Germicides (disinfection)

3. *Filtration*:
   a) Slow sands (mechanical cum biological)
   b) Rapid sand (mechanical):
     i) gravity type.
     ii) pressure type.

i) *Hygienic purification :* by storage, sedimentation. Coagulation, by use of chemicals, slow or rapid sand filtration and disinfection for providing safe water

ii) *Biological purification :* for control of algae and other nuisance or organisms.

iii) *Aesthetic purification :* by special treatment for removal of colour, taste and odour.

4. *Removal of taste odour and colour.*
5. *Removal of hardness :*
   i) Lime-soda process.
   ii) Ion-exchange process.
6. *Miscellaneous treatment:*
   a) Removal of colour, taste and odour,
   b) Removal of iron, manganese, flourides,
   c) Removal of dissolved gases.

XIII. PURIFICATION OF WATER IN INDIAN VILLAGES

Q. 8.22. What are the common methods of purification of water in Indian villages ?

The common methods of purification of water in Indian villages are as follows :

1) *Boiling.*
2) *Chemical disinfection.*
3) *Filtration.*

Generally these methods are used singly or in combination.

1. Boiling

It is the safest and quickest way of disinfecting or purifing water for house-hold purposes. Boiling for 5-10 minutes kills bacteria, spores, cysts and ova, expels the dissolved gases particularly CO_2. It, however, makes water flat and insipid which can be improved by aeration. It is a good practice to boil water in the same container in which it is stored.

2. Chemical Disinfection

The most common chemical methods are the disinfection by : (i) *Potassium permanganate,* (ii) *Lime,* (iii) *Bleaching powder and* (iv) *Chlorine tablets.*

(i) *Potassium permanganate*—It acts as an oxidising agent and destroys the organic matter preventing bacteria to grow. It is generally used for disinfecting wells, cisterns and small quantities of water. In proportion of 5 parts per million it destroys 98% of bacteria in 4 to 6 hours. Usually 3 gms. is required for a well 2 ft. in diameter and containing about 8 ft. of water or 200 gallons of ordinary water. It generally kills cholera vibrio but is of little use against other organisms. It also alters the colour, smell and taste of the water.

(ii) *Lime*—For purification i.e. disinfection of polluted water quick lime used. It is cheap and easily available. The amount required varies with the quantity and hardness of water. It is helpful in precipitation of iron in water. It is also used for softening both temporary and permanent hardness and takes about 5 to 24 hours to remove most of the bacteria and organic matter.

(iii) *Bleaching powder or Chlorinated lime*—It is an oxychloride of lime ($CaOCl_2$)-a whitish powder with feeble chlorine smell, widely used for disinfecting water. When freshly made, it contains 33.5 percent chlorine. On exposure to light, the chlorine rapidly evaporates. On ounce of good quality of bleaching powder is employed to disinfect 100 gallons of water. This amount gives a concentration of about 1 PPM.

(iv) *Chlorine tablets*—Halozane/zeolite sol.

Chlor-dechlor and hydro chlorazane tablets and zeolite sol. etc. are sold in the market. These are quite good for disinfecting small quantities of water and generally used for drinking water.

3. Filtration

Water can be purified in a house or on a small scale by filtering through ceramic filters such as :
i) Pasteur's chamberland filter.
ii) Berkefeld filter.
iii) Katadyn filter.

The essential part of the filter is the candle which is made of porcelain or in fusorial earth. Filter candles of the fine tipe, usually remove bacteria found in the drinking water. Filter candles are liable to clogged with impurities and bacteria. Although these are effective in purifying water, yet these are not quite suitable for general use under Indian conditions.

Three pitchers method was used in former days. As the regular cleanliness of the sand and the charcoal are never maintained, so this method is not used now.

XIV. PURIFICATION OF WATER ON A LARGE SCALE IN CITIES.

Q. 8.23. What are the methods of purification of water to supply in the cities like Calcutta and Delhi ?

For the water supply of the cities like Calcutta and Delhi, the water is purified by 3 main stages :
(1) *Storage.*
(2) *Filtration.*
(3) *Chlorination.*

1. Storage

Water is drawn out from the rivers and is stored in the artificial reservoirs. As a result of storage a very considerable amount of purification takes place. This is natural purification. Generally purification occurs by the following ways :

a) *Physical* — By mear storage the quantity of water improves, 90 percent of the suspended impurities settle down in 24 hours by gravity, and water becomes semifiltered.

b) *Chemical* — Certain chemical changes take place during storage. The aerobic bacteria oxidize the organic matter present in water, the concentration of free ammonia is reduced and the nitrates rise.

c) *Biological* — A tremendous drop takes place in the bacterial count and the pathogenic organism die out.

2. Filteration

It is the second stage of the purification of water, 98-99 percent of the bacteria are removed by filtration and many other impurities are also eliminated.

There are two types of filtration which are used—the Slow sand and Rapid sand filter. Generally slow sand filters are used for purification.

(a) Slow Sand Filter

For large scale purification this is the method of choice. The stages of operation are as follows :

Collection of water from the river into settling tanks and sedimentation for 1-3 days → Coagulation and precipitation of colloidal and colouring matters by adding aluminium sulphate or alumino ferric (alum containing 1% ferric sulphate) followed by storage for 3-4 weeks which renders the water pretty safe prior to filtration due to destruction of organic matter, ova, cysts, spores, and other bacteria to a large extent by oxygenation, ultraviolet rays of the sun and by the aquatic and plant life present in the water → passing of water into the filter beds. After filtration the water grvitates into the bottom of the filter beds for collection where it is chlorinated by Patterson's Chlorinating plant before discharging in the main for distribution.

3. Chlorination

Chlorination kills the pathogenic bacteria and renders water safe from the bacteriological point of view. It is a supplement and not a substitute to sand filters chlorine. Being oxidizing agents, it oxidizes iron, manganese and hydrogen sulphide and destroys taste and odour producing compounds. The chlorine is added in sufficient amounts so as to meet fully the chlorine demand of the surface water.

The presence of free residual chlorine for at least 20 minutes is considered essential to ensure destruction of pathogenic organisms in water. The goal is to maintain a free residual chlorine of 0.2 PPM at the end of 30 minutes contact.

Methods of chlorination are :
  i) Chlorine gas.
  ii) Chlorimine.
  iii) Perchloren.

(Chlorine gas is the method of choice as it is cheap and quick in action, efficient and easy to apply.)

N.B. : For the various processes for the removal of hardness of water see Q.8.31.

PURIFICATION OF WATER

Large Scale
- Storage
- Filtration
  - Slow sand or Biological filters
  - Rapid sand or Mechanical filters
- Chlorination

Small Scale
- Household Purification
  - (a) Boiling
  - (b) Chemical disinfection :
    - i) Bleaching power
    - ii) Chlorine solution
    - iii) High test hypochlorite.
    - iv) Chlorinization by solution or tablets.
    - v) Iodine
    - vi) $KMnO_4$
  - (c) Filtration.
- Disinfection of well sand Tube wells

XV. FILTERATION OF WATER

(Slow Sand Filter and Rapid Sand Filter)

Q. 8.24. Describe a slow sand filter with its working principles.

Slow Sand Filter (Description)

For large scale purification of water this method is generally followed :

The *stages of operation of this are as follows :*

Collection of water from the river into settling tanks and sedimentation for 1-3 days →

Coagulation and precipitation of colloidal and colouring matters by adding aluminium sulphate or aluminoferric (alum containing 1% ferric sulphate) followed by → storage for 3-4 weeks which renders the water pretty safe prior to filtration due to destruction of organic matter, ova, cysts, spores, and other bacteria to a large extent by oxygenation, ultraviolet rays of the sun, by the aquatic and plant life present in the water→

Filter beds : The slow sand filter beds consist of a water-tight rectangular basin usually made to masonary 60 x 40 x 15 ft. The bottom being sloped into the middle with a channel to carry filtered water into the collection pipes. The bed is made of two layers of bricks with spaces for channel, on which gravel, coarse and fine sands are laid from bottom to top as follows :

(i) 6"-12" of gravel (3/4" size).

(ii) Coarse sands 3-4 ft.

(iii) Fine sands-1 ft.

(iv) Open space- 5 to 6 ft. to fill with water from the last storage or sedimentation tank. Generally the filtered water from the filter bed goes into a well in which the level of water is maintained at 1" lower than that of the filtered ; this difference in the level of water is known as *filtration head or working head.* The rate of filtration is 50 gallons per sq.ft. per day. After filtration the water gravitates into the bottom of the filter beds for collection where it is chlorinated by Patterson's chlorinating plant before discharging into the main for distribution.

Modes of Action :

Generally water is purified by :

        (i) Physical,

        (ii) Chemical, and

        (iii) Biological processes.

(i) **Physical** : Filtration by mechanical obstruction of impurities in the interstics of the filter.

(ii) **Chemical** : Oxidation of organic matter by the organisms in the sand layers.

(iii) **Biological** : A vital layer consisting of algae and slimy deposit, colloidal slit, aquatic plants, protozoal and other organic matters formed on the surface of the sand layer in 2-3 days to act as a biological film for purifying water. When this layer becomes thicker it slows down the rate of filtration. Every 6-8 weeks it becomes necessary to scrape out this layer for fresh deposit of vital layer. Every three years the entire bed required to be renewed. For an effective filtration the rate of filtration should not exceed four vertical inches per hour.

Q. 8.25. (a) What do you mean by rapid sand filter ? (b) Describe Paterson's gravity rapid filter.

(a) Rapid Sand Filter (Mechanical filter)

In *Rapid sand filteration* water filters at a rate of about 3 vertical inches/min. or about 2 gallons/sq.ft./min. or 125 million gallons/days i.e. at a rate about 40-60 times greater than that of slow sand filter. It consists of a intake and raw water pump or gravity line, plain sedimentation basin, mixing and coagulation basin, actual filters and clear water reservoir, chlorinating devices and high lift pumping sets.

Rapid sand filter is of two types—*Pressure type* and *Gravity type*.

(i) In the *Pressure filter*—the chamber is closed and the coagulated water is driven through the sand under its own head of pressure which is greater than atmospheric pressure.

(ii) In *Gravity filter*—the water is passed through a coagulating basin to open filters through which it gravitates at atmospheric pressure and then led to the clear water tank. In this process of rapid filtration the following steps are involved :

    a) *Coagulating and formation of 'floc'.*
    b) *Filtration.*

In this system, the place of the vital layer of slow sand filter is taken by a filtering layer artificially made by producing a flocculent ppt, which with colloidal silt settles on the surface of the sand and fills up the sand inter spaces.

There are varieties of rapid filtration but the important one is *Paterson's Gravity Rapid Filter.*

(b) Paterson's Gravity Rapid Filter

It comprises five distinct processes which are as follows :

1. *Addition of chemicals.*
2. *Mixing.*
3. *Coagulation and sedimentation.*
4. *Filtration.*
5. *Chlorination.*

1. Addition of Chemicals

Raw water is first pumped into settling tanks where heavier silt is deposited and a certain amount of natural purification takes place. From the settling tank it is continously led into the plant through a measuring gear and addition of aluminium sulphate solution in proportion of 1-4 grs/per gallon.

2. Mixing

The water then passes down a mixing trough provided with baffle plates when the solution of alum is mixed thoroughly with raw water.

3. Coagulation and Sedimentation

Water is then led into a sedimentation tank divided usually into compartments. The coagulant hastens the deposition of suspended matter and produced an artificial surface film 'floc' in the tank before actual filtration. It also effects decolouration. Here water is allowed to remain for 3-6 hours, which varies depending more or less upon the prevailing season and the quality of water required.

4. Filtration

Water treated in this manner is passed through mechanical filters. The filters are contained in ferro-concrete about 7 ft. deep. The filtering medium consists of quartz or sand 33 inches supported on broken pieces of stones of pebbles 18 inches deep. The removal of the coagulated impurities and bacteria is carried out by rapid filtration.

5. Chlorination

From the filters water passes through an automatic regulating gear into a chlorinating chamber where chlorine gas is added and water is sterilised.

Cleansing of Filters

As the rate of filtration is high the filtering medium becomes loaded with micro-silt, organic matter and bacteria which interferes with the efficacy of filters. So it requires frequent cleansing, which again depends upon quality of water and season. Cleansing of filter is done by shutling the inlet valve and passing reverse current of filtered water from the clean reservoir through the bottom of the sand by means of rotatory metal arms, rakes, or a blast of compressed air. The wash water flows away to the waste over the top. A thorough cleansing of filter takes place within 15-20 mins. and a satisfactory film is formed in another 20 mins. and the filter becomes ready for service again.

Q. 8.26. Compare Slow Sand Filter and Rapid Sand Filter ?

1. The name indicates that the rates of filtration of rapid sand filter are more than 100 times faster than slow sand filters.

2. Methods of cleaning are different. Slow sand filter is cleaned by scraping the surface layer where as the rapid sand filter is cleaned by upward flow of water or compressed air.
3. Slow sand filter does not require expert supervision for operation.
4. The filtration head in rapid sand filter is higher than the slow sand filter.
5. Slow sand filter has greater reliability for bacteria removal and its cost of operation is less.
6. Slow sand filter functions very efficiently when feed water is low in colour and turbidity.
7. The demerits of slow sand is that it occupies larger space and is kept out of commission for longer period. During cleaning it requires larger volume of sand. So the capital cost of the plant is high.
8. In both types of filtration water after filtration and chlorination should be bacteriologically tested to ensure bacteriological purity.

XVI. HARDNESS OF WATER

Q. 8.27. What do you mean by hardness of water ?

OR

When water is to be considered as hard ?

Hardness of water means the soap destroy power of water. It is expressed in term of milli equivalents per litre (mEq/l). One mEq/l of hardness producing ion is equal to 50 mg $CaCO_3$ (50 ppm) in one litre of water. Though the main cause is the presence of calcium and magnesium salts in solution in the form of bicarbonates, chlorides and sulphates.

Iron, manganese and aluminium compounds also cause hardness but as they are present in small amounts, they do not consider as hard.

Q. 8.28. What are the various types of hard water ?

Hard water is of two types, namely :

(1) *Temporary*, and (2) *Permanent*.

Water containing calcium and magnesium bicarbonates are *temporary hard* and presence of sulphates and

WATER

chlorides of calcium and magnesium make water *permanent hard*. But the temporary hardness due to magnesium bicarbonate is sometimes also considered although it is very rare.

Q. 8.29. What are the different level of hardness of water ?

Different Level of Hard Water

Hardness of water is expressed in term of milli-equivalents per litre (mEq/1). One mEq/1 of hardness producing ion is equal to 50 mg $CaCO_3$ (50 ppm) in one litre of water.

According to *hardness, water is classified* as follows :

Classification	Level of Hardness (mEq/1 litre)
1. Soft water	Less than 1 (50 mg/1)
2. Moderately hard water	1-3 (50-150 mg/1)
3. Hard water	3-6 (150-300 mg/1)
4. Very hard water	Over-6 (over 300 mg/1)

N.B. : * Softening of water is recommended when the hardness exceeds 3 m Eq/1 (300 mg per litre).

PPM — parts per million. One ppm corresponds to be hardness caused by one million of calcium carbonate or its equivalent in one litre of water.

Q. 8.30. What are the bad effects (disadvantages) of hard water ?

Bad effects of hard water are as follows :

1. On Health

(a) Recent studies showed that hard water causes different types of cardiovascular diseases like arteriosclerotic heart disease, hypertension, degenerative heart disease etc.

(b) Due to the presence of magnesium sulphate, it gives rise to gastro-intestinal troubles like dyspepsia and diarrhoea etc. in persons who are not accustomed to drinking hard water.

(c) Bathing in a very hard water for a long time causes roughness of the skin and various types of skin diseases.

2. On Household Work

(a) Hardness of water causes great wastage of soap and detergents.

(b) Hard water adversely affects cooking. Food cooked in hard water changes the natural colour and appearances, and certain foods such as pulses are difficult to soften.

(c) Fabrics washed with soap in hard water do not have a long life.

(d) Requires more fuel, due to high boiling point.

3. On Industrial Purpose

(a) When hard water is heated the carbonates are precipitated and bring about furring or scaling of boilers. This leads to greater fuel consumption, loss of efficiency and may sometimes cause boiler explosions.

(b) If used in industrial process it gives rise to economic losses as it requires more fuel in engine etc.

(c) Hardness of water shorten the life of pipes and fixtures.

Advantages

Moderately hard water is good for drinking as it contains the essential minerals in it.

XVII. REMOVAL OF HARDNESS OF WATER

Q. 8.31. How hardness of water can be removed in (a) Domestic and (b) In large scale water supply ?

The following are the methods by which the hardness of water can be removed :

1. Temporary Hardness

(a) Boiling.

(b) Addition of lime (Clark's process).

(c) Addition of sodium carbonate.

(d) Permutit process.

2. Permanent Hardness

(a) Addition of sodium carbonate.

(b) Base exchange process (permutit process).

A. For Domestic Purpose

For domestic purpose generally temporary hardness is removed by boiling.

Total hardness is that which is present before boiling, and that which remains after boiling is called permanent hardness. Generally temporary hardness of water occur due to the presence of bicarbonate of calcium and magnesium and the bicarbonates of calcium and magnesium are soluble in water and these are formed in water containing carbon-di-oxide. Therefore, this hardness is removed by boiling.

1. Boiling : By boiling—CO_2 gas is removed and the carbonates precipitates. Generally the reaction is reversible and is as follows :

i) $Ca(HCO_3)_2 \xrightarrow{Heat} CaCO_3 + CO_2 + H_2O.$

ii) $Mg(HCO_3)_2 \xrightarrow{Heat} MgCO_3 + CO_2 + H_2O.$

The removal of non-carbonate hardness is done by the addition of *sodium carbonate* (Na_2CO_3) and the removal of magnesium, non carbonate hardness is done by the addition of *both lime and sodium carbonate.*

B. In Large Scale Water Supply

When the hard water is used for the large scale water supply of a city, the hard water is commonly soften by the addition of lime. Because the boiling of such a huge amount of water is not practicable. Removal of hardness by lime is known as Clark's Process.

(1) Clark's Process

In this process lime as [$Ca(OH)_2$] is used to remove the hardness due to magnesium and calcium bicarbonate. Generally 10 percent of milk of lime or in sufficient amount are thoroughly mixed by a mechanical regulater and after sedimentation, upper part of clear and soft water are drawn out. In this process chemical reactions are :

$Ca(HCO_3)_2 + Ca(OH)_2 = 2CaCO_3 + 2H_2O$.
$Mg(HCO_3)_2 + Ca(OH)_2 = MgCO_3 + CaCO_3 + H_2O$.
$MgCO_3 + Ca(OH)_2 = Mg(OH)_2 + CaCO_3$.

2. Porter Clark's Process

As the Clark's process is comparatively slow, the suspended particles of chalk are removed by filtering through coarse linen cloth under pressure. This method has, therefore, the advantage of rapidity and removal of suspended matter effectively.

** Permanent hardness of water can be removed by the addition of caustic soda precipitating sulphate of soda, which are as follows :

$CaSO_4 + Na_2CO_3 = CaCO_3 + Na_2SO_4$.
$MgSO_4 + Na_2CO_3 = MgCO_3 + Na_2SO_4$.

3. Stan Hope System (Lime soda process)

In case of water containing considerable permanent as well as temporary hardness a mixture of both lime (CaO) and caustic soda (NaOH) is employed. This lime and soda mixture process known as "Stan Hope System".

4. Zeolite softening or Base exchange process or Permutit Process :

The softening of permanent hard water is done on a large scale or for domestic purposes by filtering water through *permutit.*

Generally the permutit contains a water softener i.e. a closed cylindrical tank in which a chamber present upper portion where salt solution automatically prepared for regeneration purposes, although a specified quantity of dry salt are placed at fixed interval. The lower part contains a bed of *Permutit medium* i.e. *Synthetic zeolites contain sodium and aluminium silicate. Generally natural zeolites are green sand or gluconite found in nature.* When artificially prepared, they are called permutit. It contains sodium aluminium silicate (Al_2O_3, 10 SiO_2, 10 Na_2O) and it has got a property to inter-change their sodium for an equivalent quantity of a Ca or Mg element from water. As Na take their places from Na-zeolite (NaZ) the hard water becomes soft.

The reactions are as follows :

(i) $Na_2Z + Ca(HCO_3) + Mg(HCO_3)_2 = CaZ + MgZ + 2NaHCO_3$.

(ii) $Na_2Z + CaSO_4 + MgSO_4 = CaZ + MgZ + Na_2SO_4$.

(iii) $Na_2Z + CaCl_2 + MgCl_2 = CaZ + MgZ + 2NaCl$.

So the efficiency of permutit gradually lessen; by exchange of 'Na-base. But its functions are restored by passing a strong solution of NaCl through the medium. Then Ca or Mg given out the Zeolite again becomes Na-zeolite. The reaction is as follows :

$CaZ + MgZ + 2NaCl = CaCl_2 + MgCl_2 + 2Na_2Z$ (Z = zeolite).

So the mechanism of zeolite softening or base exchange. Purmutit process is simply a filtration through the permutit bed.

Advantages

1. In this process Ca and Mg chlorides are discharged to washes, the total amount of minerals are not reduced but only the Ca and Mg salts are placed by an equivalent amount of Na salts.

2. It is also seen that in this process a zero hardness of water is produced and the alkalinity of the water is not changed as the carbonate and bicarbonate of Na is present instead of Ca and Mg.

Disadvantages

1. As the effluent from a zeolite softner has a zero hardness, it is very corrosive to pipes, therefore the usual practice is to soften a protion of the water and mix it with

sufficient raw water to give a hardness of 50 to 100 ppm. The pipes can also be protected from corrosion by the addition of soda ash or sodium silicate to the softened water.

2. This method is suitable for household supplies and manufacturing requirements, but for town supply the cost is more than that of lime and sodium carbonate (Stan Hope system).

3. Also it cannot be used successfully if the water contains an excess of sodium salts, free acid and iron.

XVIII. HYDROLOGICAL CYCLE

Q. 8.32. What is meant by hydrological cycle ?

The *hydrological cycle is the central focus of the science of hydro- logy, which is concerned with the waters of the earth, their occurrence, circulation, distribution, and chemical and physical properties.* The hydrological cycle is not a simple link but rather a group of paths through which the water in nature circulates and is transformed from one state to another. These paths penetrate through the entire hydrosphere that surrounds the earth; they extend upwards to about 15 kilometres (nine miles) in the atmosphere and downwards to an average depth of one kilometre (0.62 mile) earths crust.

The cycle has no beginning or end, and many processes are involved. As water evaporates from the oceans and the land, it becomes a part of the atmosphere (*the evaporation process*). The evaporated moisture is lifted and carried in the atmosphere until it finally precipitates to the earth, either on land or in the oceans (*the precipitation process*). The precipitated water may be intercepted or transpired (emitted as vapour from the surface of land parts) by plants (*the interception and transpiration processes*), may flow over the ground surface (*the overland-flow process*) or down the ground slop with in the soil layers (*the thorough flow process*) and into streams (*the run off process*), or may infiltrate into the ground (*the infiltration process*). The water remaining on the ground fills in depressions, where it is stored for later evaporation (*the retention process*) or later run off (*the detention process*).

Much of the intercepted and transpired water and the surface run off returns to the atmosphere through evaporation. The infiltrated water may percolate to deeper zones (*the percolate process*) to be stored as ground water. It may later flow out as springs or may seep into streams, finally flowing to the sea and evaporating into the atmosphere to complete them hydrological cycle. Thus the hydrological cycle consists of various complicated processes of *precipitation, evaporation, interception, transpiration, infiltration, percolation, retention, detention, overland flow, thorough flow,* and *run off.* The hydrological cycle is also composed of numerous cycles of *continental, regional* and *local magnitude*—all of which are interrelated components of the global system.

CHAPTER-IX

DISPOSAL OF HUMAN EXCRETA, REFUSE

DISCUSSION FOR LEARNING

I. Disposal of human excreta :
   A) in villages.
   B) in towns and cities.
II. Septic Tank.
III. Disposal of Refuse.

I. DISPOSAL OF HUMAN EXCRETA

Q. 9.1 (A) What are the disadvantages of indiscriminate defecation?

The main disadvantages of indiscriminate defecation are :

1. *soil pollution.*
2. *propagation of flies.*
3. *contamination of water.*
4. *contamination of foods*, resulting serious health hazards and epidemics diseases like typhoid, paratyphoid fever, dysenteries, diarrhoea, cholera, hookworm, ascariasis, infective hepatitis and many other diseases.

Q. 9.1 (B) What are the essential points to be taken into consideration in hygienic disposal of human excreta?

Proper disposal of human excreta is of great importance, and necessary from sanitary, economic and aesthetic points of view. indiscriminate defecation results in soil pollution and contamination of water and food, often creating thereby serious health hazards and epidemics.

DISPOSAL OF HUMAN EXCRETA, REFUSE

For hygienic, disposal of human excreta the following points should be considered :
1. Suitable arrangements for the collection, removal and disposal of excreta.
2. There should be no chance of soil pollution or contamination of water.
3. There should be no any exposure to flies.
4. There would be no offence to senses of smell or sight.
5. Lastly the public should create cheap and clean latrine with easy construction by local labour and minimum materials which are locally available.

Q. 9.2. What are the common methods of disposal of human excreta ?

The common methods of disposal of human excreta are divided into two broad groups :

1. **Non Service Type**
    A. In *unsewered areas* collection and disposal of night soil are effected by sanitary latrines, like :
    a) Pit latrines.
    b) Borehole latrines.
    c) Dugwell latrines.
    d) R.C.A. latrines.
    e) Septic tanks.
    f) Aqua privy.
    g) Chemical closet.
    B. In *sewered areas* disposal of excreta and sewage is done by *water carriage system* and *sewage treatment*.
2. **Service Type or Conservancy System**
    Here human agency like sweepers, is employed for collection and disposal of night soil. The night soil is transported in "*night soil carts*" to the place of final disposal by—(i) *composting* or (ii) *burial in shallow trenches*.

They are also classified as
1. *By self removal system.*
2. *Conservancy system.*
3. *Water carriage system.*

1. Self Removal System

In this system the human excreta is removed from the latrine pan and disposed in a pit by self cleansing system. This is done in non-service latrines like :
   i) *Pit latrine.*
   ii) *Bore hole latrine.*
   iii) *Dugwell latrine.*
   iv) *Septic tank latrine.*

Night soil is disposed by a hand flash of water.

2. Conservancy System

In this system manual labour is applied for the early hours of the morning every day by the sweepers from the service latrine who empty the privy pans into collecting drums provided with lids. These are carried to the place of final disposal by night soil carts and disposal is done by :
   i) *Trenching.*
   ii) *Incineration.*
   iii) *By composting.*

3. Water Carriage System

This system is used in highly advanced towns and cities. Here night soil and urine together with the liquid waste of dwelling are carried through a system of drains and sewers by a flush of water and by force of gravity to a place outside the town. For this system plenty of water is required.

METHODS OF DISPOSAL OF HUMAN EXCRETA

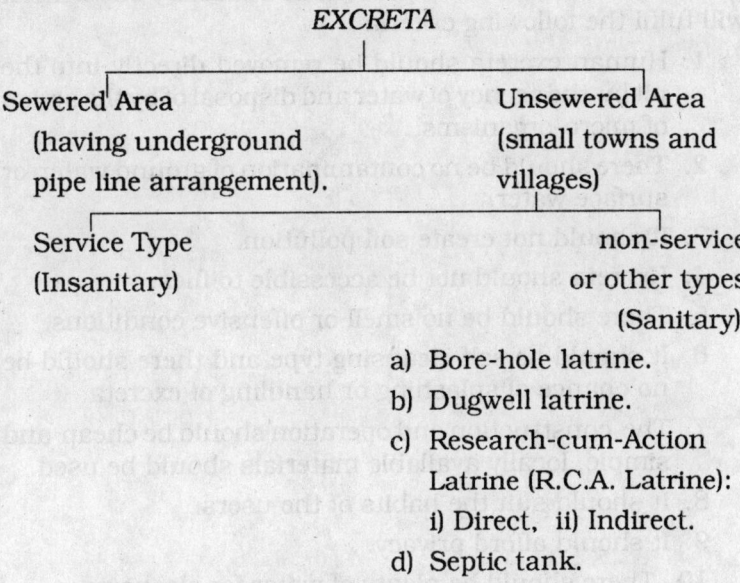

Q. 9.3. What are the common ways of disposal of human excreta in villages ?

Except few, particularly there is no arrangements in the villages for safe disposal of human excreta through privies or latrines. So most villagers for the purposes of answering nature call use the open lands or fields or banks of tanks, canals or rivers. Thus for indiscriminate defecation they usually contaminate the soil and water and become prone to the dangerous disease like hookworm and other filthy diseases. So proper disposal of human excreta in a village is utmost importance.

The common methods which are used suitably for disposal of human excreta in villages are the *Sanitary latrines*, preferably be of non-service type and one of the types of *Earth Pit Latrines* is satisfactory. But *Deep Pit Latrines*, Bore *Hole Latrines*, *Dugwell Latrines*, *R.C.A. Type of Dugwell Latrines* and *Trench* are also used for rich people, schools, and other centres of community activities of the villages.

Q. 9.4. What is meant by sanitary latrine ?

A latrine should be considered as a sanitary one when it will fulfil the following criteria :

1. Human excreta should be removed directly into the pit by the agency of water and disposal of by the action of micro-organisms.
2. There should be no contamination of ground water or surface water.
3. It should not create soil pollution.
4. Excreta should not be accessible to flies.
5. There should be no smell or offensive conditions.
6. It should be self-cleansing type and there should be no chance of splashing or handling of excreta.
7. The construction and operation should be cheap and simple, locally available materials should be used.
8. It should suit the habits of the users.
9. It should afford privacy.
10. There should be plenty of water for cleansing.
11. The site should be free from flooding. It should have superstructure to protect against rains and sun.
12. It should be far away from the sources of water supply, but would be close to the dwelling house.

Q. 9.5. What are the various types of sanitary latrines used in rural areas.

The sanitary latrines used in rural areas are of two types viz., 1. *Pit types* and 2. *Box types*.

1. Pit Types

Bore hole, Dugwell and Trench latrines are pit latrines. Here the excreta stored inside the pit undergoes dilution and decomposition in the soil. Only in porous or semiporous soils, these types of latrines can be used. These latrines are cheap and easy to construct with local labour and materials.

2. Box Types

The box types latrines are essentially digestion chambers requiring treatment of solid and liquid matter accumulated inside. They require good maintenance. They are expensive but can be constructed with proper design to suit varying soil conditions. The *septic tank, aqua privy* and *chemical closets* are the examples of box types latrines.

Q. 9.6. Describe any two methods of disposal of human excreta in the village which you think best and why ?

In *India* filth borne illnesses are the most formidable health problems in the rural areas. Recent surveys in Community Development Blocks in different states show that over 27 percent of the total mortality is due to the principal gastro-intestinal disease e.g. cholera, enteric fever, diarrhoea and dysentery. Intestinal infestation is wide-spread in the country. Hookworm, though not a killing disease, is debilitating to a considerable degree, the parasites offer a strong competition to human body in metabolising the available food.

To control these diseases, it is necessary only to provide a barrier between the sources of infection i.e. the disease producing organisms in infected excreta and the susceptible hosts, the human population. The barrier, a latrine, will prevent faecal matter from coming in contact with man or with his food or drinking water.

For individual families in rural areas, the latrine should be preferably be of non- service type and one of the types of *Earth Pit Latrine* is satisfactory e.g. *Borehole, Dugwell, R.C.A. or I.C.M.R. latrine. Septic tank* latrine may be suitable for schools and other centres of community activities and also for individual families under certain set of conditions e.g. availability of sufficient water, proper maintenance etc.

BORE HOLE LATRINE AND DUGWELL LATRINE

(R.C.A. Latrine) are the two best methods for disposal of human excreta in the villages.

1. Bore Hole Latrine

Structure : This is a circular pit made with the usual earth *auger* of 40 cm or 16" diameter to a depth of 3-4 meters (10 to 15 feet.) and even upto 6-7 meters (20-24 feet.) if the soil is not loose. Generally its depth depends on the level of the subsoil water level. It must reach 2-3 feet below the subsoil water lever. Top of the hole is covered with a *squatting* plate which is a concrete slab of about 2-9 inches in diameter. It is provided with a central slot 5½ inches wide and 12.15 inches long and is fitted with footrests on either side. The whole structure is enclosed with mud or brick wall for screening purposes. A lining of split-up bamboo is put inside the wall of the latrines hole to prevent the earth from collapsing. As an alternate arrangement a pan and a trap can be placed away from the pit and connected to the bore by burn clay pipe.

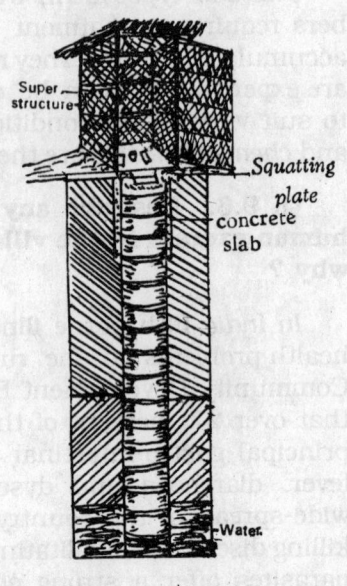

Fig. 3. Bored hole latrine

Function :— Generally the action of the disposal of excreta in the trench is biological by the nitrifying bacteria present in the soil and is eventually converted the excreta into a harmless mass. For a family of 5 to 6 people, a borehole latrine serves well for over a year, when the bore is filled up and the contents of bore hole reach 3 to 4 feet above the ground level the squatting plate is removed and the hole is closed with earth. A new hole is dug and similarly used or when the bore is filled up the pit contents can be removed and trenched and the bore can be redused. The presence of ground water, though not essential in the pit, but help for better functioning of the latrine. On the other hand if the

DISPOSAL OF HUMAN EXCRETA, REFUSE

pit is dry sufficient ablution water must be used to provide the necessary moisture needed to support the biological action.

Disadvantages—(1) This type has limited value because of this latrine gets filled up soon and new one is to be made easily.

(2) Boring with the auger needs some skill and trained person.

Advantages—But this is more popular in rural areas of India for many years as :

(i) It is in low cost to prepare.

(ii) It prevents hookworm infection and dissemination of other filthy disease.

(iii) As it reaches 2 inches below the surface of subsoil water the dilution of excreta takes place with water and helps biological purification.

2. Dugwell Latrine

It is a improvement over the *Borehole* latrine. Generally a circular pit of about 36 inches (76 cm) in diameter and 10 to 15 feet deep is dug into the ground for the reception of the night soil. It is provided with ½ inch *water seal* and the mouth of the pit is covered by *squatting plate* of about 39 inches diameter. It can be flushed with 2.27 litres or half a gallon of water. Dugwell latrine in function is similar to the bore hole latrine, but because of a larger diameter the changes of pit caving are greater than in bored holes and hence the well is preferable lined to prevent collapse. Choice of lining is guided by cost, case with which it can be used, durability and availability in the local area. The latrine of dimensions metioned above may last for about 6 years for a family of 5 to 6 members. When the well is filled up a separate well is dug and the plate is also shifted over the new well. The used well is covered with earth and left undisturbed for about 6 months, by this time the organic matter is converted into inorganic solids. The contents of the well can then be removed and used as manure. The well can be used once again to receive the human excreta. Location of pan and trap away from the well permits its connection to another dug on adjoining land. Such an arrangement will alleviate disturbing the latrine seat and super structure. Thus two wells can function alternately without requiring interruption in the use of the latrine.

Advantages : (1) It is easy to construct and no special equipment such as an auger is needed to dig the pit, (2) The pit has a longer life than the Bore Hole because of greater capacity.

Several modifications of the Dugwell latrine have been in use in the different parts of the country. Modifications are usually in the shape and dimensions of the pan and trap, lay out of the pit in relation to the pan and lining used for the pit. They have taken different names usually denoting the centres where they originated e.g. *Burdwan type., Burapalli type, Poonamallee, P.R.A.I., I.C.M.R., R.C.A.* and so on.

But now (R.C.A. Research-cum-Action) type latrine has appeared as, a readily acceptable one in rural areas considering its cost, and hygienic suitabality.

R.C.A. Latrine

The Research-cum-Action (R.C.A.) projects and organisations have evolved improved types of earth-pit latrine with *hand flushed water-seal squatting plates* which are being increasingly used in rural families. The safe distance of a latrine from a source of drinking water depends on soil, level of ground water, its slope and direction of flow and other factors. The latrines should not, as a rule, be located within 50 feet from a water source. The essential masonary parts of this type of latrine are :

(a) *Squatting plate.*
(b) *Trap.*
(c) *Lead off pipe or connecting pipe.*
(d) *Pit cover.*

DISPOSAL OF HUMAN EXCRETA. REFUSE

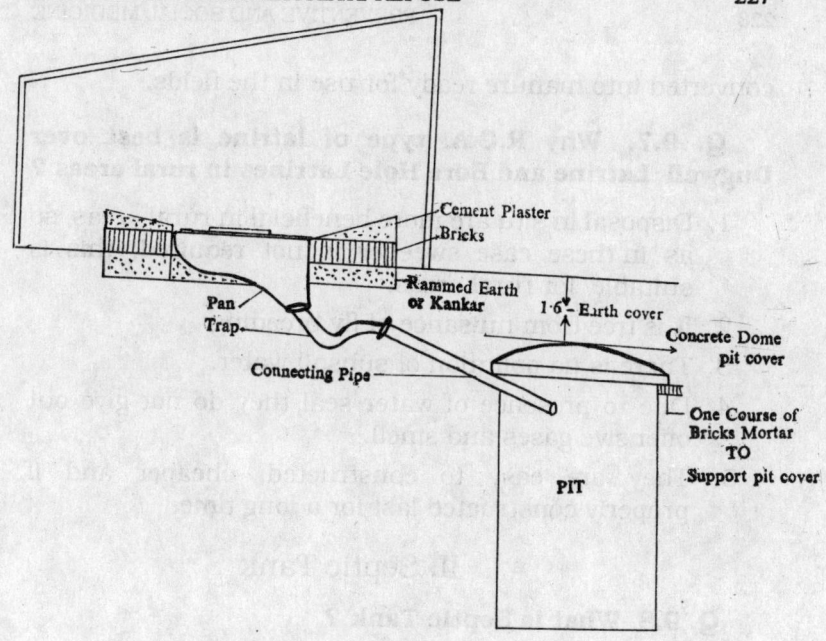

Dugwell ltrine (R. C. A. Type)
Fig. 5. Dugwell latrine

The superstructure consisting of the door walls and roof for privacy and available materials according to the amount that can be spent by the individual. The total cost of all parts including labour charges varies. A trained mason is required to fix the pan, trap and the pipe which are constructed in different centres and supplied on local demand. Preferably a site within the courtyard or adjacent to a house should be selected where two pits of 2 ft. 9 inches in diameter and at least 6 ft. in depth can be dug. In addition to the ablution water, one extra pint of water will ordinarily be enough to flush and carry to faecal mass to the pit. This water has to be added with some force for efficient flushing. All latrine pits will eventually get filled. A pit of the dimension mention above serving an average family of five, will last for nearly three years. When one pit is filled up, a second pit dug besides it. In this (RCA) type of latrine there is no disturbance of the squatting plate and the superstructure, the curved connecting pipe from the trap is turned over and fitted to the second pit. The first pit in fitted with earth and sealed. In a few months, the faecal mass is converted into manure ready for use in the fields.

Q. 9.7. Why R.C.A. type of latrine is best over Dugwell Latrine and Bore Hole Latrines in rural areas ?

1. Disposal in situ are more beneficial in rural areas, so as in these case sweeper is not required, this is suitable for rural areas.
2. It is free from nuisance of fly breeding.
3. There is no pollution of subsoil water.
4. Due to presence of water seal they do not give out offensive gases and smell.
5. They are easy to constructed, cheaper and if properly constructed last for a long time.

II. Septic Tank

Q. 9.8. What is Septic Tank ?

The septic tank is an underground, brick or concrete made tank into which house sewage is admitted for treatment and purification by biological process for atleast 24 hours.

It was first devised by *Cameron, Fowler and Clemesha* in 1906 and put forward for practice. A septic tank latrines consist of with *flushing tank, a soil pan with a trap* and chambered. Generally from the trap the sewage may pass to Comeroon's Septic Tank or Inhoff's Septic Tank or in an Oxidation Ponds. In a septic tank one or more latrines or full flushing system may be connected. A big colony houses may also drain in a Septic Tank only the size of the Septic Tank will have to be made larger.

Q. 9.9. Describe a Septic Tank with its working principles?

SEPTIC TANK

(Structure of a Comeroon's Septic Tank)

There are various designs in septic tanks. Some are double chambered and some single chambered. A single chambered septic tank has been satisfactory for small installation. Tank with more than two compartments are

DISPOSAL OF HUMAN EXCRETA, REFUSE

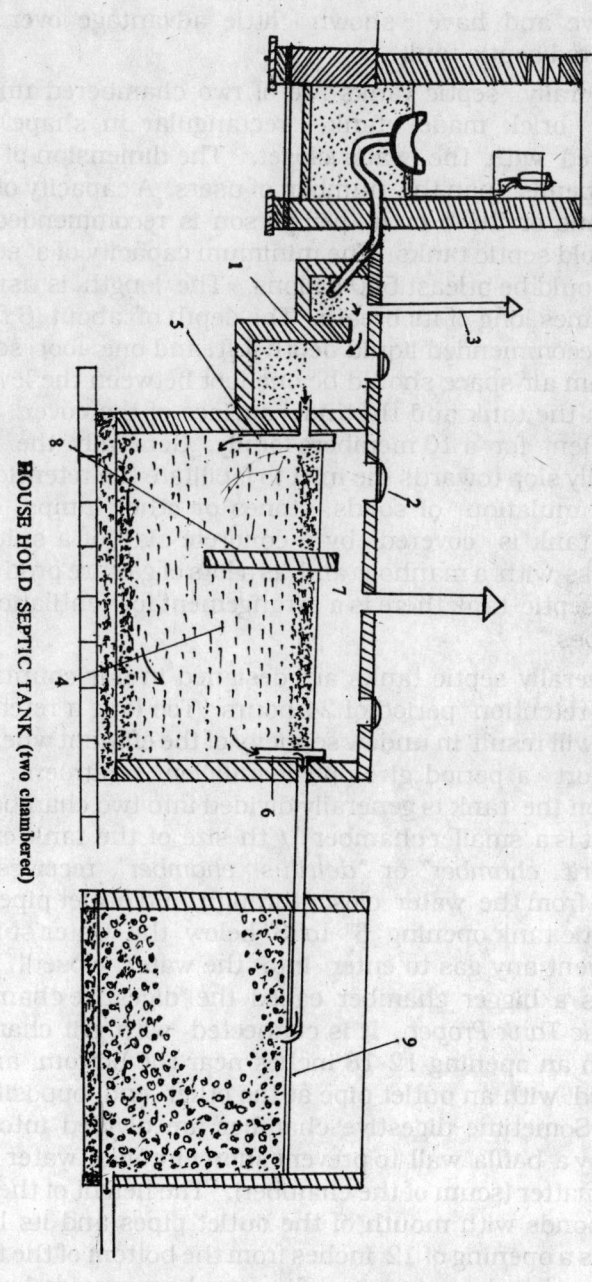

HOUSE HOLD SEPTIC TANK (two chambered)

expensive and have shown little advantage over two chambered septic tank.

Generally septic tanks are of two chambered underground brick made tank, rectangular in shape and connected with the water closet. The dimension of this tank depends upon the number of users. A capacity of 20-30 gallons or 2½-5 cu.ft. per person is recommended for household septic tanks. The minimum capacity of a septic tank should be atleast 500 gallons. The length is usually 3 to 4 times long of its breath. The depth of about 6 ft. of which recommended liquid depth 4 ft. and one foot scum. Minimum air space should be one foot between the level of liquid in the tank and the under surface of the cover. This is sufficient for a 10 members family. Generally the floor is usually slop towards the inlet to facilitate the retention or for accumulation of solids, stones or other lumps. The septic tank is covered by a concrete slab of a suitable thickness with a manhole and as a lots of gas are produced in the septic tank there is a arrangement for ventilation by *vent pipes.*

Generally septic tanks are designed in our country to allow a retention period of 24 hours. Too long a retention period will result in undew septicity of the effluent where as too short a period gives off insufficient treatment. For retention the tank is generally divided into two chamberes. The first is a smaller chamber $1/_8$th size of the tank called the "*grit chamber*" or "*detritus chamber*", receives the excreta from the water closet through and outlet pipe into the septic tank opening 6" to 8" below the water surface (to prevent any gas to enter into the water closet). The other is a bigger chamber called the "digestive chamber" or *Septic Tank Proper.* It is connected with grit chamber through an opening 12-18 inches near the bottom and is provided with an outlet pipe at the other end opposite to inlet. Sometime digestive chamber are divided into two parts by a baffla wall to prevent short circuit of water with faecal matter (scum of the chamber). The height of the wall corresponds with mouth of the outlet pipes and its lower side has a opening of 12 inches from the bottom of the tank. Both the chambers (grit and digestive) are provided with a ventilation pipe (vent pipe) and the digestive chamber with a manhole.

*** Generally in *ordinary septic* tank latrines there is no contact bed or filter bed. For one person 5 gallons of water are required for washing. Only anaerobic process is done. Sewage is put into drain after treatment with bleaching powder. As the quantity of sewages small it is diluted and may be put into the land.

*** In *rural areas* and small communities, septic tank effluent can be discharged into *soak pits*, or *utilized for subsurface irrigation*, by distribution it on the top layer of soil, by a system of loose jointed pipes. Soak pit is a pit, dug to a depth of 6 to 8 ft. in porous soil and it is 3 to 4 ft. in diameter. The pit is filled with bricks or jhamma and the effluent is made to percolate over this bed. So long as the pit is well aerated and is not choked up biological purification of sewage takes place. For *sub-surface irrigation*, open jointed tiles, or perforated types are laid is 4 feet below ground level and the effluent is allowed to drain over and area of land on which grass and other vegetation can be grown. This method is not applicable in areas of clayey soil, or ground. The absorption capacity of the soil is very important, otherwise there is chance of underground water pollution. In *areas where ground water level is high*, secondary treatment of effluent can be done by passing the effluent over sand filters, or trickling filters, before it is finally discharged. Chlorination of effluent with 1.2 to 2.0 ppm. chlorine, is recommended to destroy pathogenic organisms.

Design Features Septic Tank in Brief

1. Capacity : depends on users. Minimum capacity 500 gallons. 20-30 gallons or 2½-5 cu.ft. per person is recommended for household purposes.
2. Length : Twice the breadth.
3. Depth : 5-7 ft.
4. Liquid depth : Minimum 4 ft.
5. Air space : 12 inches.
6. Bottom sloping towards inlet end.
7. Sub-merged inlet and outlet pipes.
8. Concrete cover with manhole.
9. Ventilation pipe (vent pipe).
10. Retention period 24 hours.

It becomes one chamber or two chambers. When two chambers it contains grit chamber and septic tank proper. *Active principles—Biological treatment (Anaerobic liquifaction and aerobic oxidation by nitrifying bacteria).*

Principle Action of a Septic Tank

Generally *'anaerobic liquifaction'* takes place in septic tank proper while *'aerobic nitrification'* occurs in contact beds or percolating filters. But in case of single chamber septic tank all the action i.e. anaerobic digestion takes place inside the septic tank chamber instead of septic tank proper and contact beds or percolating filters.

In case of two chambers septic tank the raw sewage at first comes to the first chamber i.e. grit or *detritus chamber* whose capacity is one eighth of the septic tank proper. Here all the solids and heaviest particles settle down, to the bottom so there is a arrangement to take out heaviest particles time to time.

Then effluent passes to be second chamber i.e. *digestive chamber* where anaerobic digestion of sewage occurs. Here organic materials are broken up by the *anaerobic digestion process.* The anaerobic condition is due to formation of scum and not due to cover. During the process of decomposition and digestion sewage is converted into *gases, effluent and sludge.* In the digestive chamber the solids particles fall in the bottom while hard lumps of faeces float on the surface and the lighter solids including greese and fat rise to the surface to form *scum.*

Under the scum the anaerobic bacteria break down the solid masses into soluble and unstable compounds i.e. a state of fine suspension and the solid organic matter which settled down at the bottom to form *sludge.* The black deposit of the sludge accumulates at the bottom of the tank and when this becomes 8-12 inches thick it should be removed and deposited in trenches.

*** The *scum* which is a complex molecules of protein, is further digested by anaerobic bacteria into amines, amino acids etc. with liberation of CO_2, NH_3, methene and H_2S gases. These gases are escaped through the vent shaft which is present at the top of the tank.

**** The effluents which is generally dark coloured with faeced smell is drawn off without disturbing the scum. As it holds nitrogen as NH_3 it needs oxygen. So before discharge it is further treated either Contact beds or in Trickling Filter bed for conversion of different ammoniacal compounds into oxidised nitrogenous substance of harmless character i.e. nitrites and nitrates by aerobic bacteria. Usually each bed provides a period of 8 hours rest after 4 hours work in order to establish re-aeration. The final effluent is then discharged into river, stream or on the land after treating by 5 gms. of bleaching powder per gallon to disinfect it or to remove the danger of transmitting water-borne diseases.

Generally in *ordinary septic tank latrines* there is no *contact bed* or *filter bed*. The liquid effluent which consists of water used in ablution, after decomposition of organic matter passes through outlet from the septic tank digestive chamber. But as the quantity of effluent is small it passses into a *soakase pit* (having a depth of 10-12 feet) and decomposed. The liquid containing the organic materials is attacked by the soil bacteria and renders it into a stable end products.

*** *Sludge* which is a semisolid, dark brown substance, collects at the bottom of the digestive chamber of the septic tank along with the grit from grit chamber. The sludges and grits are removed once in two years or so, through the manhole provided.

Q.9.10. What are the essential points to be considered for efficient working of a septic tank ?

The following five are the essential requirements for an efficient working of a septic tank processes :

1. Abundant water supply to carry excreta to the tank.
2. Enough space should be left between the scum and the cover plate.
3. Both the chambers should be provided with ventilators.
4. Sludge should be removed at intervals.
5. No disinfectant should be used in the septic tank proper.

Q. 9.11. What are the working principles of septic tank ?

The principles of action of a septic tank is the biological methods of treatment of human excreta. Generally biological treatment does not precipitate suspended matters but reduces the complex organic substances by the action of bacteria and other micro-organisms.

Its action is a combined process and in this process two groups of organisms i.e. anaerobic and aerobic bacteria are utilised.

Anaerobic bacteria reduces organic substance into simple compound by breaking down, digesting and liquifying to a ammonia and ammoniacal compounds in the septic tank proper and then aerobic bacteria convert by the process of nitrification of ammoniacal substances into oxidised nitrogen substance of harmless character i.e. nitrites and nitrates either in contact bed or in trickling filter bed. The final effluent is generally discharged into a river or a stream or it may be treated on the land.

Q. 9.12. Under what circumstances installation of septic tank is ideal ?

Septic tank is a satisfactory means of disposing excreta and liquid water from individual dwellings, small group of houses and institutions.

The following are the circumstances for a septic tank installation :

1. There must be abundant supply of water (at least 5-10 gallons per person per day, automatic or occasional flush) to carry the excrement to the tanks and also to keep the (pan) place clean.
2. There will be no use of disinfectant in any situation of the tank. Unless the putrefactive bacteria will be died.
3. There must be plenty of space above surface of the fluid which stands in the tank to accommodate the 'scum' and the gases.
4. There should be a ventilator pipe to let off the foul gases.

5. The sludge should be removed at intervals when ever necessary.

Q. 9.13. What are the various methods of disposal of night-soil in the villages, small towns and cities ?

For the disposal of night-soil in the villages and small towns the following methods are used :

A) *Latrines*—They are of two types : *Sanitary and Insanitary*. The ones that posses health hazards are grouped under the second category. Generally speaking a latrine which does not lead to contamination of water or pollution of soil with human excrement and the ones which do not exposure the excrement to flies can be considered as sanitary latrines. Those which do not fulfil any of these criteria are insanitary latrines.

Sanitary latrines are further of the following types :
1. *Trench latrines,*
2. *Pit latrines,*
3. *Bore-hole latrines,*
4. *Dug latrines (RCA type),*
5. *Aqua privy,*
6. *Septic tank.*

In other slightly bigger towns, the following methods are used :
1. *Trenching,*
2. *Composting,*
3. *Burning.*

In bigger town or cities the system used is water *carriage system.*

Q. 9.14. What is meant by trenching ? What are its disadvantages?

Trenching

Trenching is a process of burying the night-soil beneath the surface of the soil which converts it into organic compounds of manural value by the biological action of the soil bacteria. In most of the towns in India the night-soil collected from the bucket latrine is disposed by the trenching system.

Method of disposal by trenching. Generally a plot of land is selected about 1½ miles away from the town limit and the prevailing wind, one raised ground which is not water logged during the rains. The soil should be light and porous (sandy loam) containing profusely growing nitrifying organisms which convert the organic nitrogen of the excreta into nitrates. The area should be sufficient to allow trenching for atleast 3 years without using any part twice. While one plot is used for active trenching the other two plots are used for cultivation which is absolutely necessary to prevent the soil to become *sewage-sick*.

The trenches should be 18 inches wide, 12-18 inches deep and 20-30 ft. long. These furrows are cut 6 ft. apart and are filled up with night-soil upto 1/3rd of its depth (1/4th in rainy season) and then covered with excavated earth. Shallow trenching is insanitary as it creates nuisance, bad smell and fly breeding.

Proper management :
1. Night soil should be carried in a properly constructed night-soil cart.
2. Approach roads or roads should be good and properly maintained.
3. The trench ground should be provided with (a) a cover shed for storing utensils, and (b) a water tank or a well for washing the buckets and carts.
4. No rain water should collect in the trenching ground.
5. No strong disinfectant should be used for washing the buckets as it may kill some of the nitrifying bacteria in the night-soil and soil.
6. Trench-filling with night-soil should be systematic and covered with earth to form a dome to allow for sinkage.

DISPOSAL OF HUMAN EXCRETA, REFUSE

7. Cultivation should begin three months after trenching and ploughed deep and sown first with grass, sugarcane or tobacco followed by other vegetables later.

Disadvantages :

The disposal of night-soil by trenching has the following disadvantages :

(1) Transport of night-soil and supervision of the trenching ground are difficult.

(2) Suitable soil is not always available with adjoining good water supply.

(3) With increasing population the land falls short of requirement and excess of night-soil makes trenching very insanitary creating nuisance and profuse fly breeding as the night-soil itself carries large number of eggs and larvae which develop into maggots and adult flies if trenching process becomes defective.

Q. 9.15. Describe a method of disposal of human excreta in a remote bunglow. Or Describe a Aqua Privy.

This type of latrine is the most hygienic type of latrine and is *the best for* a remote bunglow as the water supply is very small. It is also preferred in *Railway colonies* and *Labour camps*. It is best as because the latrine does not have a water seal, so there is no necessity to flush the latrine as the excreta falls directly into the pit under the water level.

Structure and Function

Aqua privy has 2 or sometimes 3 underground chambers. The super structure is over the first chamber. There is soil pan but no trap. It has a straight pipe which dips into liquid to a depth of about 4 inches. As the pipe dips in the liquid, there is no smell or fly nuisance and there is no splashing.

(a) The first chamber is called *digestive chamber.* There is no ventilation, and the anerobic germs digest and liquify the solid organic matters. The proteins are broken up to amino acids, the amino acids act on fat, and the carbohydrates are changed into simple alcohol. This type of digestion is *putrifaction by anaerobic* (i.e. nitrifying) *bacteria*. The nitrogenous, carbonaceous and sulphur containing matters are Oxygen and Hydrogen and give rise to sewage gases like CO_2, NH_3, CO, H_2S etc. and remain mixed with the liquid part (*called effluent*).

The undigestable solid portions settle down as sludge. The complete process of digestion is known as *Anaerobic digestion*.

The digestive chamber is (4½ x 4½) Sq. feet and height 5 feet. At a level of about 1½ feet from the bottom, there is an opening of two inches. Through this opening the liquid matter (i.e. effluent) together with gases, pass out in the second chamber.

(b) The second chamber is called "*classifying chamber*". The size of this chamber is similar to the first chamber. This chamber is freely ventilated by a ventilation shaft. Here aerobic digestion occurs. The gases pass out through ventilation shaft. Here minimum amount of solids in suspension are liquified. The nitrites become nitrates, sulphides become sulphates by aerobic bacteria. The sludge which falls at the bottom is removed manually once in 2 to 3 years. The effluent from the second chamber can be let out in the garden or *nala*. However, for more proper aerobic digestion, the effluent from second chamber is let in through an opening at the top by a 6 inches verticle pipe opening at the bottom of the third chamber.

The third chamber is called "*filtre*". It is filled with clinkers, stone pieces etc. The slimy growth of the surface of the clinkers contain aerobic bacteria. They further oxidise the dissolved, suspended and the colloid matters in the liquid, and the final effluent comes out from a hole at the top of the third chamber. This final effluent is clear and colourless, and is practically odourless. It can be allowed to flow in the garden or *nala*.

DISPOSAL OF HUMAN EXCRETA, REFUSE 239

Q. 9.16. What are the various stages of water carriage system ?

Various stages of water carriage system are as follows :

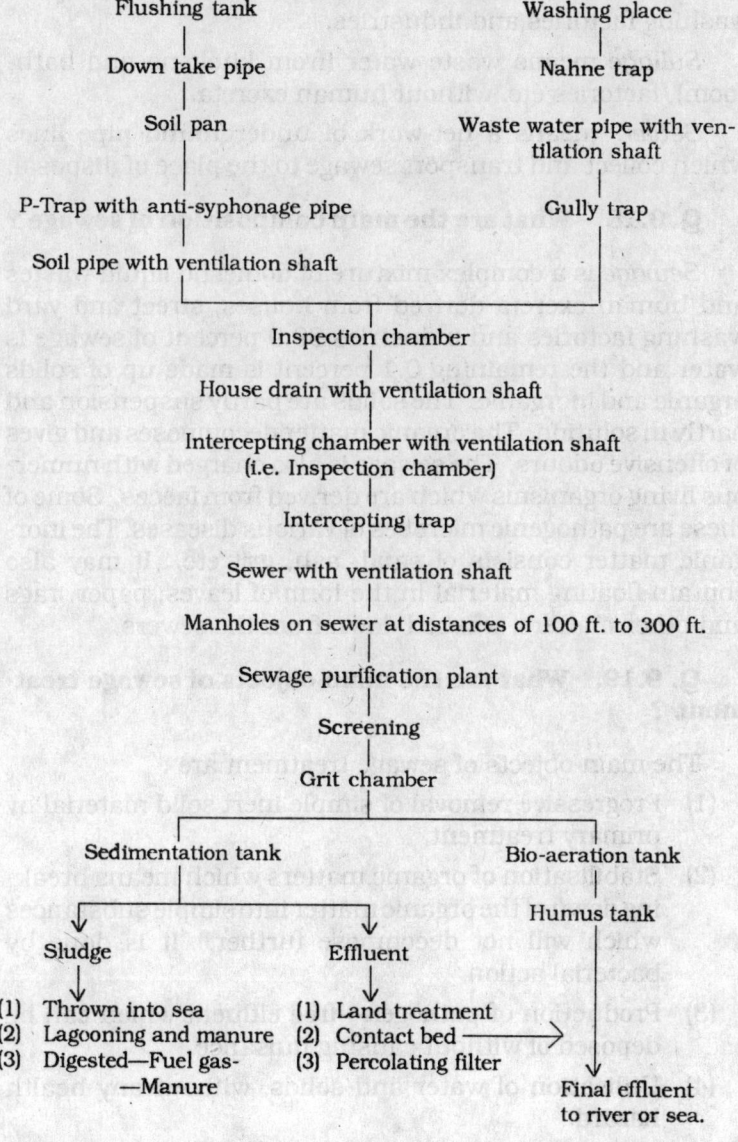

Q. 9.17. What is sewage, sullage and sewer ?

Sewage is a complex mixture of domestic liquid wastes and human excreta derived from houses, streets and yard washing factories and industries.

Sullage means waste water (from kitchens and bathroom), factories etc. without human excreta.

Sewer means a net-work of underground pipe lines which collect and transport sewage to the place of disposal.

Q. 9.18. What are the main composition of sewage ?

Sewage is a complex mixture of domestic liquid wastes and human excreta derived from houses, street and yard washing factories and industries 99.9 percent of sewage is water and the remaining 0.1 percent is made up of solids organic and inorganic. The solids are partly suspension and partly in solution. The organic matter decomposes and gives of offensive odours. The sewage is also charged with numerous living organisms which are derived from faeces. Some of these are pathogenic microbes of various diseases. The inorganic matter consists of sand, ash, grit etc. It may also contain floating material in the form of leaves, paper, rags and other matters, washed down from the sewers.

Q. 9.19. What are the main objects of sewage treatment ?

The main objects of sewage treatment are :
(1) Progressive removal of simple inert solid material by primary treatment.
(2) Stabilisation of organic matters which means breaking down of the organic matter into simple substances which will not decompose further. It is done by bacterial action.
(3) Production of pathogen—free effluent which can be deposed of without causing nuisance.
(4) Utilisation of water and solids, without any health hazard.

DISPOSAL OF HUMAN EXCRETA, REFUSE

Q. 9.20. What are different types of sewage treatment ? Describe how the sewage is disposed off ?

Treatment of sewage are mainly divided into two parts, namely (I) *Primary or Partial treatment*, and (II) *Secondary or Complete treatment.*

(I) Primary Treatment

It means progressive removal of simple solid matter from liquid part of sewage and then the solid are subjected to *anaerobic digestion.*

(II) Secondary Treatment

It means aerobic oxidation of the effluent and make them suitable for final disposal.

1. **In case of primary treatment :**
   (a) *Separation of coarse suspended and floating matter are done by :*
      (i) *Screening* (it contains pathogenic bacteria, helminthic ova etc.).
      (ii) *Bar screens* (for removal of large floating matter).
      (iii) *Fine screen* (for removal of leaves, paper etc.).
      (iv) *Comminutors* (to shred colloidal lumps into fine suspension).
   (b) *Separation of floating* oils by skimming,
   (c) *Separation of finely divided suspended matter by passing through*—**Girt chamber and Detritus chambers or Primary Sedimentation Tanks**.
      i) *Grit chamber and Detritus channels* are used for the removal of course granual solids which are periodically removed and disposed off by burial or burning.
      ii) *Sedimentation tank* : These are hopper bottomed circular tanks with redial flow, meant for removal of mineral and organic suspended solids, the sludge. It is hydrostatically removed. Sludge scrapers are provided to collect the sludge.

In Case of Secondary Treatment

Separation of finely divided suspended matter from sewage after primary settling, and separation and biological stabilisation of organic matter suspension, collidal or insoluble state of sewage are done by aerobic oxidation by any one of the following methods :

    (a) Tickling filter method.
    (b) Active sludge process into pathogen free effluent.

Final Disposal

The *effluent of* treatment plant are chlorinated to kill the pathogenic organism before discharge into small stream. But if there is large amount of dilution as well as good flow in the receiving water, further purification is taken place in the stream due to self purification of water. But all the solid i.e. *sludge* separated from sewage during the process of treatment is subjected to :

    (i) *Biological digestion resulting in partial destruction of organic matter and thickening.*
    (ii) *Drying for removal of water by air drying on sand beds.*

The solid substance of the sludge after dewatering contain mixture upto 3% or less. It can be incinerated after mixing with the garbage and combustible refuse. The sludge can be utilised as fertiliser and also as fertilizer base. The separated water from the sludge, though heavily contaminated with pathogenic bacteria is generally chlorinated before disposal into any water body. Sometimes in a complete sewage treatment plant this supernutant liquor from the sludge digestion tanks is recirculated in the process of treatment.

Q. 9.21. Notes on :

1. B.O.D./Biological Oxygen Demand :

For digestion of the organic impurities, the aerobic bacteria will take up the dissolved oxygen present in the sewage. In water or in sewage, the dissolved oxygen is 2%. *The amount* of dissolved oxygen taken up for aerobic digestion in 5 days at 20° C. is known as Biochemical Oxygen Demand (B.O.D.) of the sewage. It is measure in milligrams of oxygen taken up in one litre of sewage.

The effluent that is legally allowed to be discharged into a river or stream should be such that BOD_5 at 20 °C should not be more than 20 P.P.M. i.e. 20 mgm. per litre. This means that the discharged effluent should absorb more than 20 mgm. of oxygen but weight from one litre of the effluent.

If $B.O.D_5$ of a *sewage* is 180 P.P.M. then by some methods, the B.O.D 180 PPM should by removed, to take the BOD_5 to 20 PPM i.e, the sewage purification plant should remove (180-20)/160 P.P.M. of B.O.D.

The B.O.D. of drinking water is 1 P.P.M. and the permitted B.O.D. for the final effluent is 20 P.P.M. Hence in dilution of 1:500, no treatment of sewage is necessary (provided the nearby water is not to be used for drinking).

2. Contact Bed

They are big rectangular tanks. The bottom slopes from the centre to the sides. They are usually 6 feet deep and the capacity of tank is designed as 7 gallons of sewage per cubic foot. The tank is filled with clinkers or pieces of stones. The slimy growth on the surface of the clinkers or stones contain aerobic organisms. The aerobics oxidise the colloid and the dissolved organic impurities of the effluent. The usual time is 1 hour for filling, 2 hours for the effluents to remain in contact with the aerobic germs on the surface of the stone or clinkers 1 hour for emptying and 4 hours in the period of rest (i.e. the tank is kept empty). Thus one tank works 3 times in 24 hours. The circle works best with 4 tanks in rotation. The stones get clogged and have to be cleaned. In 5 to 8 years, renewing of the filter bed is necessary. Hence this method is costly.

3. Trickling Filters (Percolating Filtre)

It is recognised as an effective method of oxidation of sewage. It can be operated at low cost. The Trickling filter is

3 to 10 ft. deep. It may be circular, square or rectangular. The sides are of cement-concrete so that it can take the load of the primary effluent. The top is covered and has sufficient space for ventilation. The filter is filled with broken pieces of stones or clinkers etc. about 4 inches in size, or any other suitable material. The bottom of the filter is under drained, and leads to a collection channel.

The primary effluent from the sedimentation tank is distributed on the top by drop methods, or by moving distributor or spray or by any other suitable method. As the primary effluent trickles down over the broken stones, a gelatinous slime forms over the stones. The slime is full of aerobic germs, and they carry out aerobic digestion of the organic matters present in the primary effluent.

The process is continous one. There is no rest period, as the filter works better without rest. Due to the aerobic digestion, the dissolved organic matters and colloids become settleable solids. These settleable solids are called "humus'. Lastly humus pass out of the trickling filter to the humus tank.

4. Land Treatment

The land upto a depth of 3 to 4 feet has oxygen and hence the aerobic organisms, can digest i.e. oxidise the organic matters.

(a) *Intermittent downward filtration* :

Here, the disposal of sewage is of primary importance. One acre of land is required for 3,000 persons. The land is under drained by porous earthern ware pipes, at a depth of 6 feet, and the pipes are 10 feet apart. The land is divided into 4 parts, and each part receives effluent for 6 hours. The remaining 18 hours of the day is the period of aeration. The effluent is distributed on the surface by half channel drains. The effluent that comes out through the under drained pipes is harmless, and can be discharged into any river or stream. The B.O.D. removal is about 100% .

DISPOSAL OF HUMAN EXCRETA, REFUSE

(b) *Broad irrigation*:

This is also called "*Sewage forming*" i.e. *Farming by sewage*. Here, the growing of crops is of primary importance. The land required is more and one acre of land is required for 100 persons. If there is over dose of effluent, then the land will became "*Sewage sick*", and the land will not suitable for growing crops. Hence do not give over dose. By proper land treatment; the B.O.D. is completely removed.

5. Activated sludge process (*also known as Bio-aeration Process*)

This method is stated to be the most satisfactory method of sewage purification. The primary effluent from the sedimentation tank which mainly contain colloids and dissolved organic impurities is allowed to pass in the aeration tank. Aeration tank in the heart of the activated sludge unit. When the primary effluent is aerated by mechanical aeration or by diffuse air aeratian methods, the grey colour of the effluent becomes brownish, if such aerated effluent is allowed to settle, then a fine golden brownish floc, settles at bottom. The floc contains a large number of aerobic bacteria, and it called as '*Activated sludge*'. If this activated sludge is mixed with the primary effluent, the organisms in sludge utilise the dissolved and colloid organic matters in the primary effluent, and oxidise the matters with the help of oxygen, supplied through the compressed air from the bottom of the aeration tank.

The organic matters are converted to stable odourless compounds having practically no oxygen demand. The effluent is then passed to a Humus tank i.e. secondary clarifier. The sludge settles down and the final effluent is allowed to flow in rivers, streams etc. The sludge is activated sludge. 15% of it is returned to the aeration tank, as active sludge for the oxidation of the organic matters in the primary effluent. The remaining 85% is the waste sludge and is disposed off in the usual method as valuable manure. This process is easily upset by sudden change in the sewage, therefore it requires constant control and it is less adaptable to smaller communities where full-time operation cannot be provided. It cannot normaly take the shock load.

6. Oxidation pond (O-pond)

Oxidation ponds of sewage stabilizing ponds are cheap methods of sewage disposal. The principle of the working is the result of symbiosis of bacteria and algae. Oxidation ponds should be shallow with plenty of sunlight. The aerobic germs oxidise the organic carbon to carbon di-oxide. The algae by the process of photosynthesis converts CO_2 to carbon and oxygen. Carbon is used up by the algae and hence the sewage gets super-saturated with oxygen. No toxic materials should be allowed in the oxidation pond and the industrial wastes must be treated, before it is allowed to flow in the oxidation pond. It should be away from residence. Usually one acre is sufficient for 3,000 persons. Sides should be sloping. Operation depth 3 to 5 feet and free board 3 ft. The inlet is near the centre and the detention period is 7 days.

The B.O.D. removal is 60-85%. It can be made for 50,000 persons if land is available.

7. Lagooning

A *lagoon* is a shallow basin made by digging the earth to a depth of a few feet. The bottom is covered with a layer of clinkers. Sludge is pumped in the lagoon. The sludge gets dry by percolation to the underground drain and by drying. offensive smell is prevented by spreading lime or fine soil.

Subsequently the sludge is removed and used as manure. Lagoons are useful for sludge disposal.

8. Man Hole

Q. 9.22. (a) What is manhole ? What are the hazards of working inside manhole? What precautionary measures to be taken before entering manhole ?

Manholes are inspection chambers on street sewer.

For *inspection and cleaning of sewers, manholes are provided*. They are at :

a) Junction of sewer, (b) Change in the gradient of the sewer, (c) Change in diameter of the sewer, (d) On straight length at every 300 to 500 feet.

DISPOSAL OF HUMAN EXCRETA, REFUSE

Manholes have a circular cast iron cover of 20 inches in diameter. The upper position or the shaft of the manhole is a little more than 2 feet. The bottom portion is about 4 x 5 feet. Beneath is the half channel sewer.

Manholes may be :
- (a) Shallow manholes i.e. up to 3 feet deep.
- (b) Natural manholes i.e. 3 to 8 feet deep.
- (c) Deep manholes is over 8 feet deep. They have ventilating shaft of the manhole.
- (d) Drop manhole if constructed if high level sewer is to be joined to the main sewer which is at a much lower level.

The branch sewer is usually a few feet deep, but the main sewer may be much below. In such case, the high level branch sewer is connected to the low level main sewer by a gradient of about 45° angle. Such manholes are called "drop manholes".

Hazards of Working Inside the Manhole

The sewage workers run the risk of various accidents such as, asphyxiation with gas, injury from explosion drowning contracting diseases like Weil's disease (Leptospirosis), enteric fevers and other gastro-intestinal infections. Sometimes poisonous gases may kill the worker right away.

Precautions to be taken before entering a manhole :

1. The working manhole and 2 manholes on both sides are to be kept open for 2 hours.
2. A lighted lamp put in the manhole, should burn normally.
3. Work is done between sunrise to sunset.
4. Two or more workers tied in a rope enter the manhole.
5. Workers should not remain in the manhole for more than half an hour.
6. If one worker faints or feels ill, the other workers give warning, so that all the workers are pulled up.

7. Give artificial respiration or other first aid measures to the ill person, and take him to a hospital (or to a doctor).

IV. REFUSE DISPOSAL

Q. 9.22. (b) What is meant by refuse ?

Refuse means unwanted or discarded solid waste materials from houses, street sweepings, commercial, industrial and agricultural operations, arising from man's activities. An average of about 0.8 to 1.0 lb of refuse per person, per day, has been taken as a fair estimate for urban localities.

The refuse consists of :
1. *Dry refuse*—Ashes, cinders, waste paper, old iron, glass, tin, rag and fabrics etc.
2. *Garbage*— Leaves, vegetables and parings, rotten fruits, fruit skin, kitchen waste, grease etc.
3. *Stable litter.*
4. *Street sweeping*—Leaves, rags, horse and cow dung etc.

Q. 9.23. Why disposal of refuse are more important from hygenic point of view ?

Disposal of refuse are more important as they causes serious health hazard by the following ways :

(1) The organic portion of solid wastes ferments and favours fly breeding.

(2) The garbage in the refuse attracts rats.

(3) The pathogen are conveyed man through flies and dust.

(4) There is possibility of water pollution when rain water pass through deposits of fermentary refuse.

(5) This is risk of air pollution, due to accidental or spontaneous combustion of refuse.

(6) Piles of refuse are a nuisance from an aesthetic point of view.

DISPOSAL OF HUMAN EXCRETA, REFUSE

Therefore there should be an efficient collection, removal and disposal of refuse without the risk of health.

Q. 9.24. What are the sources of refuse ? Name the different methods of disposal of refuse in rural and urban areas ?

Sources of refuse :

There are various sources but from the hygienic point of view, the sources of refuse are mainly consider :

    (1) *Domestic or household refuse.*
    (2) *Market refuse.*
    (3) *Stable matter.*
    (4) *Industrial refuse.*

But there are no precise defination of these categories though :

(1) *Domestic or household refuse means*—Refuse from houses and other residential premises and they consist of ash, rubbish and garbage.

(2) *Market refuse*—These refuse are mainly refuse from retail, commercial and business premises. They contain a large proportion of putrescrible vegetable and animal matter.

(3) *Stable matter*—Collected from stable, and it contains mainly animal droppings and left over animal feeds.

(4) *Industrial refuse*—Contains variety of washes ranging from completely inert materials, such as calcium carbonate to highly toxic and explosive compounds.

(5) *Street refuse*—Consists of leaves, straw, paper, animal dropping and litter of all kinds. Generally these are collected from the street by cleansing service or scavenging.

Methods of disposal :

There is no single method of refuse disposal which is equally suitable in all circumstances. The choice of particular method is governed by local factors such as cost and

availability of land and labour. The principal methods of refuse disposal are :
(1) *In rural area*—by burning, burial or by making compost.
(2) *In the urban area*—by (a) *dumping and filling* of low land,
　　　　　　　　　　　　(b) *dumping of sea,*
　　　　　　　　　　　　(c) *controlled tipping,*
　　　　　　　　　　　　(d) *incineration,* and
　　　　　　　　　　　　(e) *composting.*

But in *Calcutta* the most solids refuses are deposited on land as *tips* or spoil heaps, or as land in fill to quarriers or as dumps containing large range of materials.

Mainly disposal of refuse is done by filling up the low lying areas-*DHAPA, the old river bed of Bidyadhari.*

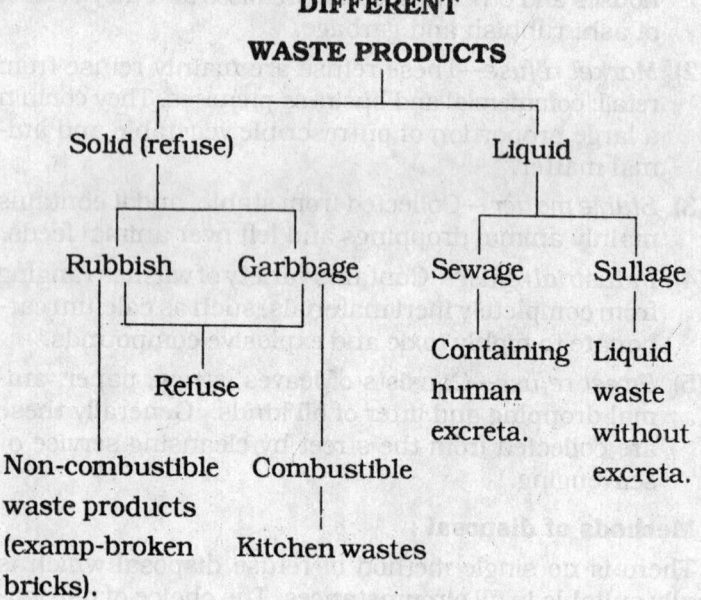

DISPOSAL OF HUMAN EXCRETA, REFUSE

Methods of disposal (solid) :
1. *Dumping*—Unhygenic.
2. *Sanitary land fill* or *Controlled tipping* :
   (a) The trench method—by trenching in level ground.
   (b) The ramp method.
   (c) The area method—in land depression disused quarries, and clay pits. Exposed surface covers with mud.
3. *Incineration*—especially for hospital refuse.
4. *Composting*—Refuse + night-soil or sludge.
   (a) Bangalore method (Anaerobic method).
   (b) Mechanical composting (Aerobic method).
   (c) Tallyguange method (for Calcutta).
5. *Manure pits*—in rural area or individual houses.
6. *Burial* for small camp.

Q. 9.25. What are the different methods of disposal of refuse in rural areas ? Describe one of them.

Generally in rural areas the refuse are disposed by *burning, burial* or by *making compost*. The procedure for composting household refuse yield a valuable manure in village without fly breeding and usual in practice. The *composting method* is as follows :

Refuse, cowdung and soil are mixed in proportion of 6:2:1 in a pit 5 x 3 x 1 feet. Generally the collections are of 14 days. The heap is watered daily and kept covered with a layer of soil. It is turned on 14th, 20th and 56th day but between the turnings the head is watered daily. The compost is ready for use one month after the last turning. After the first turnover, a second heap is started with a little of the material from the head (seed for composting) and by this way the refuse can be continually disposed off.

Q. 9.26. What is meant by composting ? Describe the Bangalore process of composting ? What are the advantages and disadvantages of composting. Describe

a method of disposal of town refuse in brief. What are its advantages and disadvantages.

Composting is a process of combined disposal of refuse and night-soil and is better than other methods because of the economic returns from the manural value of the compost. Basically it is an anaerobic biological process and also it is a process of nature where by micro-organisms convert organic matter into a more state material. The biological activity produces sufficient heat to eliminate pathogenic organisms of the wastes within a day. Actually there is triple advantage in this procedure, viz :

(i) Sanitary—it does not cause any nuisance nor it is harmful to health.

(ii) It yields manure which is valuable for agriculture.

(iii) Economic gain from the sale of compost.

Methods of composting :

The materials required are :

(1) Organic refuse from towns and farms.

(2) Adequate amount of nitrogenous material in the form of night-soil, cattle-dung, sewage and urine etc.

(3) Enough water to keep the moisture content of the compost at about 50% level.

(4) Sufficient amount of air at the early stage of decomposition.

For a large scale composting several underground trenches and pits are made for alternate use. Toward off rain some sort of a shed may be necessary. The refuse and night-soil are piled in alternate layers and materials kept moist by addition of water. Fermentation begins following fungal and bacterial activities and the temperature is raised up to 65 degree C to 70 degree C at which all pathogenic bacteria are killed and no fly larva can thrive. Several modifications of the method have been introduced at different places, of which Bangalore process is most important and usually follows in different parts of Indian cities or towns.

Bangalore Process

Usually a surface area of about 2 acres per year per 10,000 population is selected quarter mile away from the town limit. The size of the trenches varies according to the population size, being 20 x 6 x 3 feet upto 20,000 population, 30 x 7 x 3 feet upto 50,000 population and 35 x 8 x 3.5 feet for population above 50,000. The length of the pit may be compartmentalized to take up one day's supply of refuse and night-soil.

Procedure :—First, big stones, metal plates, porcelain and glass etc. are removed by hand and the rest sieved through expanded metal sheet into two portions. The one containing soil and ash is taken out. There after the following procedure is followed :

Over 6 inch thick layer of refuse night-soil is poured 2 in. thick and this alternate filling is continued till the heap rise one feet above the ground level. The topmost layer at the end of each day should be covered by 6 in. thick layer of refuse and 2 in. thick layer of soil and ash. The internal temperature rises between 65 degree C. and 70 degree C. in three days helping in decomposition of organic materials and preventing fly breeding. Following the first 5 days of aerobic action the top layer becomes dry and water is added at the rate of 2-3 gallons per foot length and the compost mass is covered with mud paste. This mass sinks to about half the depth of the trench and fresh refuse and night soil are added in the above manner and the pit tightly packed. the compost is ready for removal in 4 to 6 months as almost odourless and innocuous material of high manural value.

Advantages and disadvantages of composting :

Advantages :

1. In this process the waste volume is reduced by 50%, separated materials can be sold for recyclic or tipped and the resulting compost can be used as a soil conditioner with some nutrient value.

2. This is useful both for refuse and night-soil.

3. It can be easily put into practice and the manure is available for agricultural purposes.

4. *It is used as a manure pits* : This is useful in the rural area of India where there are no facilities for collecting and disposal of refuse. Each house can have its own disposal pits and after 5 to 6 months the refuse can be used as manure.

Disadvantages :

1. Waste pretreatment is necessary to remove materials such as metals, rubbers, plastics and glass, because they are largely unaffected by the process.

2. The end-product of composting is deficient in potash and inorganic nitrogen compared to other manure, and may contain small amount of toxic substances.

3. If used on land, it requires high rate of application, possibly augmented by chemical fertilizers.

4. It cannot be used for population more than 100,000 because of practical difficulties.

5. It is the sources of bad smell nuisance and breeding ground for the flies.

Indore Method

Under the *Indore method*, refuse and night-soil are put in alternate layers in a pit, or trench, atleast 3 feet deep and the procedure is carried out on until it is filled up 6 to 9 inches above ground level.

The material is covered by a thin layer of earth. The contents are allowed to ferment for 10 to 12 weeks, during which the pit is raked atleast 3 times for proper mixing.

Q. 9.27. How disposal of refuses done in Calcutta?

In Calcutta the disposal of refuses are generally done by Tollygunge method :

A pit approximately 45 feet x 27 feet (13.71 metres x 8.30 metres) is dug at the municipal trenching ground area by excavating 15 inches (38.10 cm.) of the soil and piling the cut earth on the untouched side, so that the finished depth is 2 feet 3 inches (0.68 metres). A 3 inches (7.62 cm) brick lining is laid in and the edges protected by a brick curb. Partition walls are constructed to make 5 compartments of 400 cubic feet (11.33 cubic metres) capacity. Besides, aeration and drainages channels are provided in the floor and the area around the pit protected with brick soiling. In one of the compartments a 6 inches (15.24 cm) thick layer of fresh rubbish is laid down and covered with a layer of night-soil, which again covered with a layer of refuse from the plot and whole is lightly mixed, till all the night-soil is taken up. A 6 inches (15.24 cm) thick layer of rubbish is again deposited and the process is repeated till the pit gets filled up. The filling of once compartment should be completed within two days. Within 5 days from the start, the pit contents must be turned to and fro by means of a long rake to ensure complete mixing. It should be turned over a second time after a further period of 10 days subsequently 2 weeks later, it can be removed and stocked and the whole process thus taking about one month. The heaps are left in the open to ripen and are ready for use at any time, after they are allowed to ripen for another one month.

Q. 9.28. What are the various methods of disposal of town refuse ? Discuss their advantages and disadvantages.

The various methods of refuse disposal are :

1. *Dumping.*
2. *Sanitary land fill (Controlled tripping)*
3. *Incineration or burning.*
4. *Composting.*
5. *Manure pits.*

Advantages and disadvantages of various methods:

Name of the Method	Advantages	Disadvantages
1. DUMPING	(a) It is an easy method of disposal. (b) Reclaimed land can be used for cultivation purposes.	(a) Refuse is exposed to files and rodents and is sources of nuisance and smell. (b) It may pollute the environment.
2. SANITARY LAND FILL OR CONTROLLED TIPPING.	Same as above.	None of the above disadvantages. So it is a quite satisfactory method.
3. INCINERATION. (BURNING)	(a) This is the method of choice where suitable land is not available. (b) It is best suitable for hospital refuse.	(a) It is expensive method and involves heavy outlay. (b) Manure can not obtained by this method.
4. COMPOSTING	(a) This is useful both for refuse and the night soil.	(a) It cannot be use for population more than 100,000 because of

DISPOSAL OF HUMAN EXCRETA, REFUSE

Name of the Method	Advantages	Disadvantages
		practical difficulties.
	(b) It can be easily put into practice and the manure is available for agricultural purposes.	(b) It is the sources of bad smell, nuisance and breeding ground for flies.
	(c) In this process the waste volume is reduced by 50%, separated materials can be sold for or recycle or tipped and the resulting compost can be used as a soil conditioner with some nutrient value.	(c) The end-product of composting is deficient in potash and inorganic nitrogen compared to other manure, and may contain small amount toxic substances.
		(d) If used on land it requires high rate of application possibly augmented by chemical fertilizers.
		(e) Waste pre-treatment is necessary

Name of the Method	Advantages	Disadvantages
		to remove materials, such as metals, rubbers, plastics, and glass, because they are largely unaffected by this process.

5. MANURE PITS :

This is useful in the rural area of India also where there are no facilities for collecting and disposal of refuse. Each house can have its own disposal pits and after 5-6 months the refuse can be used as manure.

Q. 9.29. Notes on :

1. Incineration (or Burning)

Destruction of refuse by fire is probably the safest method of disposal. This is done by "Destructor Furnace" or in Incinerator. An Incinerator consists of the following parts :

(a) A furnace of brick or concrete with fire-brick lining, grates of cast iron, ash pits and a combustion chamber.

(b) A charging door.

(c) Means of delivery of sufficient hot air into the furnace.

(d) Flues and chimney.

(e) Opening through which clinker and ashes are removed.

In *Incineration method* dry refuse is burnt inside the incinerator, during burning refuse are also thrown inside the incinerator through the above opening (hopper) time to time. The temperature required for efficient incineration is 1250 degree F. or above so it is an expensive process. Although it is an expensive method, some money can be recovered by

DISPOSAL OF HUMAN EXCRETA, REFUSE

selling the CLINKERS. Clinkers do not absorb water, so they are used for surfacing roads, making platforms of railway stations etc. The ashes are used for filling pits.

Incineration is helpful for small municipalities and townships and where large quantities of combustile refuse are produced. For melas and temporary congregation a *'Bechive incinerator'* has been found useful. It is made up of mud and iron without fire bricks. The common defect of incineration is that it gives off offensive smoke and creates a nuisance. As incinerator cause smoke nuisance, so it should be far away from the residential areas.

CHAPTER-X

DISINFECTION

DISCUSSION FOR LEARNING

I. Definition.
II. Types of disinfections—Precurrent, Concurrent and Terminal.
III. Various Disinfectants.
IV. Insecticides and Larvicides.
V. Practical Disinfection in certain situations and particular cases, like smallpox, pulmonary tuberculosis, cholera and typhoid.
VI. Certain definitions.
VII. Sanitation of a fair or mela and camp.

I. DEFINATION

Q. 10.1. What is meant by disinfection?

Disinfection means killing the germs of infection and the insects or organisms carrying the infection.

So it is one of the potent methods for the prevention of infectious diseases and is to destroy the pathogen i.e. organism, parasites and insects causing or spreading the disease, at vantage points e.g. with the sources, as they are excreted or contaminate and/or grow in the environment.

II. TYPES OF DISINFECTIONS

Q. 10.2. What is meant by concurrent and terminal disinfection ?

OR

What are the various methods of disinfections ?

Generally the methods of disinfections are of three types e.g.:

DISINFECTION

1. Pre-current disinfection.
2. Concurrent disinfection.
3. Terminal disinfection.

1. Pre-Current Disinfection

It is done as preventive measures. Chlorination of water, pasteurisation of milk, moping of floor with disinfectants are precurrent disinfection.

2. Concurrent Disinfection

Concurrent disinfection is the disinfection done when a person is ill. Its aim is to prevent the spread of infection. Disinfecting utensils, clothes, stool, sputum, urine, floor etc. are concurrent disinfection.

Examples : In *cholera* the stool, vomit, and soiled linen should be immediately disinfected with bleaching powder and buried inside the earth (in rural areas) or disposed off into the drain (in cities). The surroundings and room should also be disinfected with bleaching powder of frequent intervals. Arrangement should also be made for the disinfection of hands of the attendent and so on. Lysol and soap solution are used for concurrent disinfection in *typhoid cases*. Phenyle should also be freely used. Creosote and coal-tar derivatives are used freely for tuberculosis cases. Utensils and other materials should be disinfected by boiling or with antiseptics.

Drinking water should be disinfected by boiling or by chlorination. Bleaching powder should be applied to wells and tanks if suspected of contamination.

3. Terminal Disinfection

Terminal disinfection is done after death, recovery or removal of a patient. The idea is to disinfect rooms, clothes and other articles so that no germs of infection remain.

Examples : In *cholera or typhoid* this procedure can be carried out by bleaching powder solution, phenyle or lysol solution. Soiled materials may be burnt or buried.

In *smallpox*, the room may be disinfected by means of disinfecting agents and the beddings and linen may be sterilised by steaming or burnt away completely.

In *plague*, cyanogas is used to kill the fleas, rats and vermins, and disinfestation of beddings and bed clothes is carried out over hot sands and strong sunshine.

In case of *tuberculosis*, the room is disinfected by means of antiseptic spray and by white washing.

Q. 10.3. What is meant by disinfectants ? How they act and what are their limitation ?

Disinfectants are substances which destroy pathogenic organisms. But it does not imply that all living organisms are killed but the disinfectants are generally act :

(i) *By oxidising the protoplasm of the bacteria*, e.g. the hallogen compounds, bleaching powder and potassium permanganate liberate nascent oxygen.

(ii) *By coagulating the protoplasm of the bacteria*, e.g. the phenols and their derivatives.

(iii) *By ionic coagulation*, e.g. the metallic salts.

(iv) *By abstraction of water* (desiccation).

(v) *By emulsoid action and absorption*, and

(vi) *The dyes may act by specific combination.*

The effect may also due to :

(vii) *Poisoning of the vital enzymes system of the organism which may be brought about in several ways* viz. by inactivation of the enzyme itself, change in substrate, competitive and non-competitive inhibition. Some also act by :

(viii) *Changing surface membranes* i.e. the normal perme ability characteristic of the membrane surrounding the cell of the organism.

Limitation

Though the disinfectants are valuable for preventing diseases but there are certain limitations, e.g. :

DISINFECTION

(i) The presence of electrolytes may lower their values.

(ii) Oxidising agents give up oxygen so rapidly that they soon become inert and lastly the metallic disinfectants do not penetrate rapidly.

Q. 10.4. What are the factors which can influence the action of disinfectants ?

The factors which influence the action of disinfectants are:

(i) The nature of the invading organism and the number present.

(ii) The nature and strength of the disinfectants used and the extent to which its action is affected by the presence of organic matter.

(iii) The time taken by the disinfectant to act efficiently.

(iv) The nature of the solvent used.

(v) The temperature.

III. VARIOUS DISINFECTANTS

Q. 10.5. What are the disinfectants used in public health practice ?

Various disinfectants which are used in public health practices are :

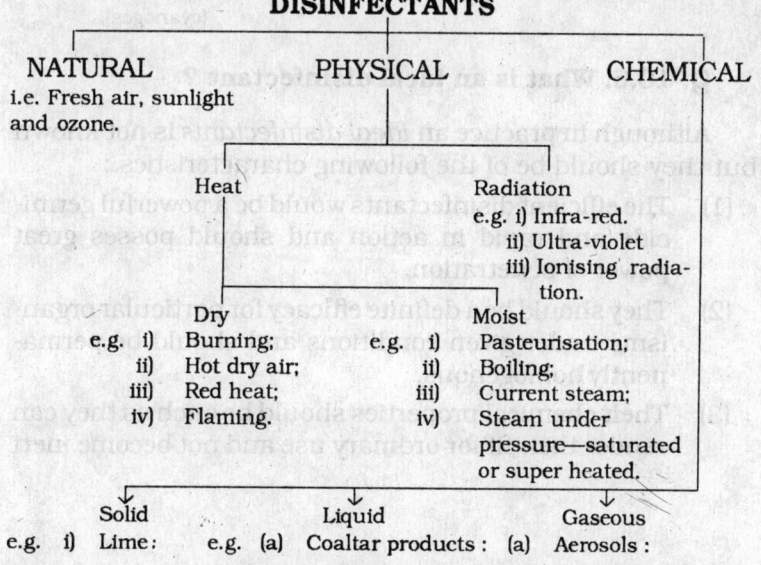

```
                    DISINFECTANTS
        ┌───────────────┼───────────────┐
   NATURAL          PHYSICAL         CHEMICAL
i.e. Fresh air, sunlight
and ozone.
                   ┌───────┴────────┐
                 Heat              Radiation
                                   e.g. i) Infra-red.
                                        ii) Ultra-violet
                                        iii) Ionising radiation.
             ┌──────┴──────┐
            Dry           Moist
      e.g. i) Burning;    e.g. i) Pasteurisation;
           ii) Hot dry air;    ii) Boiling;
           iii) Red heat;      iii) Current steam;
           iv) Flaming.        iv) Steam under
                                   pressure—saturated
                                   or super heated.
```

Solid	Liquid	Gaseous
e.g. i) Lime;	e.g. (a) Coaltar products :	(a) Aerosols :

ii) Mercury preparations perchloride of mercury; mercuric iodidte.	i) Phenol or carbolic	i) Hipochlorites
	ii) Phenyl	ii) Resorcinal
	iii) Izal	iii) Ghycocol
iii) Chlorinated lime—bleaching powder.	iv) Cylin	iv) Glycols
	v) Hycol	b) Gases
iv) Iodine	vi) Creolin	i) Formal dehyde (use in permanganate method, paraformlin methods, fomalin spray)
v) Potassium permanganate.	vii) Lysol or liquor cresotes, saponates.	
vi) Soap	(b) Formaldehyde in solution—formaline.	
vii) Centrimide Cetavion,	(c) Solution of chlorinated lime or chlorine liquid and electrolytic chlorine.	ii) Chlorine,
viii) Chiloxylenol-dettol or Roxenol.		iii) Ethylene oxide
		iv) Sulphur dioxide (use in pot method), Liquid sulphur dioxide, Clayton disinfector.)
		v) Hydrocyanic and or hydrocyanide gas (cyanoges),

Q. 10.6. What is an ideal disinfectant ?

Although in practice an *ideal disinfectants* is not known but they should be of the following characteristics :

(1) The efficient disinfectants would be a powerful germicide and rapid in action and should posses great power of penetration.

(2) They should be a definite efficacy for particular organisms under given conditions and should be permanently homogenous.

(3) Their chemical properties should be such as they can render their fit for ordinary use and not become inert

by faecal or any polluting material, i.e. they should be stable in the presence of organic matter.

(4) They should not have any injurious effects on human tissues and materials submitted for disinfection.

(5) They should be soluble in water or form an uniform emulsion in all proportions.

(6) They should be fairly cheap and should not act on metals, bleach pigment or spoil fabrics.

(7) They should have a high solvent power for grease.

IV. INSECTICIDES AND LARVICIDES

Q. 10.7. What is meant by insecticides and larvicides ?

Insecticides means which kill insects and Larvicides means which kill the larvae of insect.

Insecticides

Generally germs and insects can be killed by burning or by heat or by boiling water. But the insecticides also may be:

(1) *Stomach poison* like arsenious solution to kill house flies. *Sodium fluoride* to kill flies, rats and other insects or Paris green (aceto-arsenite of copper) to anopheline larvae. These poisons are eaten by the insects and then they die.

(2) *Contact poisons*—Here the legs, the body or the wings of the insects absorb the poison, and then the insects die. e.g. Pyrethrum, D.D.T., B.H.C. etc. They are of two types :

   a) *Knock down insecticides* like *pyrethrum* 1% in kerosene kills the germs instantly. Pyrethrum then becomes vapour and has no residual effect. Cyanogas also instantly kills rats and rat fleas.

   b) *Residual insecticides* retain its insecticide property even for months. They are chlorinated hydrocarbon group or organic phosphorus group.

     (i) The chlorinated hydrocarbon groups are D.D.T. (i.e. Dichloro-diphenyl-trichloroethane). It may be used as solution, suspension or emulsion in strength of 5%. It may be used as 10% dust, or in aerosol. On wall surface D.D.T. should be 2 gms. per square metre. B.H.C. (i.e. Benzene Hexachloride) 2 to 5% is more powerful and is used if the insects have developed resistance to D.D.T. Dieldrin 1% is more powerful and used to kill insects which are resistant to B.H.C. The residual effect lasta for 6 months. The residual effect of D.D.T. and B.H.C. is about 3 and 1 month respectively. Chlordane has hardly any residual effect. It is used as emulsion of 2.5%. Sevin and Baygon etc. are other insecticides of methyl-carbamede group.

(ii) *Organo phosphorous* groups are highly toxic and they are mostly used in agriculture, rice fields etc. They are parathion, malanthion etc.

The residual insecticides paralyse the nerves and the insect die after half to 1 hour when the respiratory muscles are paralysed.

Larvicides

1. *For killing larvae of mosquitoes* :
    (i) Prevent the breathing of a larvae by forming a layer of oil on the water surface. All varieties of larvae are killed by kerosene, petrol etc. 2 ounces for 30 sq.ft. of water surface.
    (ii) *Stomach poison*—Paris green is mixed with road dust or saw dust in proportion of 1:100 only anopheles larvae are killed as they are surface feeders.
    (iii) *Contact poisons* are D.D.T. 5% in solution or 10% as dust. Gammaxane is used in paddy field, 2 ounces in 1 gallon of water 15 gallons are necessary for one acre.
    (iv) *Gambusia fishes* will keep a well free from mosquito larvae.

2. For *killing larvae of flies* in manure, rotten vegetation, etc. :
   (i) Borax 1lb on cubic feet of manure.
   (ii) 5% cresol, D.D.T., dieldrin, chlordane, gammexane etc. are useful.

Bleaching powder and carbolic powder are of little value.

V. PRACTICAL DISINFECTION IN CERTAIN SITUATIONS

Q. 10.8. How will you disinfected the infected cloth, bed clothes and cotton garments ?

Disinfection of infected material—Infected cloth, bed-clothes and cotton garments are generally done by :

Infected clothing, bed-clothes, cotton garments are disinfected by boiling for half an hour.

For materials of bigger size and larger quantity *steam disinfector* is the best. Clothes may also be disinfected by immersing in 5 percent phenol or 10 percent formalin or in 1 in 1000 corrosive sublimate. If the clothes are soiled by blood, excreta or pus these should be soaked in antiseptic solution and then washed in soap solution (3%) at 50° C. for 3 hours and later disinfected by the usual methods. Infected rays and small pieces of clothes may be burnt.

Q. 10.9. How will you disinfect the excreta and other discharges like stool, urine, sputum, vomit etc. of a patient ?

Disinfection of excreta and other discharges :

Stool, urine, sputum, vomit and discharges from nose and throat of patient suffering from infectious diseases are disinfected by 10% carbolic acid, 5% izal, 1:100 cylin, lime or bleaching powder for 1 to 3 hours.

Sputum may be first received in spitton containing phenol or carbolic acid 1 in 10, kept for 2 hours and then disposed off. Stool may be disinfected by mixing with equal quantity of 10% formaline 1:4 lime or 3 percent chlorinated lime and allowing it to stand for one to two hours. Stool may also be brunt mixed with kerosene and saw dust.

Q. 10.10. How will you disinfect a infected room, privy and drain?

An infected room should first be disinfected by fumigation by formalin or ethylene oxide. After this the infected materials like clothing, linens, bed clothing, mattresses, infected utensils should be removed and to be disinfected. (metioned at Q. 10.8)

Indian houses made of huts are not air tight. These should be disinfected by washing with disinfectant or with 5% formalin aqueous spray (1 gallon to 400 sq. ft.). In case of smallpox 10% formaline should be used. Floor should receive particular attention. The walls and flood may be disinfected with 1 in 1000 hydrarg per chloride or bleaching powder or milk of lime. The privy and house drains may be washed and scrubbed and disinfected with cyllin or chloride of lime.

Q. 10.11. Describe the different methods of disinfection in hospitals.

Different methods of disinfection

1. *For floor*—Coaltar disinfectants emulsion of phenolic substances.
2. *For wood work*—Scrubbing with soft soap and hot water or 1 : 5000 hydrarg per-chlor or one in 1000 bleaching powder.
3. *For instruments knives, forks*—Soaking in 1% formalin or 5% lysol in 2 hours.
4. *For thermometer non-metal combs etc.*—5% solution of phenol 1 in 80 lysol or milk of lime for 1 hour.
5. *For hands*—Scrubbing with nail brush and soaps and hot water and then immersing in 1 : 500 hydrarg per-chlor or dilute lysol solution or in spirit.
6. *For books, leather articles etc.*—Formaline gas in a closed room for 3-4 hours.

DISINFECTION

7. *For sputum, excreta, vomit etc.*—Mix up with 1 in 10 phenol for 4 hours and then disposing of in drains.
8. *For face masks*—Steeping in bowls containing 1 : 80 chloroxlyenol for several hours and then boiling in water.
9. *For surgical dressings etc.*—Autoclaving in steam.

Q. 10.12. (a) Disinfection of the bedding of smallpox case.

The clothes and linen should be boiled or steam strelized or put in 10% formaline lotion. If possible linen and other ordinary clothes should be burnt.

(b) Disinfection of the room occupied by a smallpox case.

The infected room should be thoroughly disinfected with formaldehyde or sulphur dioxide. Fumigation with formaldehyde vapour for 6 hours. 500 ml of formaline plus 1,000 ml of water, is sufficient to disinfect 30 cubic metres space. The walls should be washed copiously with soap and water and left for 48 hours and exposed to direct sunlight for several hours.

(c) Disinfection of scabs from a case of small pox case.

They should be collected in a paper bag and burnt daily.

Q. 10.13. (a) Disinfection of the room of a patient died of pulmonary tuberculosis.

The room and other hard surfaces are washed copiously with soap and water and left open for 48 hours. It should exposed to direct sunlight for several hours.

Chemical disinfection of the room may be done with 2.5% *cresol*, 5 percent *phenol* or 10 percent *formaline* and left for at least 4 hours and then final washing with water is done.

(b) Disinfections of furnitures, beddings and utensils used by the patient of tuberculosis.

Books—If possible they all should be destroyed i.e. burnt.

Furniture—It should be scrubbed with soap and hot water and washed with 1:1000 bleaching powder solution.

Beddings—Beds, clothes, covers etc. should be boiled or steam disinfected. Beddings are packed in canas bads which are damped with water from outside and then steam disinfection. If no steam disinfector is available 10% formaline or 5% carbolic acid can be used.

Utensils—Knives and forks with handles are immersed in 10% formaline solution and cleaned. The solution attacks iron and steel but not copper, brass, zinc and nickle. Ordinary utensils are disinfected by boiling.

Q. 10.14 .(a) Disinfection of the stools and vomitus of cholera patients.

All dejecta and vomit should be collected in a basin and mixed with equal quantity of 5% cresol or bleaching powder solution. After two hours of disinfection, it should be buried or burnt.

(b) Disinfection of the clothings and bedding of cholera patient.

Clothes and beds of cholera patient which are of no values should be burnt. The clothes which have been contaminated, should be soaked 2½% cresol solution for ½ an hour and then washed with soap and water.

(c) Disinfection of feeding and cooking utensils of cholera patients.

These are disinfected by boiling then in water for 15 minutes of keeping them in cresol solution for ½ an hour before washing finally with water and soda.

(d) Disinfection of floor and walls of room used by cholera patient and the hands of cholera patient attendants.

The floor must be thoroughly disinfected with 5 percent cresol. The walls up to the height of 3 feet should be treated similarly.

DISINFECTION

In larger gatherings the following type of temporary construction be adopted in addition to hutments mentioned above : large waiting sheds 100 ft. x 20 ft. with cemented floors, each with a separate cooking shed for several families, atleast 3 latrines within 200 ft. and water supply within 100 ft. In case of village fair people are congregate from different areas of a localities and generally they remaind in their relatives house, so housing is not a acute problem.

3. *Water supply* :

In case of fair water supply is needed atleast 6 gallons per capita per day and should be distributed through public taps at the rate of one tap per 100 persons. it should be preferably be continous.

In case of temporary gathering of smaller congregations the water supplied should be filtered and disinfected. If necessary, potable units should be used. Each residential shelter should have minimum one water tap within a distance of 100 ft. In absence of piped water supply a sufficient number of tube-wells or protected masonary wells or tanks should be constructed for water supply.

No one should be allowed to wash or bath near the reserved water sources. If the mela is on the river bank strict guard should be placed to prevent pollution of the river on by defecation or otherwise. If water is supplied from river, water is pumped—then storage-chlorinated and supplied by taps. Soakge pit should be blow each tap.

4. *Sanitary disposal of excreta refuse and garbage* :

Generally Trench latrines or Borehole latrine are constructed 1 latrine 20 x 1 ft. and depth 1.5 ft. divided in 6 to 7 compartments of 3 feet each for 500 persons. The area should be properly lighted at night. Separate latrines for male and female, 1 sweeper for 2 latrine blocks, 10 latrine blocks for 5,000. sweeper does digging and covering nightsoil with earth. Bleaching powder 100 lbs, for 1,000 person.

Urinals 4 x 4 x 4 ft. pits filled by stone and bricks and covered with sand. It should have foot rest of stone slabs. These are soakage pits.

Refuse to be collected and put in a pit or burnt.

5. *Temporary hospital, police station, publicity office, etc. should be made.*

6. *General arrangements* :
    (a) All necessary materials like kudali, brooms, strings, lime and bleaching powder should be stored in a godown.
    (b) Duty list for the medical officer, health inspector, conservancy officer and jamadars, sweeper etc. should be ready.

Q. 10.18. What would be the duties of a Medical Officer or Sanitary Inspectors during a fair or mela ?

Medical Officer and the Sanitary inspectors and their staff are vigilant over sanitary measures and are chief authorities for arranging medical and public health measures. Their first and formost duties are :

(1) *Sanitation of water supply* :
   a) If from a reservoir water is chlorinated 1 PPM i.e. 10 lbs chlorine (30 lbs bleaching powder) for 1 million gallon.
   b) Otherwise, wells and tanks are treated with bleaching powder and they see that the required chlorine is maintained in water by pot chlorination.

(2) *Sanitation of conservency and cavenging* :
   a) They see that proper scavenging have done and the refuse are collected and disposed off properly.
   b) Fly breading is prevented by fly measures.
   c) They see that the trench latrines are maintained in a proper manner and sufficient bleaching powder and brooms are given to the staff.

(3) *Sanitation regarding food* :
   a) They destroy the unwholesome and over ripe fruits and sweets and food exposed to flies and dust.
   b) Strict supervision is kept over the food handling establishment.

c) Inspect the temporary slaughter house regarding sanitation and regarding disposal of waste from slaughter house. From slaughter house, the waste should be burried daily. Inspection of meat should be done.

(4) *Preventive measures regarding diseases* :

   a) See at check posts that all persons coming in are inoculated against cholera. If not inoculate them.

   b) Immediately cases of D and V or other cases of infectious diseases to the temporary isolation hospital.

   c) Carry out disinfection and antichlolera inoculation (if not inoculated).

   d) Medical officer must attend out-patient's clinics which have established temporarily (open day and night) for sick persons and emergencies.

So the entire area of congregation should be under the direct supervision of Health Officer and Sanitary Inspectors (sector wise). They should report daily about the public health situation of the block under them and collect information of the diseased persons who may endanger the public health of the area.

** They should also educate the people about their health which are as follows :

Health education :

(i) Do not eat food exposed to flies and dust.

(ii) Eat food when it is still hot.

(iii) Boil milk and water.

(iv) Dip vegetables (to be eaten raw) and fruits in solution of $KMnO_4$.

(v) Do not eat over ripe fruits and mela sweets.

(vi) Avoid aerated water, ice in cold drinks and ice.

(vii) Eat plenty of dahi, lemon juice, butter milk, as the acidity kills the cholera germs.

(viii) Advice every one to be inoculated against cholera.

(ix) Advice the people to use trench latrines and not open field.

N.B.—Generally food is one of the principal commodities which is responsible for the gastro-intestinal disturbances and even epidemics in the fairs. It should, therefore, be subjected to strict supervision and control to ensure supply of pure and wholesome food at a reasonable cost. State rotten, and decaying foods, fruits and vegetables should be seized and destroyed and all food should be protected from flies and bad handling. The task is not so easy. The road-side sweet-meat shops attract unlimited number of flies that carry any sort of pollution from faeces to the food. This nuisance can be controlled if the general sanitation of the area is imposed. The festival authorities and Health officers have to be very careful about the preparation and serving of holy offerings in temples. The construction of proper kitchens, the use of safe water for cooking and washing of utensils and the service of food untouched by hands are the ideals to be realised. There must be sufficient staff and workers to keep watch on every details of public health rules that are voilated by the people collected there as well by the commercial people who come to the mela for business and money.

Q. 10.19. What are the general measures to be taken after mela is over ?

After the mela is over the following general measures to be taken from sanitary points of view :

1. Rubbish and refuse should be properly cleaned and buried.
2. Night soil should be properly covered.
3. Huts for dwelling and shops and the super structure of latrines should be removed.
4. Report submitted to the chairman of the mela committee.

GANGASAGAR MELA

Q. 10.20. What arrangements are generally made during Gangasagar mela ?

During the Gangasagar mela i.e. in *Mokor sankranti* (at the last day of the Bengalee month Pous) more than 3 lakhs of people congregate at Sagardweep from the different parts of India. Generally, most of them are aged persons, poor and under nourished or half starved, and in a state of physical and nervous strain. They come unprotected against smallpox and cholera and are ignorant, particularly of health education, and as such a large majority of them are highly susceptible to these infectious diseases. So it is very essential to make proper sanitary arrangement for the successful completion of the Gangasagar mela.

Generally D.M., A.D.M., S.P., C.M.O.H of 24 Paragana and other members, like S.D.O., S.D.H.O., B.D.O., Public Health Engineers, Sanitary Inspector and other health workers of Sagardweep and Kakdweep with the help of different departments of Govt. of West Bengal and various voluntary organisations like, Ramkrishna Mission, Bharat Sevasram Sangha, Indian Red Cross Society, etc. take charge for maintaining sanitation and law and order of the Gangasagar mela and make total arrangement from accommodation to the return journey of the pilgrims.

During this mela no person is allowed to enter the mela ground unless he/she possesses any anticholera inoculation or antipox vaccination certificate. So for this purpose health authorities of the Govt. of West Bengal along with C.M.O.H. or S.D.O.H. and other paramedical staff of 24 Paragana's immunizes the pilgrims at several places like Howrah station, Sealdah station, Kakdweep, Namkbana etc. before they enter into the mela ground. First Aid centres are also arranged on several places where the pilgrims congregate first before mela days.

During the mela period several First Aid centres, Medical camps (Allopathic, Homoeopathic and Ayurvadic) along with temporary infectious disease hospital function day and night in different zones of the mela ground. For maintaining law and order 24 Paragana's S.P., S.D.O., B.D.O. and other administrative personnels with their staffs as well as several thousand volunteers of different voluntary organisations work round the clock. They also keep watch over antisocial elements and guide people accordingly. To inform people information booths, enquiry office, publicity office etc. are also made. Food Inspector inspects shops and the Sanitary Inspector is entrusted with maintaining the proper hygiene of the place.

As water of this place is not suitable for drinking purpose, it is supplied by pipes from galvanised tanks where water is maintained fresh, pure, and disinfected by chlorination. For refuse and conservancy system male and female sweepers are posted for each latrine for cleaning and filling up the used latrines. Dustbins, urinals, soakage pits etc. are also made or put in suitable places.

Generally about one month before the mela start, mela site is made clean and level and the whole area is divided into several plots according to the necessacity. It is divided to provide all sanitary and hygienic measures with that of accommodating people, shops, temporary sheds for shelter, latrines, urinals, roads medical camps etc. whole area is lightened. Above all, all put their hands in one to make the Gangasagar mela in success.

PART III

PREVENTIVE MEDICINE

"PREVENTION IS BETTER THAN CURE"

CHAPTER-XI

EPIDEMIOLOGY

DISCUSSION FOR LEARNING

I. Epidemic and Epidemiology (Definition).
II. General Principles.
III. Prevention and Control.

I. EPIDEMIC AND EPIDEMIOLOGY

Q. 11.1. What is meant by epidemic ?

An epidemic is defined as the occurrence in a community a disease or a group of diseases of similar nature, propagated or derived from a common sources in excess beyond the normal expectancy.

Although, the word 'epidemic' is a very old word dating back to third century B.C. in the writings of Hippocrates and comprises of words-*Epi*=upon and *Demon*=people. Generally the term epidemic is used for the communicable diseases like smallpox, cholera, plague etc. but now it also covers other scourage of mankind such as cancer, coronary, heart diseases etc.

Q. 11.2. What is meant by epidemic diseases ?

And what category they belong ?

Those diseases in which many persons are attacked with very similar sufferings from the same cause are known as epidemic diseases.

They belong to the category of acute diseases.

Q. 11.3. What is meant by epidemiology ?

Epidemiology means a branch of medical science which displays the general laws of epidemic diseases.

In its modern sense it is a discipline which deals principally with the study of phenomenon of diseases like origin, development and distribution of epidemic infections in man as they affect population of people. So it gives a picture of the occurrence, distribution and types of diseases of mankind, in distinct epoches of time and at various points of the earth's surface.

With the advancement of biological and medical sciences, the field included under Epidemiology has broadened considerably and is now defined :

As a branch of public health which deals with study of origin, development and distribution of epidemic infections.

Q. 11.4. What is meant by epidemiological survey ?

Epidemiological survey means the study of :

1. *Topography* i.e. Physical features and hydrography of the area.
2. *Climatology* i.e. Humidity, temperature and rainfall of the area.
3. *Geographical situation and distribution of the disease.*
4. *Occupation, economic condition, nutrition and education of the people.*
5. *Sanitation of the place.*
6. *Study of insect vectors.*
7. *Fairs and congregations, if any.*

N.B.—A spot map and the satistical data of the disease are necessary to start epidemiological survey.

Q. 11.5. Why epidemics are occurred ?

Epidemics occur due to :

1. Increase in the virulance of the germs.
2. Increased susceptibility of the people.
3. Increased facilities of transmission of disease.
4. Weather condition, nutritional condition and certain occupation lowers the health of the people and thereby predisposes the epidemic.

Q. 11.6. What is meant by epidemic curve ?

Epidemic curve :
1. Period of invation when the cases of notification rises.
2. *Period of sustenance* i.e. the cases of notification remain steady.
3. *Period of decline* i.e curve goes up and down in a declining manner.

Q. 11.7. Why do Epidemics decline ?

Epidemic decline due to :
1. Declining of the virulance of the germs.
2. Declining of susceptibility of the people.
3. Declining the facilities of transmission of the germs.
4. Increase the resisting power of the people.

Q. 11.8. What are the Primary objectives of Epidemiological investigations ?

The primary objectives of epidemiological investigations are :
1. To obtain specific knowledge of the natural happenings involving human, animal and plant populations through scientific method.
2. To arrive at generalisations regarding the cause or causes of these happenings.

The observation thus made provide us not only with the knowledge but also with the methods that can be suitably and effectively applied to control or prevent the occurrenc of those happenings which are detrogatory or non-contributory to the well-being of human population.

II. GENERAL PRINCIPAL

Q. 11.9. What are the basic Principles of Epidemiological investigation?

The basic Principles of Epidemiological investigations are :
1. Study of the reported events and current data and formulation of hypothesis on the genesis of the epidemic.

EPIDEMIOLOGY

2. Collection of all possible facts about the previous happenings of the same nature.
3. Planning and making of careful intelligent observation and recording just prior to, during and after the happening through properly trained personnel.
4. Analysis and interpretation of facts according to the logical principles so as to arrive at valid conclusions which may form the basis of administrative action or of further investigation.
5. Putting the conclusions arrived at from field observations, controlled experimental tests in the laboratory and then testing them in the field to confirm their validity.
6. Permanent recording of the observations made for future reference or further investigation.
7. *Method of approach*:

There are three fundamental approaches to the study of a disease, viz.:

(a) Clinical investigation.
(b) Controlled laboratory experiment.
(c) Epidemiological observation of a disease as it occurs under natural conditions in the whole community.

None is a substitute for the other. To have a complete knowledge of a disease in a community epidemiological approach needs to be supplemented by both clinical observation and experimental test. Epidemiological method is actually field study designed to bring clinical, laboratory and statistical procedures to the study of disease and the patients as a unified co-ordinated effort along with field observations. Field data are thereby enlarged and acquire added accuracy.

Q. 11.10. What are the sources for collecting data of an epidemic ?

Sources for collecting data of an epidemic are :
1. *Original*—specially collected during investigation.
2. *Published*—from routine recording such as :
   (i) Vital statistics,
   (ii) Meteorological data,

(iii) Sociological and economic data available from the Government Gazettes and report of central statistical organisations, National sample survey, Bhore Committee, Indian Census, D.H.S. and D.G.H.S., Health and Morbidity Survey etc.

Q. 11.11. What are the methods usually followed for collecting data ?

Methods of collection of data :
1. By personal canvassing.
2. Through agents and organisations.
3. Information through mailed cards.
4. In a well-designed schedule, the exact form of which will depend upon the requirements and size of enquiry and the methods used for tabulation and analysis.

Q. 11.12. What are the various branches of epidemiology ?

Epidemiology are divided into following branches :
1. *General Epidemiology*—General principales to study the natural history of diseases.
2. *Special Epidemiology*—Epidemiological study of specific diseases.
3. *Experimental Epidemiology*—It is undertaken to prove or disprove any hypothesis by animal experiments.
4. *Field Epidemiology*—Epidemiological investigation carried out in the field generally with the aid of laboratory and competent field investigation staff.
5. *Clinical Epidemiology*—Epidemiological studies of socio-psychological and environmental conditions of patients admitted to the hospital.
6. *Global Epidemiology*—Study of diseases affecting several countries of the world having potentialities of spread from country to country by the sea and air route by the returning army.
7. *Evaluation Epidemiology*—e.g. Health and morbidity surveys, assessment of drugs or health measures.
8. Forecasting of epidemics.

III. PREVENTION AND CONTROL

Q. 11.13. What would be the basic steps to prevent an epidemic disease ? Discuss with homoeopathic views.

In every case of epidemic, it is of primary importance to obtain information of the first cases of the disease. This will enable the sanitary officers to take effective measures against the spread of an epidemic. The carriers of the effected area are also searched out by laboratory investigations. After that the treatment and general measures of an epidemic are taken whenever possible.

Generally attention are made to lodging of the poorer class of people as they are the major source of spreading disease. Isolation of the patient is done and over crowding is prevented. Special care are taken to the excreta and other discharges of the sick. The bedding, clothing and other articles which are used by the patient are also similarly important. Proper care are taken to supply sanitary water and foods and others. Immunisation, Health Education Programme should be taken. Basically the full cooperation of the general people is the main importance to overcome an epidemic.

So to prevent the spread of an epidemic disease the common measures which are to be followed are :

(1) *Early notification.*
(2) *Investigation.*
(3) *Isolation.*
(4) *Quarantine.*
(5) *Disinfection.*
(6) *Treatment of carriers.*
(7) *Mass immunisation.*
(8) *General measures to prevent the spread of epidemic disease.*
(9) *Special control measures.*

The homoeopathic approach for controlling an epidemic is different from the routine method of individualisation of a case. Here each case is different from each other and the treatment of patient in an epidemic disease is carried on the following line :

First collection of the symptoms are made from a number of patients and the common symptoms of all such patients are chosen. Then a homoeopathic medicine is selected on the basis of common symptoms. This medicine—(Genus epidemicus) is considered as a remedy for the epidemic and at the same time it also be considered as a prophylatic one. So there is no individulisation in a epidemic disease. At different times or at different places of epidemic diseases require different medicine. As for example, in one epidemic of influenza *Eupatorium perf.* proved as genus epidemicus, in another *Gelsemium*, while in *earlier* one is *Nux vomica*.

Q. 11.14. What is meant by "Genus epidemicus" ?

Medicine which is indicated in majority of patients affected from an epidemic disease is termed as "Genus epidemicus".

The Genus epidemicus is selected after investigating thoroughly the several patients of an epidemic disease. Once selected it saves time and labour. But a Genus epidemicus for a particular disease is suitable only for that disease at that time and at that locality from which it is ascertained. The Genus epidemicus is also proved as a prophylactic remedy for other members of the family or vicinity.

CHAPTER-XII

INFECTIONS

DISCUSSION FOR LEARNING

I. Infections.
II. Various methods of infection.
III. Basic principle for control and prevention of infectious diseases.
IV. Notification, Isolation, Quarantine.
V. Vector and Vector control.
VI. Carriers—Mechanical, Biological and healthy carriers.
VII. House fly and fly control.

I. INFECTIONS

Q. 12.1. What is infection ?

The term *infection* is defined as the invasion of the body by micro-organisms and the reaction of tissues to their presence or to the toxins that these organisms produce, irrespective of weather or not the health of the person is affected.

So infection is the entry and development or multiplication of an infectious agent in the body of man or animal. The infectious agents are generally a micro-organisms like bacterium, protozoon, helminth, spirochaete, fungus or virus and are capable of producing infections, under favourable circumstances of host and environment. Thus a person may be infected but not have a infectious disease. The term *infectious disease* refers to a process caused by a micro-organisms that impairs the health of an individual person.

Q. 12.2. What are the sources of infection ?

The main sources of infections are mainly of two types namely :

1. **Homologous.** *2. **Heterologous.** **

1. **Homologous sources are :**
    (i) Active patient.
    (ii) Atypical cases.
    (iii) Carriers.

Various discharges of the patients like :
(a) Secretions of mouth, nose, throat or bronchi.
(b) Excretions such as vomitous, faeces and urine,
(c) Pus from fresh sores, scabes and scabes from skin erruption and from genital organs.
(d) Blood, are the potent sources of infection.

2. **Heterologous sources :**

Certain diseases of lower animals are also communicable to man and are the potent sources of infection. Generally the main sources are :

(A) **For Bacterial infection**
   1. Tuberculosis— Cow.
   2. Plague— Rat.
   3. Anthrax— Cattle, sheep.
   4. Malta fever— Goat.
   5. Abortus fever— Cattle.
   6. Glander— Horse, mule, ass.
   7. Salmonella infection—Rodent.
   8. Tularaemic— Rabbit.

(B) **For Viral infection**
   9. Rabies— Dog, jackal, vampire bat.
   10. Foot and mouth disease— Cattle, camel, dog, cat.
   11. Pasittacosis— Parakeet birds, pigeons, parrots.

(C) **For Spirochaete infection**
   12. Rat bite fever— Rat.

(D) **For Fungal disease**
   13. Certain form of ringworm- Cats and dogs.

INFECTIONS

(E) For Protozoal infection
14. Trypanosomiasis— Antelope, cattle.

(F) For Helminthic infection
15. Echinococcous cyst— Dog (hydratid).
16. Tapeworm— Mamals, fish.
17. Trichinois— Hog.
18. Flukes— Snails, crab and fish.

Homologous*— means another member of the same species as the victim himself.

Heterologous**—means infection derived from some other animal or plants.

Q. 12.3. What are the routes of entry of the infection in our body ?

Generally the infections enter in our body through :

1. *Respiratory tracts* (droplets infection by inhalation):
The principal diseases are Smallpox, chicken-pox, measles, mumps, influenza, diphtheria, cerebrospinal meningitis, whooping cough, pneumonia, tuberculosis.

2. *Alimentary tract* (oral route by ingestion) :
The principal diseases are cholera, diarrhoea, dysentery, typhoid and paratyphoid fevers, tuberculosis (of bones and glands), malta fevers, abortus fever, infective hepatitis, poliomyelitis, certain helminthic infections.

3. *The skin* (by inoculation or by contact) :
(a) Broken and unbroken—Anthrax, tetanus, glanders, rabies, ankylostomiasis, weil's disease.
(b) Insects bites (inoculation)—Malaria, kalazar, plague, dengue, yellow fever, relapsing fever, typhus, filaria, typanosomasis (sleeping sickness), encephalitis.
(c) Sexual contact—Syphilis, gonorrhoea, soft sore and granuloma pudenda.
(d) Unknown—(contact or respiratory)—Leprosy.

II. VARIOUS METHODS OF INFECTION

Q. 12.4. What are the various processes by which diseases are transmitted ?

Generally the diseases are transmitted by contact or by various agents which are as follows :

(I) By Contact :

A. Direct :

1. *Direct contact of diseased part with the healthy:*
   (a) *Autogenous*—skin infection- Scabies,
   (b) *Homologous*—venereal disease (syphilis, gonorrhoea) through kissing, shaking of hands, handling of infected clothes.
   (c) *Heterologous*—rabies (hydrophobia) from dog or jackal bite.
   (d) *Through patient's fingers* e.g. opthalmia.

2. *Direct contact due to close proximity.*

Air Borne

(i) *Droplet nuclei*—Pathogenic organisms from cases and carriers are ejected during coughing, sneezing and loud speaking. Actually smaller droplets may float in the air for hours. Smallpox, diphtheria, influenza, pneumonia, tuberculosis are typical examples of such transmission.

(ii) *Dust on the walls, floors and roads :*

Anthrax, tetanus and tubercle bacilli, strepto. and staphylococci are carried by the dust.

B. Indirect :

1. *Agencies acting mechanically and organisms surviving for a short time.*
   (a) *Fomites*—e.g. infected clothes, furniture, utensils etc.
   (b) *Exhaled air*—as in influenza, pneumonia etc.

2. *Agencies acting mechanically but affording protection to the organism for sometime.*

(a) *Water*— A common vehicle for germs of cholera, typhoid, polio, infectious hepatitis, lepto-spirosis, diarrhoea, dysentery etc. The sources are unprotected tanks, dobas, wells, rivers, lakes etc. and accidentally contaminated piped water supply.

(b) *Milk*— Contaminated by carriers, bad handlings or during milking or transportation. It is also vehicle for cholera, typhoid, diarrhoea, dysentery, tuberculosis, brucella infections.

(c) *Raw vegetables and fruits*—These may carry salmonella or amoebic or helminthic infections.

(d) *Cooked food*—Exposed to flies or handled by carriers may transmit salmonella and other gastro-intestinal infections.

(e) *Fish etc.*—Shell fish may carry typhoid germs and prawns cholera infection.

(f) *Flies and ants*—Generally carry infection of gastro-intestinal types on their legs and wings and contaminate food. Sometimes it may also carry tubercle bacilli from infected sputum and germs from ulcer and smallpox pustules.

II. BY THE AGENTS

Generally the agents act as an intermediate or definitive host.

1. By biting insects :

(a) *Mosquito*—Malaria, filaria, dengue, yellow fever, Japanese encephalites, haemorrhagic, West Nile fever.

(b) *Sandfly*—Kalazar, cutaneous, leishmaniasis, sandfly fever.

(c) *Ratfly*—Plague, murine, typhus.

(d) *Ticks*—Spotted fever, Q-fever, coloured fever, Russian tick types, enemic relapsing fever, tularaemia.

(e) *Mites*—Scrub typhus, murine typhus, St-Louis and western encephalitis, kyasanur forest disease.

(f) *Body louse*—Epidemic typhus, trench fever, epidemic relapsing fever.

(g) *Horse flies*—(Tabanus)—Tularaemia.

(h) *Chryop* (Mango flies)—Filariasis, loa loa.

2. **Other insect or animals :**

   (a) *Cyclops*—Guinea worm (Draincontiasis), non-biting flies- gastro-intestinal infections, Dyphyllobothrobis.

   (b) *Fish*—Tape worm.

3. **Human agency :**

   (a) As carriers of insects-body louse.

   (b) By aggregation—as in fairs and festivals, pilgrim centres.

   (c) By dispersal—carrying infection from place to place or from one country to another during incubation period and as patients and convalescents, particularly after attending fairs, festivals and pilgrim centres.

Modes of Transmission of Communicable Diseases

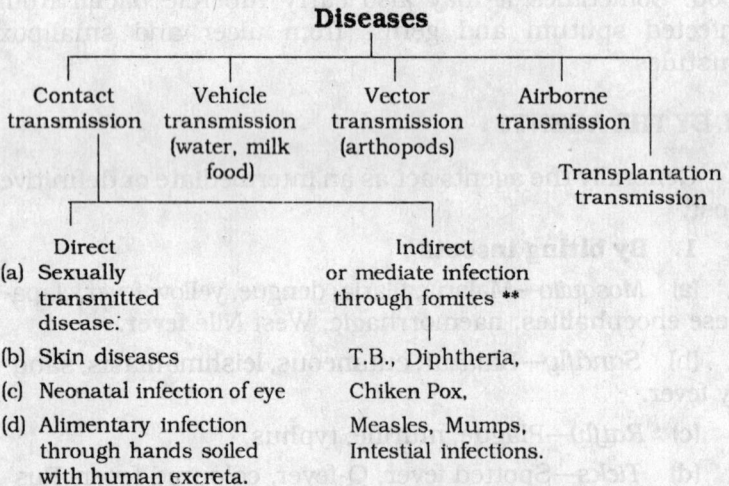

```
                    |
    ┌───────────┬───────────┬───────────┬───────────┐
 Contact      Vehicle      Vector      Airborne
transmission  transmission transmission transmission
              (water, milk (arthopods)
              food)                     Transplantation
                                        transmission
```

Direct	Indirect
(a) Sexually transmitted disease.	or mediate infection through fomites **
(b) Skin diseases	T.B., Diphtheria,
(c) Neonatal infection of eye	Chiken Pox,
(d) Alimentary infection through hands soiled with human excreta.	Measles, Mumps, Intestial infections.

**[Fomites—may be defined as an nonliving objects or substances capable of absorbing, retaining or transfering infection.]

III. BASIC PRINCIPLE CONTROL, PREVENTION OF INFECTION DISEASES

Q. 12.5. What are the basic methods for controlling and preventing any infectious disease ?

Since no communicable or infectious diseases present in the same epidemiological features, no unified method can be adopted which will be effective for control of each and every disease. But there are certain common measure to prevent the spread of communicable or infectious disease which are as follows :

1. *Notification.*
2. *Investigation.*
3. *Isolation.*
4. *Quarantine.*
5. *Disinfection.*
6. *Treatment of carriers.*
7. *Mass immunisation.*
8. *General measures to prevent the spread of communicable (infectious) disease.*
9. *Special control measures.*
10. *Organisation of communicable or infectious disease service.*

Q. 12.6. When describe a disease, what would the points of discussion ?

When describe a disease (communicable) the following points should be considered :

1. History of the disease, if any.
2. Geographical distribution of the disease, if any.
3. The causative organism.
4. How the disease is spread, i.e. ingestion, inhalation, inoculation or contact. Are there any healthy carriers?
5. Epidemiology of the disease.
6. Any relation to age, sex or occupation.
7. Any seasonal prevalance of the disease.
8. Incubation period and infective period of the disease.

9. Morbidity and mortality due to the disease.
10. Signs and symptoms of the disease.
11. Any specific treatment.
12. What are the preventive measure (i.e. Notification, Isolation, Arantine, Disinfection, Immunisation, General measures and Education.)
13. Is there any National Programme.

IV. NOTIFICATION, ISOLATION, QUARANTINE

Q. 12.7. What is meant by notification ? What are the notifible diseases ?

Notification means that a doctor who is treating a case of notifible disease must inform the health authorities so that the health authorities can take suitable measures to control the spread of the disease.

In the Municipal or urban areas, the notifible diseases or main infectious diseases are—Smallpox, cholera, chickenpox, diphtheria, meningitis, plague, rabies, leprosy, tuberculosis, whooping cough, diarrhoea and dysentery, typhoid and paratyphoid fever, typhus, relapsing fever, anthrax, measles, mumps, influenza, pneumonia, yellow fever.

In *Rural areas*—Smallpox and cholera are notifible but recently diphtheria, polio and malaria have been added.

Q. 12.8. What is meant by notification ?

Notification means that a doctor who is treating a case of notificable disease must inform the health authorities, so that the health authorities can take suitable measures to control the spread of the disease. But there is no Notifiable Disease Act in India. Only a limited number of municipalities and the Presidency towns enjoin medical practitioners to report infectious diseases. In West Bengal particularly in Calcutta the notifiable diseases are : *Cholera, infective hepatitis, plague, smallpox, cerebrospinal meningitis, diphtheria, gastroenteritis, and any other epidemic, endemic or infectious disease which the Government declare to be a dangerous one.*

Q. 12.9. What is meant by isolation ? What would be the basic criteria or requirements for establishing an Isolation hospital and home isolation ?

Isolation means that the person who is suffering from an infectious disease is isolated, so that further infection from the patient is avoided. Compulsory isolation of the patient is to be done in cases of dangerous diseases (i.e. Plague, smallpox, cholera). General hospitals cannot treat such cases and home isolation is not permitted if an isolation hospital exists.

(A) Isolation Hospital

Isolation hospital should be in every town.

Basic criteria or requirement for Isolation Hospital are :
(1) Site should be dry and well drained and over 200 yards from residential areas.
(2) There should be a compound wall.
(3) Wards should be separate for different types of diseases.
(4) Walls and floors should be impervious with round corners.
(5) Rooms should be 12 ft. high with 144 sq.ft. area for each patient.
(6) Windows should be big and preferably fly proof.
(7) Special observation wards for doubtful cases.
(8) There should be special ambulance for infectious disease patients.
(9) There should be arrangement for disinfection.
(10) Sufficient open land for putting up tents in case of emergency.

(B) Home Isolation

Home Isolation is not permitted for dangerous diseases unless there is no Isolation Hospital. A dharmasala or a school should be used as an Isolation Hospital in rural areas. *The requirements are :*

(1) The structure should be a detached one or atleast it should be a separate room in a corner.
(2) Daily mopping of the floor is to be done by disinfectant and window and door curtains are to be dipped in disinfectants daily.
(3) Proper arrangement for disposal of vomit, stool, sputum, urine etc.
(4) There should be trained attendants.
(5) Mosquito nets in cases of insect-borne diseases.
(6) No children or visitors should be allowed.
(7) Segregation and immunization of contacts.
(8) In villages, stool, urine, sputum, vomitous may be put in boiling water and then disposed off. Stools and vomits may also be mixed with saw dust and kerosene and burnt.

Q. 12.10. What is meant by Quarantine ? What are its various types ? Mention its disadvantages.

Quarantine means the detention or isolation of persons who have come in contact with infectious disease, for a period of time equal to the lowest incubation period of the disease to prevent effective contact with those not exposed.

Quarantine may be *inward* or *outward* :

(a) *Inward*—When quarantine is imposed on a healthy town for its own protection.

(b) *Outward*—When it is imposed on an infected town or village for the protection of the surrounding country. There are various types of outward quarantine, viz.:

(i) *International.*
(ii) *Scolastic.*
(iii) *Domestic.*

(i) *International Quarantine* :

It means compulsory isolation at the port, of all persons coming from an infected place (and not timely inoculated against the disease). In India this is especially imposed in cases of :

Yellow fever	—	6 days
Smallpox	—	14 days
Cholera	—	5 days
Plague	—	6 days
Typhoid	—	14 days
Replasing fever	—	8 days

(According to W.H.O. from 1951)

(ii) *Scholastic Quarantine* :

Children from an infected house during the period of quarantine should not be permitted to attend the school until the last case in the house has ceased to be infectious.

(iii) *Domestic Quarantine* :

All persons or visitors, particularly children should be strictly prohibited to enter an infected house. All members of such infected house should be kept under watch for a period equal to the incubation period of that disease. But this is not practicable, but is the best method to stop communicable disease in a house.

Quarantine has now been superheaded by *surveillance* under which the contacts are kept under close observation by health authorities for the period of quarantine instead of strictly detaining them.

•*Objections or Disadvantages* :

(i) The infective period of some disease being much longer than the period of quarantine, so only quarantine period is not enough to prevent infection.

(ii) It is distasteful to travellers and traders for longer inactiveness or interference of the quick movements, so it produces intense temptation of invasion.

(iii) Due to fear of quarantine, the disease is very often concealed, which produces increase incidence of the disease invasion.

V. VECTOR AND VECTOR CONTROL

Q. 12.11. What are vectors ?

Vectors are those insects that carry the germs of infection. They are *winged* or *wingless* insects and are mechanical carriers or biological carriers.

(a) The winged insects are :
 i) *House flies*—They are mechanical carriers, and carry germs from stools, sputum and dust.
 ii) *Mosquitoes*—They are biological carriers of malaria, filaria, yellow fever, dengue fever etc.
 iii) *Sand flies*—They are biological carriers of various diseases like sand fly fever and protozoal diseases like Kala-azar and Oriental sores.
 iv) *Tse-tse flies*—are biological carriers of sleeping sickness.

(b) The wingless insects :
(They are biological carriers)
 i) *Fleas*—carry plague, murine typhus.
 ii) *Lice*—carry epidemic typhus and relapsing fever.
 iii) *Ticks*—carry ticks typhus and a variety of other fevers.
 iv) *Mites*—carry mite-typhus, relapsing fever and scabies.
 v) *Bed bug*—There is no proof that bugs carry any disease.

(N.B. : *Ticks* and *Mites* are not insects. They are arachnida having four pairs of legs.)

VI. MECHANICAL, BIOLOGICAL AND HEALTHY CARRIERS

Q. 12.12. What is meant by mechanical carriers and biological carriers ?

  (a) **Mechanical carriers**—Carry the germs of infection by :
 i) Their leg, body or wings.

INFECTIONS

ii) They may vomit out the germs through their saliva.

iii) They may pass living germs in their stools.

N.B. : In mechanical carriers the germs neither multiply nor undergo any development.

(b) Biological carriers—Here the germs may multiply or undergo development or develop and multiply. They are of following types :

(i) *Propagative*—Here the germs multiply only i.e. the plague germs multiply in the throat of a rat flea.

(ii) *Cyclo-development*—Here only the development takes place i.e. immature microfilaria in human blood becoming mature microfilaria in the culex mosquitoes.

(iii) *Cyclo-propagative*—Here the development as well as propagation take place, i.e. the male and female gametocytes of malaria are sucked by the female anophelene mosquitoes. The gametocytes become gamets, zygot and then forms sporozoites.

[N.B. : The host on which the parasites become sexually mature is the *"Primary Host"*. On *"Intermediate Host"* the parasite thrive out do not attain sexual maturity. *Primary Host* is also known as *Definitive Host*

Q. 12.13. What is meant by healthy carrier ?

A healthy carrier is defined as a person who harbours a specific infections agent but shows no signs or symptoms of diseases. Such a person may spread the disease to others while he does not suffer himself.

Generally healthy carriers are found in the following diseases :

(a) *Typhoid and paratyphoid fevers.*

(b) *Dysentery.*

(c) *Cholera.*

(d) *Diphtheria.*

(e) *Meningococcal meningitis.*

(f) *Gonorrhoea.*

(g) *Infective hepatitis.*

(h) *Malaria.*

(i) *Poliomyelitis.*

Q. 12.14. What are the conditions affecting insect as disease carriers ?

For an insect to be an efficient *carrier* or *vector*, of a disease organism, it must be present in the correct place at the correct time and in the correct proportion with regard to the host animals. The season must be right, the temperature and the humidity suitable. The amount of winter rainfall and summer drought affects the vector population, as do the presence of shade or sun, the height of trees, and the thickness of under growth and the density of decaying vegetation, as well as the nature of living organisms in the compound—all of these factors may determine whether or not the insect vector can spread an infectious agent in a given environment. The height and duration of virus concentration in the blood of the host animal may be of critical importance. If virus is plentiful and persists for a long time in the host's blood, then whole clouds of insect vectors may become infected and able to spread infection with their next bite; if there is little virus in the host's blood and it disappears quickly, few if any of the biting insects may become infected and disease does not spread. Some biting insects are highly fastidious and will bite only one or two hosts; others are promiscuous. When humans intrude into a host vector reserve, the outcome depends on one, several, or all of these factors. Human may came to on harm, or they may contract a severe insect-borne disease such as one of the many forms of insect-borne disease.

Q. 12.15. What is meant by vector control ?

Vector control means the controlling measures for spreading insects and insect-borne disease.

To stop the spread of disease by insect-borne parasites, human adopt two main methods :
  (i) *To prevent contact between themselves and insects.*
  (ii) *To attempt to destroy insects.*

Most often both methods one used together. To prevent contact, people may site their habitations too far away from breading grounds for insects to reach them; they may clear

INFECTIONS

areas of shurb and forest in between, so that insects have no shelter to help them across. People should also still practice simple methods around the home :

The wearing of protective clothing and boots toward nightfall, screens across windows or around beds, and the use of an insect-repellent lotion on any exposed skin.

N.B. : Also see Q. No. 13.16.

Q. 12.16. Describe the principle methods of killing insects?

Methods used to destroy the insect carrier range from simple domestic procedures to major engineering schemes.

(a) *A fly trap*—is a useful method of reducing the number of flies or other carriers in a single household, but it has no effect on the total insect population.

(b) *Long lasting lethal sprays*—on walls of houses and other buildings, kill insects that invade building, but to have any permanent effect on the insect population, they must be used on a wide scale on the breading grounds as well. This may mean the spraying of lakes, swamps, and scrub land by helecopter. But there is a risk of destroying other forms of life besides the insect aimed at.

(c) *Major engineering*—projects can have massive and sometimes unexpected effects on vector life and human disease. Draining a lake or a swamp, altering the course of a river, cleaning a forest area, building a town in a rural area—all these may be done with no though of altering the balance of life in the area, but the effect may be profound, and it may be beneficial or harmful. Beneficial if it deprives disease carrier of their habitat, and harmful if it brings humans nearer to it.

Minor works may also bring changes—the fillings in of cracks in walls and floors, the draining of pools around a village, and the use of concrete instead of mud for floors or the use of stone instead of wood, for walls of huts and other buildings—all these cut down the chance of insects breading near human habitation. Major or minor, such works can alter the biological environment and carried out with fore thought, can greatly benefit human life and health.

(d) *Biological methods of control*—A knowledge of the life and habits of the insect is the basis of biological methods of control. The *tse-tse* fly of trypanosomiasis or sleeping sickness, feeds largely on the blood of big game animals, and if humans can drive these off from an area, the tse-tse flies must also disappear. *Xenopsylla cheopis*, the plague flea, depends on rats for its meals of blood, and extermination of rats brings an end of the flea and plague in the area. Some species of fish feed on malaria larvae on the surface of lake waters, and stocking the water with these fish has been successful in cutting down the number of adult mosquitoes that fly off to attack humans.

Insects are often highly fastidious in the type of vegetation that they choose as cover or refuse. Some can survive certain climatic conditions only under plants that grow close to the ground; other depend on water plants for protection and oxygen. Clearing away such plants can have a more profound effect on insect population and is more biological rational than the use of non discriminating insecticides. These biological measures may be very simple but they are derived from detailed study of all of the life of the area. At a more basic level, humans have attempted to interrupt the reproductive cycle of insects by raising large populations of males in laboratories and so affecting their reproductive organs by radiation, chemicals, or cross breeding that, when released, they are incapable of fertilizing females.

VII. HOUSE FLY AND FLY CONTROL

Q. 12.17. What are house flies ? Why they are important?

House flies are nonbiting winged insects. They live for a month or so, and can fly a distance of one kilometre. Their life—cycle is completed in 10 to 12 days, depending on the temperature and humidity. Eggs are laid in refuse dump, manure, rotting vegetables and excreta of man and animals.

Importance :

They are mechanical carriers and they carry infections by :

INFECTIONS

(i) Feet, body and wings which remain infective for a day.

(ii) By regurgitating, the flies remain infective for a week.

(iii) By passing germs in their stool, they remain infective about two weeks.

Q. 12.18. What are the various diseases spread by common "house fly" ?

House flies are mechanical carriers and they carry infections through the sputum, faeces and dusts spreading the following diseases :

(i) *From sputum*—Tuberculosis.

(ii) *From faeces*—Cholera, dysentery, gastro-enteritis, food poisoning, infective hepatitis, poliomyelitis and various worm infections.

(iii) *From dusts*—Organic dust causes allergic disease. Infective dust may contain anthrax and tetanus spores, diphtheria and tuberculosis bacillus, the ova of thread and round worms etc. which will produce the respective disease like anthraxis, tetanus, diphtheria, tuberculosis, vermicularis and ascariasis etc.

Q.12.19. What are the methods that should be followed to prevent housefly's spreading disease ?

House fly's diseases are very much contagious. They may bring about a desertrous effect in our community. So they should be prevented. Generally for preventing these diseases the following measures can be taken :

(i) *Prevention of breeding of flies.*
(ii) *Protection of food from flies.*
(iii) *Destruction of adult flies.*
(iv) *Health education to the public.*

1. Prevention of breeding flies :

(a) This can be done by prompt removal and proper disposal of all refuse including cowdung, night-soil etc.

Refuse should not be allowed to accumulate in the stables, cowsheds, slaughter houses, fish markets and garbage-dumps. They should be regularly cleaned atleast once a day and refuse should be removed in covered carts to the closed pits.

(b) The conservancy arrangements should be efficient. Construction of fly proof latrines, no cesspools, excreta cover with earth are essential.

(c) For destruction of eggs, larvae and pupae of flies in the manure, substance toxic to flies in their various stages should be used. D.D.T., gammexane, bleaching powder, etc. can be used for this purpose.

2. Protection of food from flies :

For the protection of food from flies—all arrangements should be made for proper storage and protection of food. It is advisable to screen windows and doors of home, dairy farms and kitchen and milk rooms.

3. Destruction of adult flies :

If adult flies have emerged out then they are killed by :

(i) Fly swalters.

(ii) Tangle foot *i.e.* (5 parts castor oil + 8 parts resin).

(iii) Fly bait *i.e.* (2% formaline in sugar and milk).

(iv) Sodium arsenite solution (1 oz to a gallon is sprayed over manure).

(v) Spraying D.D.T., Dieldrin, Gammaxane 5%, Pyrethrum in kerosene oil can be use. The effects last for 2-3 months).

(vi) Spraying of flit is also useful.

4. Health education :

A fly consciousness should be created among the people through health education.

Fly control campaigns should be organised and cooperation of the masses should be solicited. The people have to be educated regarding the harm done by the flies to us and the general measure should be—*Keeping the food-stuff properly*

INFECTIONS

covered, Fly proof kitchen, Eat food when it is still hot, Store food in meat safe, Do not eat food-stuff that are exposed to flies and dust, and do not eat over ripe fruits, state sweets etc.

Q. 12.20. What is meant by anti-fly measures ?

Anti-fly measure means :
(i) Prevention of breeding places of flies.
(ii) If flies are found breeding, they should be killed.
(iii) If adult have emerged prevent access of flies by the methods described above (Question No. 12.19).

Q. 12.21. What are the modes of transmission of Arthropod's borne diseases ?

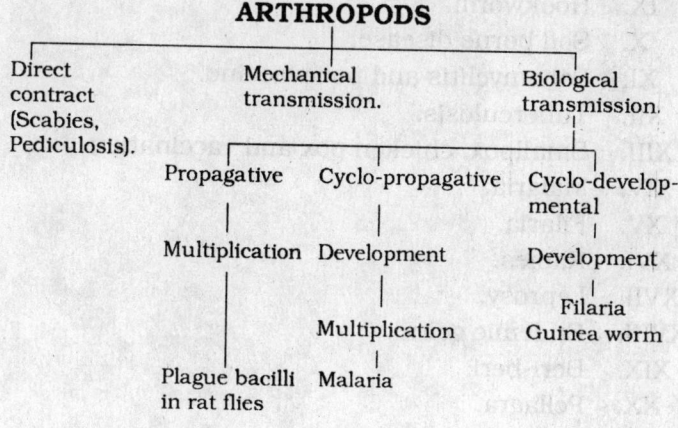

CHAPTER-XIII

COMMUNICABLE DISEASES

DISCUSSION FOR LEARNING

I. Definition of communicable disease.
II. How they occur?
III. Droplet infection.
IV. Incubation period.
V. Cholera.
VI. Gastro-enteritis, (Diarrhoea and Dysentery).
VII. Infective hepatitis.
VIII. Intestinal parasites.
IX. Hookworm.
X. Soil borne disease.
XI. Poliomyelitis and poliovaccine.
XII. Tuberculosis.
XIII. Smallpox, chicken pox and vaccination.
XIV. Malaria.
XV. Filaria.
XVI. Rabies.
XVII. Leprosy.
XVIII. Endemic goitre.
XIX. Beri-beri.
XX. Pellagra.

Q. 13.1. What is meant by Infectious disease and Contagious disease?

"**Infectious disease**" *is defined as a disease of man or animal resulting from an infection.*

"**Contagious disease**" *is defined as the disease which could be communicated by direct contact from host to host.*

Thus *Smallpox* is contagious disease. The contagion is conveyed from person to person through the air, whereas in case of *Bubonic plague*, the infection results only from bite of infected *Rat-flea*, hence it is not contagious in the sense that bubonic plague is not direct communicable from person to person.

According to modern concept, both infectious and contagious diseases are called communicable disease.

So a Communicable disease is defined as an illness due to specific infectious agent or its topics products, which are transmitted directly or indirectly to a susceptible host from an infected person or animal or through the agency of an intermediate animal host, a vector or the inaminate environment.

I. COMMUNICABLE DISEASE

Q. 13.2. What is meant by communicable disease ?

A *communicable disease* is one which arises from transference of an infecting agent—a microb, or its toxic products from the existing sources like—man, animal or soil to a susceptible host or hosts (man or animal) through a variety of transmission agents present in the environment and after a variable period of incubation depending upon the nature of the microb, manifests itself in certain types of signs and symptoms due to changes in the normal functioning of the body.

Q.13.3. What are the factors that are essential for the development of the communicable disease ?

For the development of communicable disease the following factors are essential :

(i) Caustive or aetiological agent.
(ii) Sources or reservoirs of infection.
(iii) A mode of escape from the reservoir.
(iv) A mode of transmission from the reservoir or the source of causative agent to the potential new host.
(v) A mode of entry into the new host.
(vi) A susceptible host.

Generally all the links of the chain are essential. If any of these link is missed, then the disease will not occur, even though the remaining five factors are present.

III. HOW THEY OCCUR ?

Q. 13.4. What are the various types of communicable diseases ? And how they occur ?

Communicable diseases are of following types :
(1) **Diseases by ingestion** (i.e. from eating and drinking).
(2) **Diseases by inhalation** (i.e. from breathing).
(3) **Diseases by inoculation** (i.e. from bites of insects and animals).
(4) **Diseases by contact** (i.e. from direct contact).

1. The diseases by ingestion can occur from :

(a) *Animal parasites* i.e. Thread worm, Round worm, Guinea worm, Trichinella, Tape worms, Hydratid disease and diseases due to fluke.

(b) *Bacterial or viral diseases*—i.e. Cholera, Enteric fever, Food poisoning, Dysentery, Infective hepatitis, Poliomyelitis, Tuberculosis, Diphtheria etc.

(c) *Chemical poisoning :*
  i) *Accidental* i.e. due to copper, arsenic, phosphorous, insecticides etc.
  ii) *Deliberate*—Addition of prohibited colouring matters and preservatives. Use of poisonous adultrants.

(d) *Deficiency diseases*—are mainly due to protein, minerals and vitamin deficiencies in food.

2. The diseases by inhalation can occur from :

(a) Virus diseases i.e. influenza, chicken-pox, small-pox, measles, mumps, poliomyelitis and common cold.
(b) *Coccal disease*—i.e. Pneumonia, cerebrospinal fever (Meningococcal meningitis).
(c) *Diseases by bacillus*—i.e. Diphtheria and Tuberculosis.

COMMUNICABLE DISEASES

3. **The disease by inoculation may be from :**
    (a) Bites of insects.
    (b) Bites of animal.
    (c) Germs getting access in the body by pricks, cuts or by injury of the skin.

(a) *By insects bites* :
   i) Mosquitoes causes—Malaria, Filaria, Yellow fever, Dengue fever, Haemorrhage fever and Virus encephalitis.
   ii) Sand fly causes—Sand fly fever, Kala azar, Oriental sore.
   iii) Tse-tse fly causes—Sleeping sickness.
   iv) Rat fly causes—Plague, Murine typhus.
   v) Lice causes—Typhus fever and Relapsing fever.
   vi) Tick causes—Typhus fever and Relapsing fever.
   vii) Mites causes—Scabies, Typhus fever.

(b) *Animal bites* :
   i) Rat bites causes—Rat-bite fever.
   ii) Dog bite causes—Rabies.

(c) *Germs gaining access in the body through cuts and injury* :
   i) From any animal we may get—Anthrax and Actynomycosis.
   ii) From horse we may get—Glanders.
   iii) From soil we may get—Tetanus.

4. **Disease by contacts are :**

Scabies, Ringworm, Trachoma, Yaw, Leprosy, and Venereal diseases like Syphilis, Gonorrhoea, Chanceroid etc.

Q. 13.5. (a) What are the common diseases carried by insects ?

The common diseases which are carried by insects are :

1. *Mosquitoes*—Malaria, Filariasis, Yellow fevers, Dengue, Encephalitis.

2. *Fleas*—Bubonic plague, Endemic typhus and Chiggerosis.
3. *Lice*—Epidemic typhus fever, Indian relapsing fever, Trench fever.
4. *House flies*—Typhoid fever, Cholera, Dysentery.
5. *Tse-tse flies*—Sleeping sickness.
6. *Sand flies*—Sand fly fever, Oriental sore and Kalazar.
*7. *Ticks and Mites*—African relapsing fever, Rocky—Mountain spotted fever, Tick typhus.

* (Not insects but Arachnida.)

III. DROPLET INFECTION

Q. 13.5. (b) What is meant by droplet infection ?

Droplet infection means that the germs of diseases are travelling, through droplet of sputum or saliva. These diseases are the diseases from the throat and the lungs. When a person is talking, coughing, sneezing or even when breathing, germs are thrown out with droplets of sputum etc. Smaller droplets can travel about 20 to 30 feet. Larger droplets travel only about 3 feet. The size of droplet varies from 15 to 300 microns. The minute droplets lose the watery part by evaporation, and the germs (mainly virus) remain suspended in the air for a long time and can travel long distance. They are called *"droplet nuclei"*.

Def.—*If a Susceptible person is within the range of spray of infected droplets come out from the saliva of the mouth or nose and throat of a person into the atmosphere during sneezing, coughing, laughing or talking, he is likely to inhale some of those droplets before falling and cause diseases, then this type of infection is called Droplet Infection.*

Q. 13.6. What are the diseases spread by droplet infection ?

Diseases spread by droplet infection are :
(1) *Smallpox*, (2) *Pulmonary tuberculosis*, (3) *Diphtheria*, (4) *Chicken pox*, (5) *Measles*, (6) *Whooping cough*, (7) *Mumps*, and (8) *Influenza*.

COMMUNICABLE DISEASES

Q. 13.7. How can we prevent a disease from droplet infection?

Prevention can be done by :
1. *Avoiding over crowding.*
2. *Proper sweeping and swabbing.*
3. *Use of ultraviolet light.*
4. *Guarded mouth by handkerchief or by clothes during coughing and sneezing.*
5. *Maintaining personal hygiene.*

Homoeopathic View

Generally psora and susceptibility are the basic requisites in the subject before he/she can be infected. So if the susceptibility of the subject is controlled or changed better results can be observed.

IV. INCUBATION PERIOD

Q. 13.8. What is meant by incubation period ? What are its importance ? What is infective period ?

Incubation period is defined as the time interval between the entry of the disease agent and the onset of clinical manifestation of the disease. During the incubation period, the disease agent undergoes multiplication in the body of susceptible host. When a sufficient density of the disease agent is built up in the body, the body defences are overcome and the equilibrium of the health is distrubed and the disease results. The length of duration of the incubation period is a characteristic of each disease. It may be be from few hours to many days or weeks. The duration of the incubation period depends on the host parasites relationship.

Infective period is the period during which time an infected person can transmit the disease to another person. It is also known as *"period of communicability"*.

Generally the period of incubation and the period of communicability (Infective period) of some common diseases are as follows :

Infection enters our body through	Name of the disease	Incubation period	Infection period or period of communicability
I. Ingestion	1. Cholera	A few hours to 5 days	2 weeks or so long as *vibrios* are present in stool.
	2. Typhoid	12 to 14 days	6 weeks or as long as organism is found in stool.
	3. Infective hepatitis	30 days	3 weeks, until stool culture are negative.
II. Inhalation	1. Small pox	12 days	Till last scab fall off.
	2. Measles	8 to 15 days	During the period of catarrhal symptoms and about a week after rash.
	3. Chicken pox	14 to 15 days	2 weeks or till last scab fall off.
	4. Mumps	12 to 26 days	2 weeks.
	5. Diphtheria	2 to 7 days	2 weeks or until virulent bacilli disappear from secretions i.e. till 3 swabs are negative.
	6. Poliomyelitis	14 days	2 weeks after recovery.
	7. Tuberculosis	Long	As long as germs are in sputum.

Infection enters our body through	Name of the disease	Incubation period	Infection period or period of communicability
	8. Influenza	1—3 days	First 3 days of fever.
	9. C.S. fever	2—10 days	The infection is by carrier.
	10. Scarlet fever	2—3 days	Rare in India.
III. Inoculation	1. Plague	3—6 days	As long as rat fleas are on the patient (3 weeks).
	2. Yellow fever	3—6 days	Infected Ades in first 3 days of fever.
	3. Typhus fever	7—12 days	Infected lice as long as the disease exists.
	4. Relapsing fever	7—12 days	Infected lice, ticks, mite in disease period.
	5. Virus encephalitis or Dengue	5—6 days	Infected mosquito for 8 to 11 days.
IV. Contact	1. Leprosy	Long	As long as he is lepromatous.
	2. Puerperal fever		During child birth.

Importance

1. Incubation period is of fundamental importance in epidemiological studies. By a knowledge of the incubation period, we can estimate the onset of infection and thereby search for the sources of infection.

2. It is also useful in determining the quarantine period which may be advised.

V. CHOLERA

Q. 13.9. What is cholera ?

Cholera is an acute and highly infectious gastro-intestinal disease due to *vibrio cholerae* with high morbidity and mortality occuring mostly in the Asiatic countries, particularly in India, Pakistan and Bangladesh.

Clinically, it is manifested by sudden onset of diarrhoea followed by vomiting, copious, painless, pouring of watery stool generally rice water in colour is the main initial symptoms of the patients ; other symptoms are attributable to dehydration or loss of fluid, muscular cramps, suppression of urine, fall of blood pressure followed by uraemia and other complications.

The disease usually becomes fatal, if the dehydration is allowed to continue, unchecked without proper rehydration in time.

Q. 13.10. How cholera is spread ?

*How cholera is spread in a village ?

1. *Direct*—Cholera is mainly a water-borne disease. Generally the cholera is transmitted directly to a person when he drinks contaminated water or eats contaminated cooked food or unwashed fruits, vegetables or other raw or uncooked food.

2. *Indirect*—This disease is also spread indirectly by using, eating and drinking utensils washed with contaminated water, or through flies which carry infection both mechanically and vitally.

COMMUNICABLE DISEASES

3. *Contact*—Contact infection are also found, especially in over crowded dwelling without proper sanitary facilities. In case of careless handling of vomitous, dejected and infected linens facilitate this way of infection.

*Secondary facors in the spread of cholera are : Fairs and festivals (aggregation disposal), flood, famine, drought and earthquake (natural calamities), rainfall and humidity, (environmental factors), starvation, fatigue, debility, ignorance, illiteracy (social factors) etc.

Q. 13.11. How it can be prevented and controlled ?

*(Describe in brief the measures to be adopted to prevent out break of cholera in a city or village mentioning both the personal and general prophylaxis. or What preventive measures you would advise in the face of a cholera epidemic ?)

Cholera being an emergency disease. Its control measures are directed with equal importance towards the sources of infection, transmission factors as well as the host. **The fundamental principles of control of cholera are :**

1. *Notification of the occurrence of the disease to the authorities concerned in taking preventive measures within shortest possible time.*
2. *Mobilisation of the forces and means of defence to the effected area or to the spot of infection.*
3. *Measures directed to prevent the spread of infection from the sources.*
4. *Measures directed against the transmission factors.*
5. *Increase the specific resistance of the community at risk.*
6. *Prevention of importation or spread of infection into a locality where there is no cholera.*
7. *Legal provision for ensuring prompt action in fighting epidemics of cholera.*

1. Notification of the Occurence

As cholera is an infectious disease, for successful combating early recognisation of the cases and immediate notification to the health authorities concerned are utmost important. All cases of purging, vomiting and symptoms of dehydration should be reported to be suspected cases of cholera and attempts should be made for the confirmation by bacteriological diagnosis, and by stool culture. Some of the acute gastro-enteritis cases though bacteriologically negative may be treated as cholera on the basis of the clinical findings.

*Generally an outbreak of cholera in a village should be notified immediately to the Medical Officer Incharge of P.H.C. and the M.O.I./C. of P.H.C. notified to the District Health Authorities, State Health Authority and the National Health Authority.

2. Isolation and Treatment

The second and the most important step is isolation of suspected cases. Isolation and augmentation of early treatment is generally serve two purposes viz.:

(i) Reduced mortality, and (ii) Prevent further spread of infection. Generally no hospital or a doctor can treat a cholera case, if an Isolation Hospital exists. The case must be removed to the Isolation Hospital as per the Municipal Act.

*But in village where there is no Isolation Hospital or during a flood, the Medical Officer of the Primary Health Centre arrange for Isolation, in primary school or mobile medical teams are immediately organised, temporary hospital are started in available accommodations and then starts to giving intravenous saline to the patient. Mere giving of intravenous saline will prevent 90% of deaths.

3. Disinfection

Concurrent and *Terminal disinfection* are carefully done in relation to the excreta disposal and soil clothings of cholera

COMMUNICABLE DISEASES

patients. Disinfection of stool and vomit is done by 1 oz. of bleaching power in a pint of cholera stood or by 5% Izal.

Soiled clothes are put in boiling water. Useless rags are burnt. Floors, walls and furnitures are disinfected with phenyl. Privies, house gullies etc. are disinfected with phenyl. Utensils are boiled or scalded. Hands are dipped in lysol or detol solution.

*In villages, if disinfectants are not available then boil the stool and vomitous before disposal.

N.B. : *Cholera dead* bodies should never be allowed to be thrown in rivers, so they are properly disposed by burning or burial.

4. Immunization

It is done by anticholera vaccine. As immunity is produced after 9 days, so for the first 6 days (i) A teaspoon of essential oil mixture is given twice a day, (ii) Bili-vaccine i.e. 1 pill of bile on empty stomach followed by one tablet of vaccine after 15 minutes. Immunisation should not only be done to the contacts but also mass immunisation must be carried out.

Towns and villages :— On the down stream of a river, should be immunised against cholera in anticipation before floods. It is better to immunise all villages, before the monsoon starts. Anticholera inoculation gives immunity only for 6 months. Recovery from an attack of cholera does not give any immunity.

5. Long Term General Measures

(a) *Sanitary measures* :
  i) All measures of drinking and domestic water supplies should be chlorinated with adequate dose in order to have desirable residual chlorine.*
  ii) Removal of refuse to prevent fly breeding.
  iii) Antifly campaign.
  iv) Proper disposal of excreta.
  v) Boiling of feeding and cooking utensils.

vi) Ensure proper sanitation in eating houses, sweet and meat shops, aerated water factories, milk shops etc.

vii) Destroy stable and rotten foodstuff and food exposed to flies and dust.

viii) Try to trace out carriers
*(Generally in fairs or melas the sanitation is often not quite satisfactory. A healthy cholera carrier contaminates the water or food and starts the epidemic of cholera. So a proper sanitary arrangement can prevent cholera in case of village fairs or meals).

(b) *Health education or propaganda :*

How the disease occurs and how it can be prevented by various measures if propagated to the public by various propaganda or placard this will be best method for prevent cholera. *Generally the propaganda should be* :

(i) To boil water and milk.

(ii) Avoid ice and cold drinks.

(iii) Wash vegetables and fruits that are to be eaten raw, in solution of potassium permanganate.

(iv) Advice people not to remain on empty stomach, and take dahi, butter milk, sour lime etc. as acidity in food kill the *cholera vibiros*.

(v) Eat food when it is still hot and stored food in a meatsafe or keep the food properly covered.

(vi) Don't eat food exposed to flies and dust.

(vii) Proper cleaning of hands before eating or handling food.

(viii) Advice all people to take anticholera vaccine.

Conclusion—Fairs, melas and pilgrim gatherings are often the sites for starting cholera epidemic. As proper sanitation cannot be ensured in such gatherings, a healthy cholera carriers start cases of cholera and then the disease flares up. Cholera becomes an epidemic, specially if the sources of drinking water supply is contaminated by *cholera vibiros*, as happen in cases of floods.

Chlorination of water can prevent water-borne epidemic of cholera, but unfortunately only 75% of our urban population and 3% of the villagers, gets chlorinated water supply. So *boiling water* in the villages is the only thing that can prevent cholera epidemic.

N.B. : *Legal provisions for ensuring prompt action in fighting epidemic of cholera :*

1. Quarantine

Quarantine of ships and airships may be done, and the ships are disinfected. The persons not having valid cholera innoculation certificates are quarantined till the incubation period of the disease is over, and are given cholera vaccine. International quarantine period is of 5 days. In cities or villages, segregation and surveillance of contacts are also done.

2. National Cholera Control Programme

There is an epidemic disease act in the states for the legal and promptaction in fighting epidemic of cholera. But it does not operate between states. As such it has been recommended by the Expert committee on smallpox and cholera, that a central Infection Disease Act should be promulgated to ensure uniform process all over the country in respect of cholera. So *National Cholera Control Programme* was started in 1970-1971 in Endemic Areas.

There are 4 types of cholera workers at the Block level together with other staff. The duties of cholera workers are :

1. Regular disinfection of drinking water.
2. Collection of sample of stool and send to the samples to the laboratories, in bottles Rectal Swab method or blotting paper or gauze, dipped in stool and sealed in plastic packets to prevent drying.
3. Surveillance of the contacts.

In *Urban* areas the Local Health Authorities control the diseases by usual methods of notification, segregation and surveillance of contacts. Disinfections of stools, vomits and formities, mass immunisation and general measures like chlorination of water supply and wells, control of fly breeding and sanitation of the food premises. But in rural areas through the principles of cholera control are same, the method of implementation differs due to vast surroundings, poverty of the people, illiteracy, primitive habits of the people. Generally the Medical Officer Incharge (M.O.I./C.) of P.H.C., can mobilize all his staff for the control of the infection and sends reports to S.D.H.O. So that the control measures will be started in other P.H.C's. also.

VI. GASTRO-ENTERITIS

(Diarrhoea and Dysentery)

Q. 13.12. What is meant by Gastro-enteritis ? What would be the steps for prevention and control of this disease ?

Generally *Diarrhoea* and *Dysentery* in epidemic form are known as *Gastro-enteric disease*. The causes of diarrhoea and dysenteries are numerous and varied. Generally they are determined as a group of infectious diseases caused by various types of organisms bacterial, protozoal, helminthic or viral in nature producing clinical manifestations of loose motions with or without much and/or blood in stool. They have a common epidemiological feature of transmission through faecal contamination of food or drink. They are prevalent throughout the world and mostly associated with low standard of hygiene. The common ailments of human gastro-enteritis groups are :

1. *Amoebic dysentery*—due to Entamoeoba-hystolytica.
2. *Bacillary dysentery*—due to Shigalla Bacilli.
3. *Diarrhoea*—due to Giardia Intestinalis.

Prevention and Control Measures

1. Generally they are not notifiable in India, no special control measures are needed, only attempt to be made to improve personal hygiene, particularly in defaecation, washing of hands and food handling.

COMMUNICABLE DISEASES

2. The patient should be given effective treatment as early as possible to reduce the risk of his becoming a carrier. Isolation if possible should be done in hospital until the patient is free from the organism.
3. The faces should be treated with strong disinfectant before disposal.

In Epidemics

Reports of epidemics (Gastro-enteric diseases) institutional or localised in an area, have special importance from control point of view. During an epidemics, all cases of diarrhoea and dysentery (Gastro-enteric disease) should be treated accordingly with a precaution. The most important measures of protection of the community are safe water supply and sanitary disposal of night-soil and garbage.

(A) Sanitary Measures

1. If water is of doubtful purity, as a temporary measure it should be used after boiling or by mixing halozen tablets or zeolite liquids.
2. If fly nuisance is present, it should be delt with by treating fly breeding places with insecticide viz. Benzene Hexachloride (Gemmaxane) etc.
3. Food should be protected from dust and flies by keeping it screened and cover.
4. Raw vegetables should not be eaten unless well washed and then dipped in boiling water or potassium permanganate solution.
5. All food-stuff should be protected from flies and cooked and other servants should be trained to handle food after washing hands very well.

(B) Health Education

1. For controlling diarrhoea and dysentery in the community improvement of environmental sanitation and health education should be given the highest priority. As for examples :
   (a) The simple mechanism of infections processes may be taught to the mothers and other members of the family from antenatal stages, viz.
      i) How the infecting organisms escape from the body in the faecal matter and infectious agents enter through oral route.

ii) Foods and drinks including milk and water are the most common vehicles. Food handlers if unclean may carry infective agents in their fingers.

iii) Uncooked food and food allowed to remain in dirty utensils and uncovered are often responsible for transmission of infection.

(b) Regarding diet— mother should know the infants and toddler's diet, stage by stage. There must be optimum protein intake along with other proximate principles, vitamines and trace elements for satisfactory and uneventual growth of the child.

(c) In areas where fresh human faeces is applied to crops it should be composed and stored enough at the prevailing temperature to ensure the death of the cysts.

(d) Latrine must be provided and water if not already purified should boiled.

(e) There is no immunoprophylaxis against the disease.

*Sometimes *Homoeopathic Medicine* as a prophylaxis may be recommended for a known exposed group of persons.

VII. INFECTIVE HEPATITIS

Q. 13.13. What is meant by hepatitis ?

Jaundice is the main symptom of hepatitis, or inflammation of the *hepar*, or *liver*. Serum hepatitis has been shown to be caused by a virus, called *Hepatitis B virus*. Infectious hepatitis is probably also caused by a virus, called *Hepatitis A virus*. Another common cause of hepatitis has not been isolated, andfor lack of better name, is called *Non-A, non-B hepatitis*.

Infectious hepatitis spreads easily from person to person by the fecal-oral route. It is a disease of close personal contact but can also spread in food and water. *Serums hepatitis* is more commonly injected into the body, straight into blood stream via a vein or, less directly, via the subcutaneous tissues. The virus floats in the blood serum of an infected person and can get out on the point of a syringe needle or other instruments. If the syringe is then used unsterilized on another person, enough virus is injected to infect that person. Blood given in transfusions, for example, may be contaminated with the virus, and serum hepatitis is a hazard of all of the manipulations in which the blood of one person passes into the body of another.

COMMUNICABLE DISEASES 325

Q. 13.14. What is the difference between serum hepatitis and infectious hepatitis.

The two diseases are similar, *Infectious hepatitis*, which is more often mild, frequently attacks children, in whom inflammation of the liver may be so mild that jaundice is absent. Older people suffer more severely. Serum hepatitis is more commonly a fairly serious illness. In both diseases, the effected person suffers from weakness and sluggishness, with loss of appetite, headache, some fever, and some generalized aches and pains. Jaundice, the main feature, may range from a tinge yellow in the conjunctivas to a deep orange dyeing of the whole skin. Itchinges of the skin is troublesome when jaundice is severe. After a week or two, recovery begins, although it may several weeks before the patient is back to normal. Of persons jaundiced with infectious hepatitis, probably not more than one or two per 1,000 die, but, in elderly persons with serum hepatitis, moratality may rise to 20 percent.

It is not always easy to decide whether a person has *infectious hepatitis* or *hepatitis B*. A history of contact with another patient or of an injection, or transfusion may help to decide. A blood test is of some value, for patients with serum hepatitis often have a substance in their blood called *Australia, or hepatitis B, antigen*, whereas patients with infectious hepatitis do not. Infectious hepatitis can be controlled by strict personal hygiene and by the provision of safe food and water supplies. The incidence of serum hepatitis can be lessened by serupulous attention to aseptic technique and by screening of blood donors for *hepatitis B antigen*.

Q. 13.15. What is meant by infective hepatitis ? How can we prevent it ?

The disease formerly known to be eatarrhal Jaundice is designted, at present, as *Infective Hepatitis* of viral origin. On account of its different modes of infection and spread the disease viral hepatitis is further classified into two types viz. *Infective Hepatitis* and *Serum Hepatitis* ,of course, clinically these two varieties can easily be differentiated. The infection is manifested by *anorexia*, nausea, malaise, abdominal discomfort and fever and generally followed by jaundice with high coloured urine in which bile is usually detected. There may be infection without jaundice. Such cases are often missed and can be recognised by liver function tests.

Infectious Hepatitis is also a notifiable viral disease. The germs are generally present in the stool as well as in blood. Commonly the disease spreads by contamination of water, milk, food etc. The Icteric case are mainly spread the disease. This disease is also spread by flies. Some time by injection needle, use for an icteric patient, also spread the disease.

Incubatiod Period is shorter in infectious hepatitis varying from 10 days to 40 days, whereas in case of serum hepatitis, it is never less than 6 weeks usually being 12 to 14 weeks and the longest incubation period may be upto 6 months. Case fatality is generally very low being nearer 2 percent.

Boiling do not kill the virus. Filtration of water and then chlorination with 4 P.P.M., chlorine will kill the virus.

Prevention and Control

1. *Individual protection* :

There is no specific therapy. Chemotherapeutic agents and antibiotics are not effective. Rest, high caloric diet and symptomatic treatment by homoeopathic medicine are advocated with glucose or fructose orally or intravenously, is very helpful.

2. When faecal as contamination of the environment appears to be responsible for the spread, improvement of sanitation and personal hygiene would reduce the incidence of outbreak. When community water supply is suspected to be contaminated, measures must be taken correct the supply as early as possible. In the mean time the people should be asked to use water after boiling.

3. The virus of infectious hepatitis has not yet been cultivated in tissue culture, as such it has not yet been possible to prepare a vaccine or active immunization of contacts of population at risk, otherwise, can be done with *immune serum globulin 0.01 ml.* per pound of body weight as early as possible after exposure.

COMMUNICABLE DISEASES

4. Special precautions in sterilising syringes and needles should always be taken to avoid serum hepatitis. It can be prevented also by screening blood donors and eliminating all these giving history of jaundice. Liquid plasma if stored for 3-6 months appears to result in the smallest incidence of serum hepatitis. The pool size of plasma donors should reduced to minimum if not avoidable.

5. Above all :
    a) *Super chlorination of water.*
    b) *Food sanitation,*
    c) *Antifly measures,*
    d) *Educate people to boil water and milk and explain that personal hygene plays an important part in controlling the infection, are the basic for prevention of infective hepatitis.*

VIII. INTESTINAL PARASITES

Q. 13.16. What are intestinal parasites ?

The various common intestinal parasites are :

1. *Ascaris lumbricoides* (Round Worm)
2. *Oxyuris vermicularis* (Thread Worm)
3. *Trichinella spirallis.*
4. *Ancylostoma duodenale* (Hook Worm)
5. *Taenia solium* (Tape Worm)
6. *Taenia saginata.*
7. *Dibothriocephalus latus.*
8. *Hymenolepis nana.*
9. *Schistostoma japonicum* etc.

These are mainly living in the intestines and are totally dependent on the body for their nutrition and living.

N.B. : Dr. Farington has given a beautiful homoeopathic view regarding worms. Just as insects cannot attack a healthy apple, similarly worms cannot exist in a healthy person. So if the body is free from psoric tint, the worms will not be found a congenial soil and have no footing. So for the treatment of intestinal parasites antipsoric treatment is very effective.

IX. HOOK WORM

Q. 13.17. What is meant by hook worm infestation or Ancylostomiasis ? Or What do you know about the hook worms ?

Ancylostomiasis or *hook worm infestation* means a disease caused by *Ancylostoma deuodenale*—a common parasite of our intestine.

(*A. deuodenale* is an old species, and *Necator americanus* is a new world species.)

Ancylostoma deuodenale the hook worm infection is wide spread in the tropical and subtropical countries. It is highly endemic in most of the states in India as noted by survey. About 70 percent of the workers of the coal mines and of villagers of West Bengal and Bihar are infested, though many of them are without showing any hook worm diseases infestation.

Clinical Characteristics

The infection causes a chroic debilitating condition with generally very vague symptoms depending on the extent of infection and the nutritional status of the patient. Hypochromic microcytic anaemia is the commonest manifestation. Infected children may be retarded in physical and mental development. Occasionally dermatitis or ground itch may develop at the place of entry of infection. The diagnosis of the infection depends on finding the typical eggs in stool.

Q. 13.18. How does the disease occur ? What are the modes of infection of the disease ancylostomasis or Hook worm ? or Describe the life cycle of hook worm. or How do people get infected by hook worms?

The adult worms are about one centimetre long. Both males and females have hooks and they remain attached to the duodenum. Man is the only host and the sole reservoir of infection. They frequently change the site, so that there are marks of injury in the duodenum. The worm sucks about 5 drops of blood daily and the injury marks also bleed.

COMMUNICABLE DISEASES

There may be hundreds of such worms on the wall of the duodenum.

The female discharges even two million eggs. If stool is passed on the open field, the eggs become *rhabditiform larvae* and then become mature *filariform larvae*, and are then ready to penetrate the skin. They live for about 2 months on the moist earth or on grass blades. *When a person walks bare footed, the larvae come to the skin and then penetrate the skin through hair follicles, sweat glands, cut in the skin or even unbroken skin.*

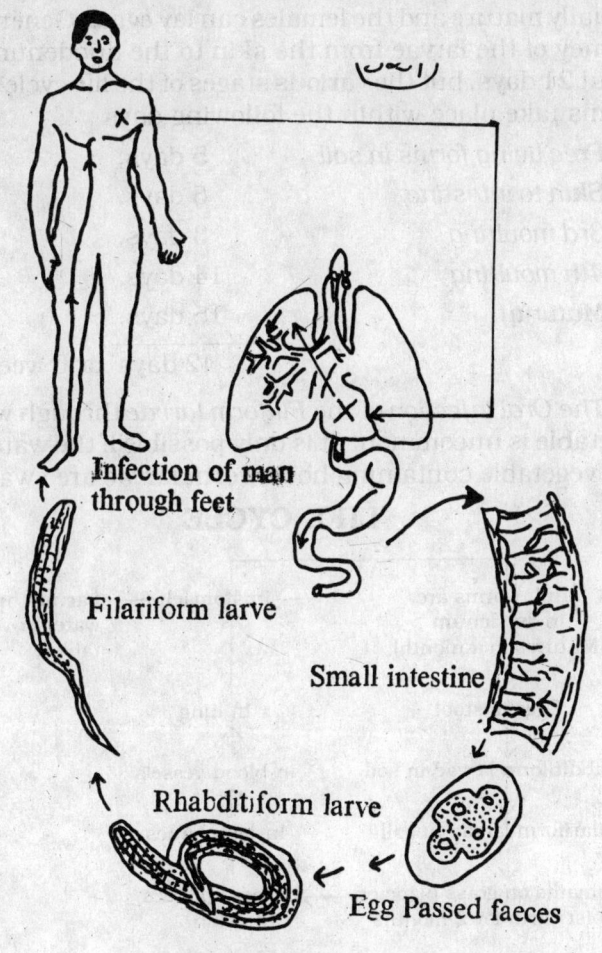

Life cycle of Hook worm

At the sit of entry, "ground sore" occurs. The larvae then pass through the lymphatics and come to the circulatory system and then, to the capillaries around the alveolus of the lungs.

They penetrate into the alveolus, and comes up to the throat with the sputum. The sputum when swallowed, the larvae go to stomach and then to the duodenum (small intestine), by this time, they undergo *third moulting*. Also in the intestine, they acquire provisional buccal capsules and after 3 weeks the worms undergo *fourth moulting* in order to develop permanent buccal capsule after which they become sexually mature and the females can lay eggs. Generally the journey of the larvae from the skin to the duodenum takes about 21 days, but the various stages of the life cycle of hook worms take place within the following days :

Free living forms in soil	5 days.
Skin to intestine	5 days.
3rd moulting	3 days.
4th moulting	14 days.
Maturity	15 days.
	42 days or 6 weeks.

The *Oral infection* of the *Filiform larvae* through water or vegetable is uncommon. It is only possible if the water, food and vegetable containing hook worm larvae are swallowed.

LIFE CYCLE

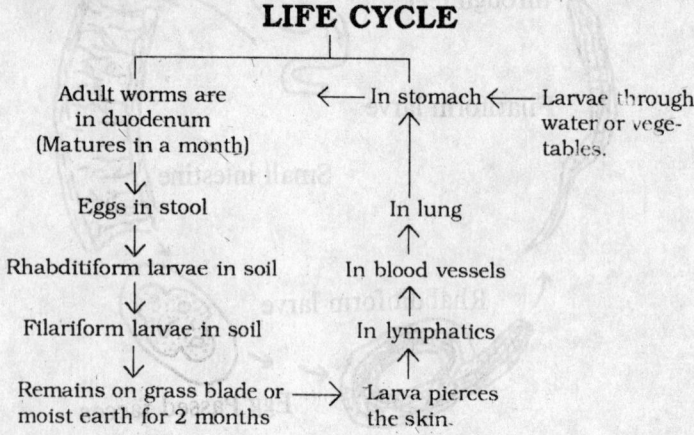

Q. 13.19. How we can prevent and control the disease of hookworm ?

Theoretically, prevention of hookworm disease is an easy matter, as it's cause is known and all characteristics of the parasites are understood. But in practice it is one of the most difficult disease to handle owing to its extensive prevalence, enormous reproductive power of the worm, rapid development of the ova in the infective stage, and because the infection is the direct result of careless and filthy habits.

1. The *first step* in the prevention of this disease is to stop it in those already affected. Accurate diagnosis, careful treatment on modern lines followed by examination of the faeces will reduce the source of infection and the possibility of fresh infection. But there still remains another source of danger through "carriers" who present no special symptom or symptoms so mild as to pass unnotice, but who harbour from a few to a couple of hundred worms, which lay eggs in large numbers all the time. These carrier should be isolated and properly treated.

So the treatment has two aspects : *Individual treatment* aiming at radical cure of the patient and *Mass treatment* to reduce the intensity of infection and frequency of transmission.

1. (a) *Individual treatment*—In individual treatment, the condition of the patient, especially anemia should be taken into consideration. If anaemia is severe, it should be treated first with iron before specific anthelmentic treatment.

   (b) *Mass treatment*—For mass treatment, the anthelmentic drugs should be used with great caution. Unless there should be side effects.

2. *Other measures* :

   (a) *Removal of the source of infection*—For removal of infection, periodical examination of all persons living infected localities and under conditions favourable to the existence of larvae is necessary. In mills, factories, plantations, etc. all workers should be similarly examined and any one suffering from dyspepsia or anaemia more carefully examined, and if any one ancylostomes are found in the faeces they should be segregated and properly treated.

(b) *Prevention of soil infection* :

i) It is generally done by sanitary latrines. Particularly attention should be paid to providing easily accessible privy accommodation, especially where a large number of men congregate and work e.g. in mills, factories, etc. Septic tank latrines, or in their absence borehole or dug-well latrines may be constructed in village.

(ii) Where night soil are used as manures, the storage of the night soil, for atleast 6 weeks, is often advocated. In order to kill the infective larvae of the hook worms in night soil addition of salt or lime 1:5000 dilution is more effective.

(c) *Health education* :

Considering the fact that infection and dessemination of the disease are mainly due to the ignorance and uncleany habits of the people, the essential steps should be taken to educate the people.

The Basic Steps

1. They should not eat unwashed fruits or vegetables and should not drink muddy water or water from dirty receptacles.

2. All water for drinking purpose should be purified. Everyone living in hook worm areas should be taught the essential facts about worm and its effects.

3. Cultivators and other workers in mills, factories, plantations etc., where the disease prevails, should be told of the danger of the going about bare footed. So they should wear shoes. In rural areas, where people work on the fields, the use of shoes by the cultivators is unknown, and during the rainy season when the fields and roads are sloppy or partly inundated, the utility of using boots and shoes, and in their absence cheap wooden sandles (kharrams), as a means of reducing and preventing infection should be impressed on the people.

COMMUNICABLE DISEASES

Main preventive measures for water and soil borne intestinal diseases like Hook worm, Giardia, Ascariasis etc. :

1. Proper disposal of night soil by aqua privy, septic tank latrine, bore-hole latrine etc.
2. Educate people not to pass stool on the open field.
3. Do not walk bare footed, better use boots in infected areas.
4. Boiling or chlorination of water.
5. Dip vegetables and fruits in solution of potassium permanganate.

Q. 13.20. What are the influence of soil on hook worm infestation?

Augustine experimentally shows that 3 percent moisture is the minimum amount in which the larvae of hook worm can live in a sandy loam containing some humus and a little clay. But acidity of soil does not influence the incidence of hookworm infestation. Even when the soil is heavily impregnated with salt, and defaecation is indiscriminate and ground saturated with strongly brackish water there is no hook worm infestation. So the hook worm infestation depends upon the suitability of soil. Generally when the people pass stools in or about the dwelling, open land or on the banks of rivers and tanks, the larvae are scattered by rains and all traces of faeces are lost, but the porous earth becomes permeated with larvae in the encysted and infection stage. Moist earth, *especially if sandy so as to retain moisture, or shadded by vegetation, offers ideal conditions for the life of lavae.*

X. SOIL BORNE DISEASES

Q. 13.21. What is soil ?

Soil is a mixture of disintegrated material of underlying rock, deposit of transported sand and slit mingled with decayed vegetable and animal matters (humus). The upper layer (few inches to several inches) is generally called the mould of humus formed out of decayed animal and vegetable substances and the subsoil consists of decayed primitive rock (few feet to hundred feet).

Q.13.22. What are its public health utilities ?

It is well known that carcasses of animal and human dead bodies, are buried inside the earth for final disposal. Soil is also used for disposal of night soil in the trenching ground and in the various types of latrines, namely *trench latrines, well latrines* etc.

The bacterial content of the soil, particularly the anaerobic and nitrifying bacteria carry out this function of safe disposal of dead animals and decaying vegetable matters. Some diseases are also occur from contaminated soils, so this is also a most public health importance for prevention and control of these diseases.

Q. 13.23. What are the soil borne diseases ?

The diseases which are associated with the soil are :
1. Diseases caused by spore bearing pathogenic bacteria as their natural habitat e.g. *anthrax, tetanus* and *gangrene*.
2. Diseases due to soil pollution with human excretion—*enteric fever, cholera, diarrhoea and dysentery*—the organisms contaminating the soil for a short period and eventually the water sources, vegetables and food.
3. Disease caused by animal parasites *hook worm* and other helminthic infections through ova, eggs and larvae which are deposited on the soil in human excreta.
4. Diseases facilitated by the dampness of soil are :
   Respiratory diseases, tuberculosis and rheumatism.

Thus soil sanitation is an important measure for health protection and prevention of diseases.

XI. POLIOMYELITIS

Q. 13.24. What is meant by poliomyelitis ?

Poliomyelitis is an infectious disease, epidemic and endemic throughout the world and caused by one of the three types (type I, II & III) *of an ultramicroscopic enterovirus.* It is principally an infection of the human alimentary tract but may affect the central nervous system resulting in irreversible flaccid paralysis. Man is the source of infection. The usual mode of transmission is the *"faecal-oral route"*. The infection period (time between infection and onset of disease) is about 7-14 days.

Clinically, it is characterised by—fever, malaise, headache, stiffness of neck and back and moderately increased cells and protein in the cerebrospinal fluid. Paralysis of voluntary muscles most commonly of the lower extremity occur in severe cases; involvement of respiratory nerves control is quickly fatal. In many cases infection, however, does not result in paralysis and are mild and some of them simulate the Aseptic Meningitis Syndrome, others have vague symptoms with no sings referable to the central nervous system. It is estimated that for every clinical case there will be atleast 100 sub-clinical infections. It can be diagnosed if paralysis of muscles set in.

Q. 13.25. How we can prevent and control the disease poliomyelitis?

Strangely, improved standard of living and poliomyelitis are co-related. The disease is less common amongst people with primitive habits and overcrowded localities. The virus is in the pharynx and is also present in the faeces. Thus the diseases can be spread by ingestion or inhalation. The seasonal prevalence of the disease is summer and monsoon. The preventive measures of poliomyelitis are same as other diseases but after care treatment for poliomyelitis is very important. By proper exercise, the paralysed part regain strength. The *1st step* of prevention is *Notification*.

1. *Notification*: The disease should be made notifiable in every state of the country.

2. As the cases are highly infectious during prodormal and early stage isolation has a very limited value. But bed-side nursing and clinical care are essential to restrict development of deformities and to some extent to reduce spread of infection.
3. Paralytic as well as non-paralytic cases should be designated as poliomyelitis in order to faciliate epidemiological analysis.
4. *Mass immunization*—with oral poliovaccine should be undertaken at the earliest indication of an outbreak. But there is no substitute for routine immunisation. In India, all children upto 5 years of age should be immunised as a routine procedure.

*Oral polio-vaccine is generally given in 3 doses to infants i.e. at the age of 4th, 5th and 6th months, but in children, the oral polio is given in 2 doses.

Passive protection of immediate contacts within 2 days of exposure with gamma globulin has been found to prevent attack in exposed family members.
5. During an outbreak children should be avoided close contact with persons of other family.
6. During an outbreak in an area, operation of nose and throat, and parental inoculation should be avoided and postponed except in emergent conditions. Unnecessary travel and physical strain after known exposure should be avoided.
7. Patients with residual paralysis should be brought under care of a specialised polio clinic to provide maximum recovery through rehabilitation therapy and proper exercise.
8. *International measures* :

This disease is not notifiable internationally as cholera, smallpox, plague, yellow fever, typhus and relapsing fever etc. But it is desirable that occurrence of epidemic should be communicated to World Health Organisation (WHO) at Geneva. WHO has established reference laboratories in different centres for the identification of poliomyelitis and relative viruses and for advising on all investigative work on the disease. At the international symposium on poliomyelitis control held in March 1983 in Washington, the possibility of eradicating polio on a world wide basis was considered within the century by immunization through Global polio eradication programme. Recently UNICEF has sponsored field study to introduce the new "high potency" Salk Vaccine in India. Till the results of the above study are known, it should be remembered that OPV is still one of the safest vaccines in use and has got the recommendation of the WHO.

Q. 13.26. What are main problems of polio vaccination in India ?

At present the OPV is wholly imported and even after fourth decades of independence, it has not been possible to manufacture this life-saving vaccine in the country. Under the national EPI programme, OPV is administered to infants from the 3rd month in 3 doses of monthly intervals and a booster doses is given at 1½ years to 2 years of age. In urban areas the vaccine is provided through hospitals, maternity homes and health centres, and in rural areas through PHC. Besides, many voluntary organizations have periodically helped in organizing immunization camps.

Despite the availability of adequate quantity of OPV, vaccination coverage is about 42% of the proposed target. However, this is not due to poor acceptability of the OPV but due to other factors which include :

(i) *Ignorance about the availability of the vaccine.*

(ii) *Inconvenient scheduling of the vaccination services.*

(iii) *Inadapt handling of the vaccine logistics by the health staff.*

(iv) *Poor mobilisation of community participation in immunization services.*

(v) *Poorly developed and frequent breaks in the cold-chain system.*

(vi) *Lack of initiative and drive on the part of the health staff to adapt vaccination strategies to suit situations and achieve targets. Besides other factors, like frequent power-cuts, which in many parts of the country have* become almost a daily feature would adversely affect potency of heat-sensitive vaccines which is normally stored in refrigerators in PHC's.

The current situation of polio vaccination is not very encouraging and now efforts are being made to ensure success of polio vaccination programme.

POLIO VACCINES

Q. 13.27. What do you know about Polio vaccine?

Polio vaccine is once again the news. There are two types of vaccines available : an *Inactivated* (killed) *Polio Vaccine* (IPV) or *Salk vaccine* and the other live attenuated (rendered safe) *Oral Polio Vaccine* (OPV), or *Sabin vaccine*. In 1955, Jonas Salk announced the development of his effective polio vaccine. Between 1953 and 1957, Sabin developed his vaccine. He thoroughly tested his vaccine on monkeys and human including himself and members of his family. Both the vaccines proved to be safe and highly effective. Though safe and effective vaccines have been available for the past 20 years, it is unfortunate that poliomyelitis continues to be a major public health problem in most countries of the world.

The *World Health Organisation* (WHO) recently recommends OPV for use in its expanded programme of immunisation (EPI) and it has been widely used in India. But endemic poliomyelitis has almost been eliminated in several countries with either OPV (e.g. the USA) or IPV (Finland, Sweden). There is no clear consensus about which type of vaccine is more effective, although most people would favour OPV because of its perceived ability to confer greater herd immunity. The contrary view that IPV exerts a profound herd immunity effect has been thoroughly reviewed and presented by Darell Salk.

Q. 13.28. What are the differences between Sabin and Salk vaccine of poliomyelitis?

*Comparison between OPV and IPV

Sabin Vaccine (OPV)	Salk Vaccine (IPV)
1. Live attenuated virus.	1. Killed formalised virus.
2. Administered orally as "Drops".	2. Given intramuscularly or subcutaneously as an injection.
3. Induces both intestinal (local) and humoral (circulating) antibodies.	3. Induces only circulating antibodies.
4. Prevents intestinal infection by wild polio virus.	4. Does not prevent intestinal infection by wild strains.
5. Highly effective in controlling epidemics.	5. Not helpful in controlling epidemics.
6. Cheap (about 50 paise per dose).	6. Expensive-about 10 times costlier than OPV.
7. One of the most heat-sensitive.	7. Relatively heat-stable.

XII. TUBERCULOSIS

Q. 13.29. What is Tuberculosis ?

Tuberculosis is a specific communicable disease caused by the acid fast bacillus Mycobacterium tuberculosis. The germs may be of human, bovine or avian variety.

(a) The *human variety* mainly affects the lungs, but may also occur in any part of the body i.e. from the skin to the bones.

(b) The *bovine variety* is more common in cattles. The milk of tuberculosis cows, goats etc. may produce bovine type of tuberculosis in the intestinal glands. However in India, bovine strain is not noticed either in pulmonary or non-pulmonary tuberculosis lesions. Human variety of tuberculosis can affect cattle or other animal.

(c) The *avian variety* i.e. of birds are extremely rare in man. Thus, as per as India is concerned the infection is by human variety of tuberculosis. KOCH discovered the bacillus in 1982. It is also known as *phthisis* which is a Greak word meaning "I waste". In tuberculosis, the persons get eirly tired, there is loss of appetite, loss of weight, evening rise of temperature, pain in chest, suppressed cough due to pain, and coughing of blood in sputum in the chronic stage.

Q. 13.30. How do the diseases spread ?

OR

What are the modes of infection of the disease Tuberculosis.

Generally the disease tuberculosis spreads by (i) *Inhalation*, (ii) *ingestion* and (iii) *direct implatation*.

Among these, inhalation is the commonest. Sputum of an open case is the greatest source of infection :

(1) So the disease mainly spreads by inhalation through '*droplets*' ejected during coughing, sneezing, laughing, yawning or by speaking loudly.

(2) *Droplet nuclei* i.e. dried sputum through 'dust' also transmit the disease.

(3) Tuberculosis is or also can spread by ingestion due to food, contaminated by tuberculosis germs from any infected person, or by flies or infected utensils etc. Consuming infected meal will also give rise to the disease by ingestion.

(4) Sometimes inoculation into the skin and mucous membrane (during injection) causes transmission of disease.

There is no carriers, and the germs do not form spores. Even then the germs are very hardy and can remain in the dust for months. But by whichever method the germs enter into the body, ultimately through lymphatics it enters into the blood stream. The phagocytes engulf the germ and usually the primary lesion heal, but the regional lymph glands remain as reservoir of infection for many years. In 5% of the cases the lesions do not heal. The brunt of infection falls on the lungs and hence the pulmonary tuberculosis is the most common.

COMMUNICABLE DISEASES 341

Q. 13.31. How can we control and prevent the disease Tuberculosis ?

The prevention and control of the disease Tuberculosis generally done by the following measures :

(1) Measures to raise the general resistance by :
   a) *Improvement of standard of living.*
   b) *B.C.G. vaccination.*

(2) Measures to reduce infection by :
   a) *Case finding and investigation of contacts.*
   b) *Isolation of patients.*
   c) *Dis-infection and proper disposal of sputum etc.*
   d) *Treatment—Chemotherapy and antibiotics.*
   e) *Chemoprophylaxis.*
   f) *Rehabilitation.*
   g) *Health education.*

1. Measures to raise the general resistance :

(a) *Improvement of the standard of living :*

This involves improvement of socio—economic conditions, with better housing, better nutrition and facilities for rest and recreation etc. which are generally done by :

   i) Improving the quality of food.
   ii) Pasteurisation of milk.
   iii) Antifly campaign.
   iv) Destroy food exposed to flies and dust.
   v) Inspection of meat.
   vi) Well lighted, well ventilated, damp proof rooms.
   vii) Broad roads, parks, play-grounds are the "lungs of the town".
   viii) Industries to be away from residence. Stone crushing, glass manufacturing, sand blasting, textile mills, coal mining industries etc. are of special importance as they are the important prediposing causes of tuberculosis.

(b) ***B.C.G. Vaccination :

As immunisation is done to a person who has no germs of tuberculosis in the body, hence immunisation is done to the infants within first 7 days of birth by B.C.G. vaccine and then again at the age of 5 years. The older children may be immunised by B.C.G. after tuberculin (i.e. Mantoux) test. Positive mantoux test suggest, that there are germs of tuberculosis in the person and B.C.G. vaccination is not to be done.

** B.C.G.

B.C.G. means *Bacillus Calmette Guerine*. (According to the name of its discoverer Drs. Calmette and Guerine the two French scientists, who subcultured a bovine tubercle bacillus in bile-potato medium continuously for a period of 14 years (1908-1921). It is a living bovine stain of tuberculous bacilli, whose power has been attenuated by growing the germs in bile for years. *B.C.G. contain attenuated live tuberculosis germs freeze dried vaccine*, B.C.G. vaccination is generally given intradermally in the skin of the arm, just below the shoulder joint. The strength of the vaccine is generally 0.5. to 1.0 mgm. per ml. The dose is 0.1. ml. containing 0.075 mgm. B.C.G. or made up freeze-dried vaccine is given intradermally to all successive persons. Within 10-14 days an induration develops at the site of inoculation, which increases gradually into nodule with pus formation leading to an ulcer. This heals within about 4 weeks leaving a scar. the vaccinated person becomes tuberculin positive within 10-12 weeks after vaccination so immunity against tuberculosis is produced.

2. **Measures to reduce infections :**

(a) *Notification* :

1. Tuberculosis is a notifiable disease so early detection of cases and investigation of contacts is the first and most important to control tuberculosis. It is generally done by clinical symptoms, routine X-ray examination, sputum test, tuberculin and mass x-ray examination. This is supplemented by investigation of contacts by physical examination and X-ray so that

suspects can be given prophylactic treatment and the non-tuberculin reactors protected by B.C.G. vaccination.

(b) *Isolation of patients* :

Isolation is a need for infective cases till they are bacteria free by drug treatment. This may be done at home by nursing supervision, strict personal hygiene, disinfection of sputum and covering nose and mouth in coughing and sneezing, indiscriminate spitting should be completely prohibited.

Generally the patients should have separate room, separate spoons, cups, etc. Spitting is in a spittoon containing 5% *carbolic acid solution*. They should avoid to come in contact with children or kiss the children and they should take treatment regularly.

(c) *Disinfection and proper disposal of sputum etc.* :

Sputum should be collected in covered spittoon containing *phenol* or *5% carbolic acid solution*, and should be disposed off by burning in fire or burying it deep into the soil. Articles including hankerchiefs, cloth and eating utensils should be regularly disinfected by boiling water. Bedding should be exposed to sun. Concurrent disinfection of room is done with 2% phenyl. The room is mopped. Sweeping is avoided as it will cause infected dust to fly in the air and spread infection.

(d) *Treatment with antibiotics and chemotherapeutics drugs* :

The specific antimicrobial therapy of tuberculosis has opened a new avenue for the control of tuberculosis. The object is to render the infected cases or non-infectious as quickly as possible and thereby cut down the transmission of infection. The cases must be treated adequately for a sufficiently long duration, atleast for minimum period of one year.

Generally proper chemotherapy can cure more than 90 percent cases. Improper or irregular treatment leads to drug resistance.

** Generally the drugs are used classified into two groups : namely—'first line' or standard or major drugs, and the 'second line' or minor or reserve drugs. The first line drugs are *Isoniazid or INH, streptomycin, paramino salicylic acid or PAS and Theacetazone (TH)* and the second line drugs are *Ethionamide, pyrazinamide, cycloserine etc.* First line drugs are used in case of newly diagnosed cases and second line drugs are used for so called drug failure cases.

(e) *Chemoprophylaxis :*

Contacts and suspected are treated with antitubercular drugs to prevent development of T.B. Isoniazide i.e. INH is the drug of choice. The dosage recommended is 10 mg./kg., generally given for a period of one year. Young close contacts of known infectious cases, new borne babies sucked by tuberculosis mothers, hyperallergic individuals giving false reaction, silicotic and siderotic miers may be given this chemoprophylatic treatment.

**Chemoprophylaxis and vaccination are complementary and can be used simultaneously with vaccination.*

[Dr. Kent has suggested *Tuberculinium* 200, 1M and 10M at intervals of a month, three doses of each potency causes immunity to tuberculosis.]

(f) *Rehabilitation :*

Rehabilitation is needed for those cases that are not enable to treatment but are infectious and others who though cured, have been crippled or disabled as a result of disease and are not capable of carrying on their old occupation. Such cases are rehabilitated by providing them an alternative occupation in the public or private sector. Some of them can be rehabilitated in rehabilitation colonies.

(g) *Health education and promotion :*

(1) Health education is given to the patients as how to avoid being a source of infection to others, how to ensure a healthy and sanitary living.

COMMUNICABLE DISEASES

(2) Health education is given to the public regarding the disease process i.e. its aetiology, source of infection, methods of prevention etc., through talking, postering or cinema show etc.

Mainly advice are given to :

(i) Put handkerchief over the mouth when coughing or sneezing.

(ii) Don't spit indiscriminately.

(iii) Spit in spittoon containing 5% carbolic lotion.

(iv) Children are not to be allowed to go near a person suffering from tuberculosis.

(v) The patient is isolated and concurrent disinfection of the room, clothes, spoons etc. are to be done.

(vi) As the poverty i.e. malnutrition, ill lighted, ill ventilated, over crowded, damp room (which lack of sunshine) are the predisposing factors to prevent and controlling disease; good food, fresh air, sunshine are utmost important; pardah system is not healthy system, avoidance of smoking and drink alcohol are important.

(vii) Health promotion is generally done by creating a suitable environment based on the personal and family hygiene and general well-being of the community. The standard of living, education, economic status and social security should be raised. The general resistance of the community should be improved by adequate and balanced diet, good housing and good sanitary environment.

Q. 13.32. What would be the preventive measures in industrial establishments.

1. Proper housing with sanitary arrangement for the workers.
2. Proper location of industries and placements of machine in the factories.

3. Tuberculin testing and B.C.G. vaccination of the susceptible rural recruits.
4. Arrangement for early detection and domiciliary treatment for the diseased. This can be well-organised as the community involved is compact and under better control.

N.B. : Tuberculosis in the rural areas can be largely controlled by controlling the disease in the industrial areas as workers are mostly drawn from the rural areas and those who are attacked with tuberculosis return to the village spread the infection. Even control of tuberculosis being ordinarily difficult in rural areas in comparasion to urban, rural and collieries.

Q. 13.33. What are the homoeopathic views about this disease ?

Tuberculosis can be acquired or inherited. In a case where it is acquired, syphilis will be traced at same stage. Inheritence presupposes susceptibility.

Homoeopathy regards tuberculosis as flared up psora. Some regard syphilitic miasm as also bonded with psora.

Syphilis in a parent means tuberculosis in the children. Thus *syphilis plus psora from the miasmatic constitution of tuberculosis.*

Treatment :

Kent has given a positive curative course for children susceptible to tuberculosis, and that is *Tuberculinum bovinum —1M, 1OM, CM, two doses of each to be administered at long intervals.* In a patient suffering from tuberculosis, tuberculinum alone is seldom curative, although it may be a intercurrent medicine. The useful medicines are (choose according to symptoms) :

Ars alb, Cal carb, Cal phos, Hep, Iodium, Kali carb, Lyco, Phos, Sangunaria, Sep, Silicia, Spongia, Stanum, Sulph etc.

COMMUNICABLE DISEASES

Q. 13.34. Describe the National Tuberculosis Control Programme.

1. Main objectives :

i) To deal with the tuberculosis problem through integrated health services.

ii) To arrange for detection and treatment of all definite cases of tuberculosis with a view to decrease the pool of infection.

iii) To cover the entire country with B.C.G. vaccination of susceptible population to protect them from the danger of uncontrolled infection.

Basic principles :

The basic principles of the National Programme for the Control of Tuberculosis are :

(1) To give B.C.G. *vaccination* to healthy children below the age of 19 years without doing "Tuberculin test".

(2) *Sputum examination* is to be done at any primary health centre, if there is a microscope at the centre.

(3) *Domicillary treatment* of Tuberculosis cases by INH and PAS or INH and Thiacetazone (TH).

(a) In the Rural Areas :

i) **At District level**, the patients are diagnosed by X-ray and sputum examination and free drugs are given for 18 months.

ii) **At Block level**, the district tuberculosis centre trains the staff of P.H.C. regarding the method of collection and staining of sputum and giving anti-tuberculosis drugs.

iii) **B.C.G. team**—They carry out B.C.G. vaccination to healthy children under the age of 19 years. The schools are also covered up by this staff.

iv) **Sanitary inspector** has also a role for controlling T.B. He can collect sputum, prepare smear and stains. He distributes medicines to the patients. He motivates the patients for taking full treatment. He helps B.C.G. team by advance publicity in village. He also gives health education.

v) **Health education :**

(1) Tuberculosis spreads from person to person by coughing.
(2) Children are more susceptible.
(3) Children can easily be protected by B.C.G.
(4) The tuberculosis person should cover his mouth when coughing.
(5) He should spit in spitton containing 5% carbolic lotion.
(6) Tuberculosis can be treated at home effectively.
(7) Every patient must take treatment for at least 18 months.
(8) All persons having fever and cough for more than two weeks, must get themselves checked at the nearest PHC.

(b) In the Metropolitan Cities, there is a network of chest clinics with facilities for diagnosis, treatment, domiciliary services and B.C.G. vaccination programme, under one T.B. centre. There is one clinic for a population of about 2 *lakhs*. At each municipal of government maternity homes, the infant is given B.C.G. vaccination before the mother leaves the maternity home.

Q. 13.35. What is meant by housing ? What are the basic principles and fundamental needs of housing ?

Housing : Next to food men's primary quest is shelter. *La-corbusier*, the famous French architect defined house as a "machine to live in". According to WHO housing is *"the physical structure that man uses for shelter and the envious of that structure including all necessary services, facilities, equipment and devices needed or desired for the physical and mental health, social well being of the family and individual.*

COMMUNICABLE DISEASES

Principles and needs : *So the basic principles and the fundamental major needs of healthful housing are :*

(1) Fundamental physiological needs.
(2) Fundamental psychological needs.
(3) Protection against weather conditions.
(4) Protection against contagion and infection.
(5) Protection against animal attacks, insects and accidents.
(6) Maintenance of privacy and security of life and property.
(7) Attainment of efficiency and comfort of living.

Also housing has an intimate relationship with health and it influences morbidity and mortality in an indirect way. More than 50 percent of the day's period is spent in homes and more so for house-wives, children and women-folks. It is a family abode and all the functions of the family, e.g. biological, social, religious and cultural are performed here to make into a *"sweet home".*

Q. 13.36. What are the essential components of a good house ?

The essential components of good house are :

Living rooms according to number of inmates, drawing room, store room, kitchen and dining room, bath room, good water supply, safe and sanitary latrine, open space and yard, kitchen, garden, and trees, fire protection devices and security measures; (and cattle shed and tanks, if possible).

XIII. SMALLPOX AND CHICKEN POX

Q.13.37. What is Smallpox ?

It is highly contagious viral disease with diphasic febrile episodes accompanied typical skin eruption caused by Variola virus.

Characteristics : The onset of the disease is sudden with predormal symptoms of fever, malaise, headache, abdominal pain and prostration, ordinarily of 3-4 days duration with limits of 1-5 days. The temperature then falls commonly to normal. The eruption appears on the third day of illness and pass through successive stages of *macules, papules, vesicles* and *pustules* and finally *scabs* which fall off about the end of third week leaving a scar. The lesions are deeper seated than those of chicken pox. *The key to identifications* is the distribution of the lesions. This is usually symmetrical and general, more profuse of irritated areas, prominences and extensor surfaces than on the protected areas, depressions and flexure. Most abundant and earliest on the face, next on forearms, and wrists and favouring the limbs than trunk ; more abudant on shoulders and chest than on joints or abdomen. Lesions are sometimes so few as to be overlooked. Synonym : **Variola.**

It is of three types:

(a) *Haemorrhagic variety* : Where the vesicles contain blood and there is bleeding from the nose, intestine etc. It is usually fatal.

(b) *Coufluent variety* : Where several vesicles are combined. It is also often fatal.

(c) *Discrete variety* : Which are the usual cases.

Q.13.38. What is the usual course of Smallpox ?

1. *The usual course of the disease unmodified by vaccination is as follows :*

After an incubation period of 12 days, there is sudden rise of fever with severe backache and headache. The fever becomes down on *third day* and *macular* spots appear. In 2 to 3 days, it becomes *papule* in the skin. After 3 days it becomes multilocular umbilicated vesicle. After 3 days it becomes pustule. Then there is secondary rise of temperature and the patient may die or after 12 days scab forms. After a further period of 12 days or so the scabs fall off.

2. *The course of the disease modified by vaccination is as follows :*

The incubation period of smallpox is usually 12 days but it may vary from 5 to 21 days depending on the partial

COMMUNICABLE DISEASES

immunity existing in the person or due to the virulence of the germs. The infective period is from the day of onset of the fever, till the last scale falls off.

Differences Between Smallpox and Chickenpox

Small pox and *Chicken pox* are both diseases in which virus enters by the respiratory route, multiplies in the internal organs, and at the height of infection, causes a rash on the skin. The rashes are at a first glance similar. In each the first thing seen is a flat spot, or *macule*; this changes into a clear blister, or *vesicle*; the contents become turbid, and the blister is then called a *pustule*. The pustule dries up, forming a *scab*, and the scab separats, leaving a *scar*, or *pock*. Although the diseases are similar, there are *two great differences*.

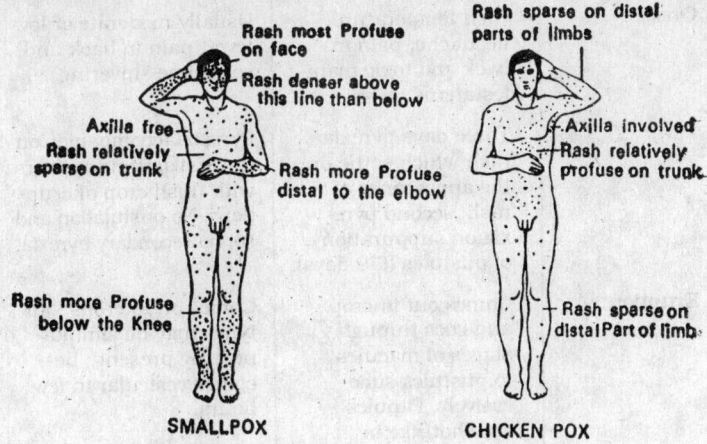

Difference between smallpox and chickenpox

In *Chicken pox* the rash is heaviest on the trauk and on the upper part of the limbs; it has a centre-seeking, or *centripetal* distribution. In Smallpox the rash is heaviest on the face and on the lower parts of the limbs; its distribution is *centre-freeing*, or *centrifugal*. The other fundamental difference is in the rate of progression from macule to pock.

In *Chicken pox* the progression is so rapid that the early stages are often not noticed; with in a few hours, the macules have changed to vesicles, and by the end of 24 hours the first scabs have appeared.

In *Small pox* a macule takes three days to change to a vesicle, and it is eight days before the first scab is formed.

No one can say why the two rashes behave so differently, but it is fortunate that they do, for it is usually possible to diagnose the two disease by examination of the rash. The viruses can be distinguished in the laboratory.

Q. 13.39. What are the differentes between Small pox and Chicken pox.

Differential Characters of Smallpox and Chickenpox

		Small pox	Chicken pox
1.	Prodormata	Severe	Slight or absent
2.	Onset	High temperature, headache, pain in back and toxic manifestations.	Usually moderate or low fever, pain in back and sometime shivering.
3.	Fever	Three days pyrexia rash which settle on the appearance of rash; second pyrexia on suppuration of pustules (6-9 days).	Pyrexia accompanies on the first day and appears with fresh crop of eruptions. No pustulation and so, no secondary pyrexia.
4.	Eruption	Comes out in crop and goes through stages of macules to pustules successively. Papules are shot-like in hardness, deep seated, becomes vesicular on 5th or 6th day of illness.	Comes on in crops; all types may be simultaneously present; becomes vesicular in few hours.
5.	Distribution of rash.	*Centrifugal spots,* are abudant on the face, forearms, wrists and palm than on abdomen, chest and loins; affects extensor surfaces generally.	*Centripetal, spots are* copious on the chest and abdomen and fever on face, affects flexor surfaces generally.

	Small pox	Chicken pox
6. Character of eruption.	Centre of vesicle umbilicated.	Centre of the vesicle is rounded.
7. Complications or sequelae.	Likely to have severe complications and sequelae. Even death is 50% to 80%	Nil or very rare. Death is practically nil.
8. Skin scar	Eruptions leave pits, often dee and cause permanant disfiguration.	Pitting occasional and slight as a rule. No permanent disfiguration.

N.B. : Vaccination prevents small pox but vaccination will not prevent Chicken pox.

Q. 13.40. What are the methods that the family members should adopt to prevent and to spread of small pox when a child of their family is suffering from this disease?

Preventive measures are to be considered in two main headings :

        I. General Measures.

        II. Specific Measures.

I. General Measures

    (A) During Attack of an Individual :

    1. *Early diagnosis :*

This is the first step for checking the spread. After diagnosis the drugs are administered to ally headache, backache, chill and fever. But there is no specific drug yet found effective. During the erruptive stage and removal of crusts, symptomatic treatment by homoeopathic medicine is more effective. Nursing care is also more essential.

    2. *Other measures :*

Other measures like (i) Prompt notification, (ii) Isolation of the case, (iii) Surveillance of contacts for 12 days ; (iv) Disinfection room with 10% formaline or formaldehyde and other articles, (v) Contact and mass immunisation, and (vi) Antifly measures are done which are *same as follows during a outbreak of smallpox epidemics.*

[Also see *Q. no.—13.41*]

Q. 13.41. How we can prevent the spread of Small pox in a village ?

Preventive measures are to be considered in the two headings :

            I. General Measures.
           II. Specific Measures.

I. General Measures

(A) During Attack of an Individual

Early diagnosis of treatment :

This is the first step for checking the spread of small pox. Clinical diagnosis is easy when the cases are large but difficulty arises when the cases are few. Laboratory methods for diagnosis of small pox should be adopted. Generally after diagnosis the drugs are administered to ally headache, backache, chill and fever. But there is no specific (allopathic) drugs yet found effective. During the eruptive stage and removal of crusts symptomatic treatment by homoeopathic medicine is more effective. Isolation of the patient nursing care, disinfection of room, clothes etc. are also more essential.

(B) During an Outbreak

During an outbreak of small pox the principles measures which should be followed are :

    1. *Notification.*
    2. *Isolation.*
    3. *Surveillance of contacts and personal protection.*
    4. *Disinfection.*
    5. *Care of the corpses.*
    6. *Mass immunisation.*
    7. *Health education.*
    8. *Other measures like—Quarantine and other legal measures.*

1. Notification

During the outbreak of smallpox prompt reporting is absolutely essential to health authorities locally, nationally and internationally.

2. Isolation

Then the patient and suspected person should be transfered to a smallpox hospital or an isolation hospital or isolated room in a home until all scabs are separated from the body. Generally the room is darkened with red light and the patient is kept under mosquitos curtain. Persons attending must be well protected by vaccination and revaccination.

3. Surveillance of contacts and personal protection

Besides being vaccinated, physicians and nurses, neighbours or visitors or well wisher when visiting a smallpox patient should wear a long over all fitting cloth along the wrist and neck. After visit they should change their clothes or garments. Then these garments and clothes should be immediately removed and placed in a airtight receptacle and disinfected with formline vapour. The hands should be thoroughly washed with soaped water and then again washed in some strong antiseptic solution. Generally all persons who have come in contact of the patient without vaccination should be vaccinated unless they should be kept under surveillance for 21 days after the last contact of the patient.

4. Disinfection

(a) *Sick room :*

The contagion of smallpox harbours in carpets, beddings, clothings etc. and therefore these and all unnecessary furniture and other articles which are capable for harbouring infection should be taken out of the sick room. Articles or furniture that have already been exposed to infection, should not be removed unless these are disinfected. The room should be ventilated, 10% solution of formaline may be advantageous if it is kept in the sick room in a vessel. Generally rooms are disinfected by fumigation with formaldehyde or sulphur vapour for 6 hours. The room may also be washed copiously with soap and water and left for 48 hours and exposed to a direct sunlight for several hours.

(b) Clothes and linen should be boiled or stem sterilised. All scabs should be collected and burnt.

(c) As the nose and throat are liable to harbour the virus of smallpox, so they should as far as possible be cleansed and the throat gargled with some disinfectant.

(d) Case of convalescents— No person after recovery from smallpox should be allowed to go out and receive visitors until every scab, crust and scale has disappeared and there is no sore on the body. The hair should be carefully brushed to remove all particles adhering to the scalp and the whole body should then be thoroughly washed with soap and water. The convalescent may have a bath with some antiseptic lotion and clothing should be thoroughly disinfected.

So disinfections both concurrent and terminal of patient's excreta and used material are essential.

5. *Care of corpses* (or care of the dead body) :

All persons dead from smallpox should be wrapped in sheaths soaked in 40% solution of formaline and should be burnt or buried without any delay.

6. *Mass immunisation* :

For the control of spreading smallpox mass immunisation by vaccination is the best and is known as specific measures.

So the specific measures which are adopted to control and prevent the spread of smallpox are immunisation. It is of two types : (i) *Active* and (ii) *Passive*.

(i) *Active immunisation*—by vaccination is the oldest immunisation method adopted in public health work and is most effective in protecting the susceptables and in controlling the spread of the disease in the community.

(ii) *Passive immunisation*—with antivacinial gamma globuin is used only in a limited measure but is specially valuable in protection of risk groups e.g.

Hypo-gamma globulinaemia. Beta-thiosemi carbazon was found in the field trial at madras to be effective in preventing the development of smallpox to persons exposed to the diseases but is not safe for general use. Homoeopathic medicine—*Variolinum, Malandrinum* and *Vaccininum* used as a oral vaccination and act as a both preventive and curative in case of smallpox.

7. *Health education :*

In India people have some superstitious beliefs and practices in respect of smallpox, arising out of severity of the disease and absence of specific treatment. There are some people who are concientious objectors of vaccination. A regular health education compaign through audiovisual and other methods like handbill, public pamphlets etc. are highly desirable. They should know how to protect themselves against smallpox.

PREVENTIVE MEASURES IN BOTH NATIONAL AND INTERNATIONAL LEVEL

1. Quarantine

Under International sanitary regulations of a traveller who comes from or has passed through an infected area should have a valid smallpox vaccination certificate. If the person is not vaccinated and refuses, a quarantine period of 16 days is reasonable safe guard against the spread of infection. So seaport quarantine procedure is compulsory vaccination of persons moving out of endemic areas or infected seaport is best for preventing smallpox. The validity of International certificates of vaccination extends for 3 years after successful primary vaccination and is effective from 8 days after vaccination or revaccination.

2. Lagislation (Legal measures)

An appropriate legislation for compulsory vaccination and revaccination with necessary powers to the health authorities to take action should be promulgated by the central legislature to be uniformly.

II. Vaccination in Case of Smallpox

Smallpox vaccination means the introduction of cowpox germs (i.e. vaccina virus) in man.

Q. 13.42. What are reactions to primary vaccination ?

Generally the reaction of *primary vaccination* are follows :

1. After inoculation of cowpox virus, on third day a papule appears.

2. On 5th day it becomes multilocular umbilicated vesicle with areola. Upto 10th day the areola increase in size. There is fever from 5th to 10th day, and the fever becomes normal by 13th day.

3. On 11th day the vesicle become cloudy but not purulent.

4. By 13th day scab is formed. the scab falls off by 21st day. Such successful primary vaccination affords protection against smallpox for 5 years. The multilocular, umbilicated vesicle with areola on 8th day is stated as successful primary "take".

In case of revaccination the papules occurs on 2nd day and the vesicle subside within 5 to 7 days. In immune persons, papule occur on the 18th day, and fades away in 3 days.

[N.B.—*As per International Sanitary Regulation, revaccination against smallpox is held valid for 3 years only.*]

Q.13.43. What is the age for primary vaccination ?

The usual age for primary vaccination is within 3 months of birth, but as the children are highly susceptible to smallpox, neonatal vaccination has been started. (The Ministry of Health in England in 1962 has stated that the "preferable age for vaccination is second year" due to the risk of post vaccinal encephalitis amongst infants.

Q. 13.44. What are the contra indication for vaccination ?

COMMUNICABLE DISEASES

1. Do not vaccine if the person has fever or skin disease or within 3 months of pregnancy.

2. Persons suffering from asthma or other allergic conditions should be de-sensitized before vaccination is given.

*Causes of failure of vaccination :

(i) If the vaccinated part is kept to the rays of the sun.
(ii) Using the needles when they are still hot.
(iii) The prick is too superficial.
(iv) The potency of lymph is lost.

Q. 13.45. In what parts of the body or where the vaccination is done ? Give the technique of vaccination.

In infants, the usual site is the outer side of the arm or thigh. Revaccination is done on the forearm.

Technique :

1. Prepare the vaccine if it is freeze dry vaccine.
2. Clean the part with acetone or with warm water.
3. Dipthecool sterile bifurcate needle is used for vaccine.
4. For primary vaccination give 10-20 superficial punctures at one place. In revaccination give 15 superficial punctures at one place. The prepared freeze-dry vaccine is not to be used on the next day.

Q.13.46. What are the complications which occurred from vaccination ?

1. Normally in primary vaccination there will be fever and pain at the site of vaccination. Nothing should be applied. Only after the "take" sterile boric ointment, sandlewood or boroline may be applied around the vesicle, to prevent itching sensation.

2. Application of infected ointments or contamination of the vaccine lymph may give rise to tetanus or septic infection.

3. In some cases, local or generalised rash may occur within 10 days of vaccination. There is no cause for alarm and these rashes rapidly fades away.

4. *Post vaccinal encephalitis* may occur 1 : 2,00,000 primary vaccination mostly in infants. After 10 days the infant vomits and passes to coma. It may be a rare disease, but the death-rate is extremely high. The cause is still not known. It does not occur after re-vaccination.

5. *Generalised vaccination* is another dangerous disease. It occures after 10 days of vaccination. It may be due to vaccination done with skin disease or may be autoinoculation by scratching the vaccinated part and transfering the virus to other part of the body.

Q. 13.47. What is meant by vaccination ?

The term *'Vancination'* though originally applied to the method of immunization against smallpox, is a now a general term for producing active immunity artifically and the material used for vaccination called *'Vaccine'*.

Sir *Edward Jenner* in 1788, first pointed out that the inoculation of man with cowpox (vaccinia) cofers immunity from subsequent attacks of smallpox, in the same way that an attack of smallpox does to a patient. Since then many experiments were made to confirm these results and the practice of vaccination has become general. Where it is done on a person not previously vaccinated, it is called *primary vaccination*, and when it is done on a person who has been previously vaccinated it is called *secondary vaccination*.

Q. 13.48. What are the principle methods of vaccination ?

Generally smallpox vaccination is done by, (i) *puncture method*,(ii) *incision methods*, (iii) *scarification method* (iv) *rotary method*, (v) *multiple pressure method*. The number of insertions are three in case of primary and one in case of revaccination. They should be 1½ inches (38.10 mm) apart so as to prevent them from joining together. The part of the body where the vaccination is done in infants, the usual site is the outer side of the arms or thigh. Revaccination is done on the fore-arm. Besides this vaccinations are also done *intrademally* (B.C.G.), or *subcutaneously* (typhoid, plague, cholera etc.), injection or through the oral route (billi-vac-

COMMUNICABLE DISEASES

cine). In case of live attenuated virus or bacterial vaccine only a single inoculation is enough while in case of vaccine made of killed organism or toxoid generally multiple doses (atleast two), are needed e.g. typhoid, plague, cholera etc. though in emergencies only a single dose may be used. It takes a minimum of 7 to 8 days to detect the noticeable response, the optimum generally reacting weak after the second dose. In case of triple or polio vaccine three doses are necessary given at monthly intervals, the peak of immunity reacting the optimum is not earlier than the fourth month. The degree and duration of immunity vary considerably in different types of vaccines. Those made up to toxoid give more or less durable protection as in tetanus and diphtheria. With living attenuated organisms used as a vaccine the duration and quality of immunity is stronger and more lasting (e.g. smallpox, yellow fever, poliomyelitis etc.) and so is the natural active immunity compound to the artificial active immunity. A *'booster'* dose of vaccine i.e. vaccine at intervals of several months after the first application always enhances the immunity level against that particular antigen. (In case of smallpox it is called secondary or revaccination.)

Q.13.49. What are the bad effects of vaccinations and their curative Homoeopathic Medicines ? Or What are the complications of vaccinosis ?

The following are the bad effects or complications of vaccinosis and their remedies or currative medicines :

1. Fever—*Aconite* 30.
2. Pain, swelling, burning and stinging— *Apis mel* 30.
3. Septicemia—*Malandrinum* 200, *Pyrogenium* 30.
4. Unhealthy dry, scrufy or pustulating skin—*Malandrinum* 200 and *Gun powder* (6x).
5. Ersipelas—*Vaccinenum* 200.
6. Deep pits—*Variolenum* 200.
7. Large and angry looking vesicles, very painful with high fever—*Belladonna* 200.
8. Diarrhoea—*Antim tart* 30.

9. Irritation of the part during and after heating—*Sulph* 30.
10. Nervousness, impatience and irritability—*Vaccininum* 200.
11. Red pimples on various parts—*Vaccininum* 200.
12. Bilotches most evident when warm then restlessness—*Vaccininum* 200.
13. Flatulent dyspepsia— *Thuja occidentalis* 200.
14. Nuralgia— *Thuja* 200.
15. Extreme debility, sallow skin warts— *Thuja occidentalis* 200.
16. Incipient tuberculosis—*Tuberculinum* 200.
17. Abscess in axilla—*Silicea* 200 and *Kali mur* 30.
18. Conjunctivitis—*Silicea* 20.
19. Jaundice—*Cortalus horridus* 30.
20. Itch like eruption deriving the child of sleep—*Mezefum* 30.
21. Asthma—*Thuja occidentalis* 200.
22. Imbecility of mind—*Thuja occidentalis* 200.

XIV. MALARIA

Q. 13.50. What is malaria ?

Malaria (from Italian, "bad air") is one of the most serious environmental disease. Although it has nothing to do with bad air, it does rise from still bodies of water and spread across the surface of the land. Heat and cold, and the moisture of the air affect its movement, and even twilight, darkness, and dawn mark the rise and fall of this infection. But the cause of the disease is a unicellular parasites called *Plasmodium*, and it is conveyed to humans by the female *Anopheles* mosquito.

Malaria is a group of specific parasitic disease due to infection with any one of the four human species of sorozoa of the genus **plasmodium** *(P.vivox, P. ovale, P malariae, P. falciparum).*

Caused by the bite of an infective female anopheline mosquito, and is characterised principally by *intermittent fever* (recuring bouts of fever and shake the suffer with alternating shivering and sweating), *secondary anaemia and enlargement with cachexia supervening in untreated cases.* According to the rate in which asexual parasites multiply and berst out of the patient's red blood cells, these attacks may occur every day (*quotidian malaria*), every third day (*tertian malaria*), or every fourth day (*quartan malaria*); but often different cycles of sporulation are going on the person's RBC's at the same time, and the periodicity of the shivering attacks is blurred.

***Plasmodium falciparum* tends to sporulate in 36 rather than 48 hours, and the attacks come on more quickly than every *third day*; the disease is then called *subtertian malaria*, or more often because of its severity, malignant tertian. Malaria can mimic almost any other disease. The infected person becomes anaemic from loss of red blood cells and may be jaundice, have gastroenteritis, slow signs of bronchitis, have a hectic, continued fever, or even collapse and be cold, with no fever at all. Any ill person who may have been exposed to infection must be regarded as malaria until proved otherwise. In most persons the attacks come to an end even without treatment, though they recure latter. But when *P. falciparum* is the parasite, the fever is often mild for a day or two, with headache, aches and pains, and a little vomiting or diarrhoea, and then changes with treacherous suddenness to an overwhelming illness, with signs of liver, kidney or respiratory failure, or with coma from invasion and blocking of small blood vessels of the brain, a characteristic of cerebral malaria. Persons with these symptoms may die unless they can have the most urgent and skilful medical attention, and it is one of the tragedies of malaria, which is easily treatable, is so often not identified until the unmistakable but desperate stage of cerebral malaria sets in.

Q. 13.51. How malaria parasites are devlieoped ?

The *mosquito begins* its life as an *egg* deposited on water. The larva hatches out in two or three days and spends the next few weeks near the surface of the water. It feeds on micro-organisms in the water and breathes in oxygen from the atmosphere through a spiracle, or breathing office, at one end of its body. After molting four times it changes into *a pupa*, and from the pupa emerges after a few days the *adult mosquito*. The young mosquito floats for an hour or so on the

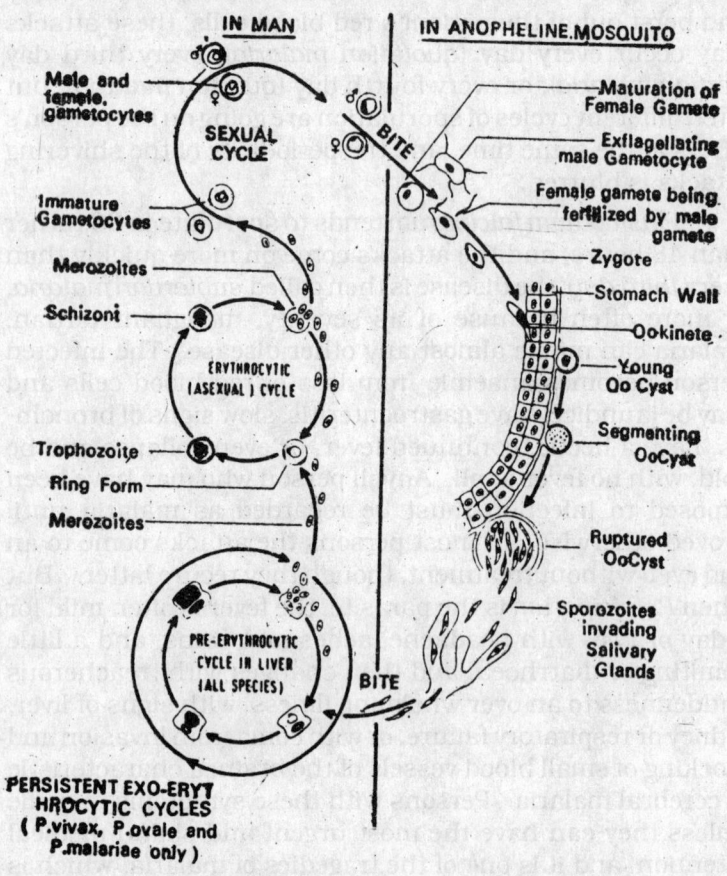

Life Cylee of Malaria Parasites

pupa case until its wings dry and harden, and it flies into the air, where the adult female is soon matted by a male. The pairs then separate, the male to seek plant juices as its food, the female to feed on human blood. She is armed with mouth parts, specially adapted for cutting into human skin which she pierces in her search for a blood vessels ; at the same time, she squirts some saliva into the wound. When she has had her fill of blood, she flies off to rest, but, if plasmodium, the malaria parasites, were present in her victim, some will have entered her stomach as she sucked the blood. The sexual forms of the parasite, *gametocytes*, mate in the mosquito's stomach, and the fertilized female gamete (sex cell) encysts in the stomach wall. After one to three weeks the cyst bursts open, and a large number of young sexual parasites, the *sporozoites*, emerge.

These find their way to the salivary glands of the mosquito, and the next time she bites she will inject some of these parasites into her victim. The parasites multiplying in the victim's liver for a week or so and spill into the blood stream, in the form called *merozoites*, and enter many of the red blood cells (R.B.C.). There they multiply, or sporulate, asexually; after two or three days they burst out of the red cells that they have destroyed and enter some more, repeating the cycle over and over again, detroying red blood cells each time. Eventually some sexual forms emerge, the gametocytes, they do not multiply or mate in the human body, but if the victim is bitten again, they get sucked into the mosquito's stomach, and the life cycle of the malaria parasites begins again.

Q.13.52. How we can prevent and control the disease malaria ?

OR

What measures are needed to prevent the spread of malaria ?

Malaria is not a *notifiable* disease, but it is helpful. Isolation, quarantine, and disinfection are of no value. There is also no immunization against malaria, however,prophylactic measures are sometime useful. But the general measures are most important and they are as follows :

Generally the prevention and control measures of malaria are divided into four main heads :

1. *Measures directed against the parasites and reservoirs of infections.*

2. *Measures directed against the vector species.*
3. *Measures directed against man-made malaria.*
4. *Control of man community i.e. health, education and other measures.*

1. Measures directed against the parasite and reservoir of the infection, or if a person suffering from malaria. (i.e with positive blood slide) :

It is done by treating the malaria parasites with various antimalarial drugs. Treatment in the acute stage of the disease destroys the parasites and prevent formation of gametocytes which play an essential role in the transmission of disease. However, practical experience made it clear that no drug in safe doses is fully effective against any parasite and malaria cannot be eradicated by distribution of drugs of malaria as a chemoprophylaxis.

2. Measures directed against the vector species (Antimosquito measures) :

A three prolonged attack is generally aimed out :

(A) *Anti larval.*
(B) *Anti adult.*
(C) *Protection from bites as a measure of personal protection.*

(A) Anti larval measures i.e. prevention of creating breeding places of mosquito.

It is done by (a) *Natural*, (b) *Mechanical* and (c) *Hydrotechnical methods.*

(a) Natural methods :

(i) Altering flora i.e. removal of *pistia*, growth of *wolffia, lemna, and azolla* inhibits anopheles breeding.

(ii) Altering exposure to sunlight or shading, as some species avoid sunlight and some species *(a.minimum)* shading.

(iii) Polluting by herbage packing, but there is danger of *culicine* breeding.

(b) Mechanical methods :
  (i) Screening, cleaning, channelling of water collections i.e. by providing proper drains to the natural flow of water.
  (ii) Proper drainage by the construction of open drains, subsoil drains etc.

(c) Hydrotechnical measures :

Flooding, agitating, stagnating, river training, impounding, sweetening or freshening, salinifying, intermittent drying, flushing, mudding the water etc. are appropriate antilarval measures for local situation and habitats of the mosquito species.

Inspite of above measures, if mosquitoes are breeding, then the larvae are killed by use of larvicidal oils, paris green, kerosene oil, D.D.T. or others by suffocating, toxic or drowning action.

Augmentation of natutual enemies particularly fish, such as *gambusia* which feed on larvae are also used.

(B) Adult Control

Inspite of antilarval measures if adult mosquitoes have emerged out, then they are killed by the following methods, namely :
  (i) *Destruction by hand*—by using hand nets or swalters.
  (ii) *Catching by trap*—different type of traps are used.
  (iii) *Fumigants*—sulphur burning, SO furmigants etc. only give temporary effects.
  (iv) *Spray killing.*
  (v) *Genetic control*— (recent advancement).

***Spray killing :

(a) *Systemic spray killing* of adult mosquito now the method of choice for malaria control and eradication measures. If the mosquito is destroyed within 10 days after the original blood feed, it cannot transmit malaria. The method of residual DDT spray has thus been devoid. Two substances which have been used for the purpose are *pyrethrum* and *D.D.T.* (Dichloro-Diphenyl-Trichloroethane) with kerosene, recently commercially it is known as Flit. i.e. 3 ounces of 4% pyrethrum + 1 ounce D.D.T. + 1 gallon kerosene oil.

(b) *Gammexane* (BHC or Benzyl Hexa-Chloride) are also used for spray killing of adult mosquitoes but it is not as effective as D.D.T.

*(Generally spray operation with synthetic insecticides is done according to the well-defined time schedules, usually two rounds of spray operation each with 100 mgm D.D.T. per square feet are given on the inner side of the walls of human and cattle dwellings).

****Genetical control :

Genetical control of mosquitoes are now in the experimental stages. There are several theories like radiation theory, incompatibility theory, gene control theory etc. Examples :

(i) If some male mosquitoes are caught and made sterile by radiation and then they are set free. The theory is that the female mosquitoes with whom such sterile males mate, also become sterile.

(ii) As per incompatibility theory, certain male mosquitoes of one area are incompatible with female mosquitoes of another area. The mating of such males with incompatible female mosquitoes will make the female mosquitoes sterile.

(But these are on experimental level.)

(C) Protection From Bites

Inspite of killing mosquitoes if still there are mosquitoes then prevention from being bitten by mosquitoes are done by mosquitoes nets, mosquito proof rooms or by application of mosquito repellants like *eucalyptus oil, citromella oil, sandle wood oil, di-methyl-phthalate, dibutyl-phthalate, odomos* etc.

3. Control of man and man-made malaria :

As now the man-made malaria are prevalent (specially in Calcutta i.e. West Bengal), recently the best way to control malaria in situations created by man is to anticipate such happening before any project is undertaken. In this field both engineers and medical men should work in intimate cooperation. The main principle would be :

(a) Prevention of erection of borrow pits, brick field and quarry pits.

(b) Clearance of jungle may have adverse effect in regard to malaria.

(c) Embankment across the line of drainage may be allowed if a natural drainage is maintained by bridges and channels.

(d) In constructing of roads, highways and railways, the borrow pits created should be provided with proper drainage.

(e) In the construction of dams and barrage care should be taken to avoid leakage, see-pages and overflow and if they occur their collection and drainage provision should be maintained so long as the danger of malaria exists.

(f) Similar precautions should be taken in the irrigation system (or in Metro rail of Calcutta) in which accumulation of water in low lying areas and depression should be prevented subsoil drainage with proper outfall should be established if water logging ensues.

4. Control of man and community :

Health education :

(a) Isolation and quarantine of gametocyte carriers and segregation of healthy individuals away from the infected have only limited value. But health education on personal and community health and on the basic appreciation of sanitation and cleanliness and as the causation, transmisson, and prevention of malaria is a great helpful in prevention and control of malaria.

(b) Prevent being bitten by mosquitoes by driving away the mosquitoes by burning "*katal*" or similar products and use of mosquito repellants like "*odomos*" etc. and finally by the use of mosquito nets are the basic health education.

5. Other measures :

Legislation to provide adequate power to health authorities to take antimalaria measures and to impose certain responsibilities on people themselves not to undertake any action which will increase mosquito are necessary.

Conclusion :

Thus the prevention of malaria can be tackled in two main ways :

(i) *By trying to break contract between humans and mosquitoes.*

(ii) *By administering drugs to persons exposed to bites to prevent the onset of the disease.*

The mosquito can be attacked in the larval and adult stage. Antimalaria drugs, if taken regularly, prevent the onset of the disease. But malaria prasites resistant to drugs have appeared in several malarious areas. Combinations of old and new drugs have been tried to combat this, more than 100,000 possible drugs have been listed in the allopathy along in the search for an effective one. The struggle against malaria is not over. However with the aid of WHO and other international agencies, India has attained conspicions success in the National Malaria Eradication programme since 1953, but still it needs to be followed up by vigilance and concerted efforts to carry out the maintenance phase properly.

Malaria National Eradication Programme

1. Objectives :

1. To prevent deaths due to malaria.
2. To maintain the green and industrial revolutions.
3. To consolidate the gains achieved so far.

COMMUNICABLE DISEASES

2. Services :

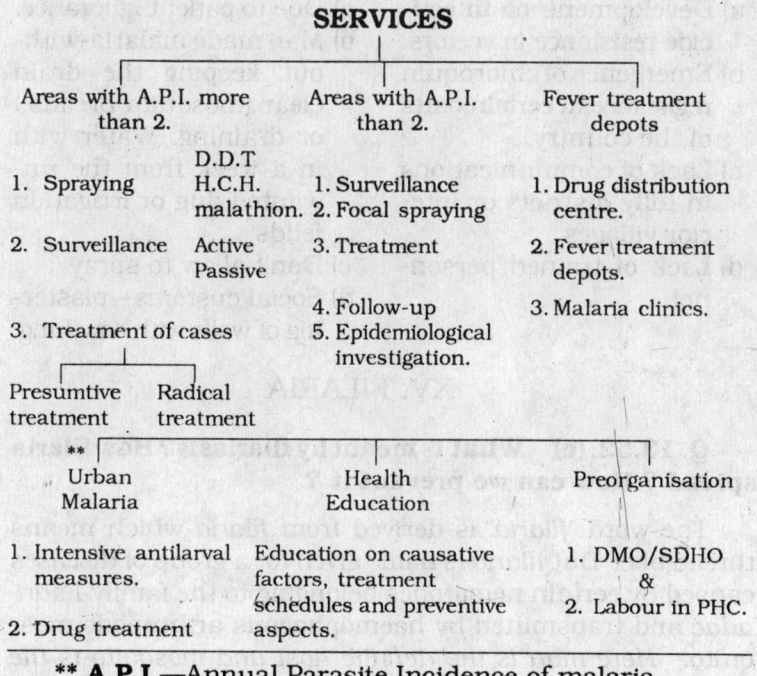

** **A.P.I.**—Annual Parasite Incidence of malaria.

$$A.P.I. = \frac{\text{Confirmed cases during year}}{\text{Population under surveillance}} \times 1,000$$

Q. 13.52. (b) What are the causes of reappearance or setback of malaria in India ?

Causes of Reappearance or Setback of Malaria

Administrative
(a) Shortage of insecticide
(b) Shortage of man power
(c) Shortage of finance
(d) High price of insecticide

Operational
(a) Lack of sufficient transport
(b) Migration of labour population.
(c) Habits of new-plastering of houses.
(d) Refusal of spraying on religious grounds.

Technical

Social

Technical	Social
a) Development of infecticide resistance in vectors.	a) Due to patient ignorance.
b) Emergence of chloroquin registance in certain parts of the country.	b) Man made malaria-without keeping the drain clear (mosquito breads,) or draining. Water with in a week from the unwanted dug or irrigation feilds.
c) Lack of communications in hilly districts or interior villages.	c) Don't allow to spray.
d) Lack of trained personnel.	d) Social customs—plastering of walls with cowdung.

XV. FILARIA

Q. 13.52. (c) What is meant by filariasis? How filaria spread ? How can we prevent it ?

The word '*filaria*' is derived from *filaria* which means thread like. But *filaria* is name given for a group of diseases caused by certain nematodes belonging to the family *Filariadae* and transmitted by haemophagous arthropods mosquito. *Here man is the definite host and mosquito is the intermediate host.* In India only known vectors of filariasis are *Culex fatigans* for brancroftian filariasis and *Mansonoides* for B. malayi infection.

Generally in India, the term filariasis commonly used to designate the disease caused by *Wucheria bancrofti* and *Brugia malayi* which are the parasites found in India. The disease is characterised by both acute and chronic clinical manifestations, e.g. lymphangitis, lymphadenitis, filarial fever, elephantiasis of the genitals, legs or arms, hydrocele etc. though this disease is not fatal but responsible for prolong suffering and desiability. characterised

*Main difference between Bancroftian and B.malayi :

Genital lesions are rare or absent in *B.malayi* infection, but genital lesions like hydrocele, elephantiasis of scrotum or penis and the mamnae in addition to elephantiasis of the extremities are common in bancroftian infection. But in both cases the lower extremities are affected more than the upper limbs.

Transmission or spreading of the disease filarisis :

Culex fatigans and Mansonides mosquitoes are the only known vectors of filariasis in India. The sources of infection are cases and carriers. The microfilariae are present in lymphatics and glands of the infected persons. The lymph containing the microfilaria reach the circulation and are picked up by the female mosquitoes during their blood meal. Further development takes place inside the mosquito. Each microfilaria develops into infective stage in mosquito and transmits it into another human host at its subsequent feeding. Thus the disease spreads from one individual to another.

Prevention and control :

Filariasis is of great public health importance in India, next only to malaria among the mosquito-borne diseases. The disease is prevalent in all the states except those of Western and some far Eastern regions. Heavily infected areas are Uttar Pradesh, Bihar Aandra Pradesh, Orisa, Tamil Nadu and Kerala.

Generally main preventive and control measures are :
(a) Against the parasites and (b) Against the vector.

(a) **Against the parasites** : Early detection and prompt treatment of the infected persons both on individual and mass scale with filaricidal drugs is the only effective and safe method against all filarial infection. At present *Diethyl carbamazine* (Hetrazan) is the only of choice for this purpose. But there are various types of toxic effect of which common are :

(i) *Toxic effects due to drug itself* e.g. headache, nausea, vomiting, dizziness, sleepness etc.

(ii) *Allergic reactions due to destruction of microfilaria and adult worms* e.g. pyrexia, local inflammations around dead worms, pruritus etc. These reactions are observed particularly after the first dose, 24 to 36 hours after administration.

Due to these side effects Hetrazan's use for mass therapy has not been a practical success.

(b) Against the vectors :

N.B. : Same as malaria.

XVI. RABIES

Q. 13.53. What is rabies ?

"*Rabies*" means "madness",especially madness in the rabid dog, and humans have always associated rabies with dogs. The dog is still regarded as the main source of rabies, and as far as rabies in humans goes, this is true,but rabies virus depends for its survival in nature on the constant and widespread infection of smaller animals, and the diseases in foxes, jackals, wolves, and dogs is a mere occasional overspill from this deeper pool of infection in mongooses, polecats, and related animals and among martens, ferrets, skunks, weasels, and bats.

Generally rabies is defined as an acute, rapidly fatal neurotropic, viral infectious disease, communicated from a rabid animal to a susceptible animal through wound usually produced by biting. Man acquires it only from an animal, usually a dog.

Reservoir of rabies virus :

Dogs act as a major source of human infection in India. Rabies virus is maintained in nature in stray dog population by a dog to dog cycle. Though, it also exists in wild fauna (Jackles, foxes and wolves etc.), the role of such animals in causing human rabies is of little significance.

Rabies virus gets localised in the brain and salivary glands of a rabid dog. As a result, transmission to man takes place by the bite of a rabid animal, with the desposition of the virus into the skin through saliva. Licks of a rabid animal on abraded skin and on fresh wounds also serve as a means of human infection.

Q. 13.54. Rabid dog. What happens when a dog gets infection by the bite of other rabid dog ?

The incubation period of the disease in the dog is between 3 weeks to 3 months. After the incubation period

COMMUNICABLE DISEASES

is over—a dog infected with rabies shows restlessness, loss of appetite and a desire to hide. Then, it usually runs away from home, attacks passers-by all of a sudden without a warning bark. It tries to swallow inedible objects (pieces of wood, racks and dirt, etc.), and suffers from excessive salivation. Gradually, it becomes depressed, paralysed and dies on the fifth or seventh day of the disease.

A dumb froms of rabies develops in some dogs, which lacks the excitement stage described above. Such dogs directly enter into the paralytic stage, but the infectivity of the saliva is the same.

The saliva of a rabid dog may be infective 6 days prior to the onset of the symptoms and remains so during the course of the disease till its death. Because of this fact, a dog is kept for 10 days under observation whenever suspected to be rabid. It may usually develop clinical disease and die of rabies during this period.

Q. 13.55. What happen, when a person is bitten by rabid dog ?

The incubation period is 2 weeks to 2 months or longer. The incubation period is short, if the bite is on the neck or on face. It is long, if the bite is on the hand or leg. The incubation period depends on the distance of the bite from the brain. The virus travels through the lymphatic vessels around the nerve. Once the virus reaches the brain, he gets the disease of rabies (hydrophobia). Nothing can save him and he must die in about 4 days or so. Anti-rabid immunization is the only method to prevent the disease and death of man.

Rabies symptoms in human—begins with vague symptoms of malaise, headache, and fever, but in a day or two the stage of excitement comes on. The person becomes anxious, sleepless, and fearful. The muscles of the throat become paralyzed so that he cannot swallow or drink and this lead to dread of water, or *hydrophobia*. The mental state varies from maniacal excitement to dull apathy, but soon the person falls into coma and is usually dead in less than a week.

Q. 13.56. How we can prevent and control the disease rabies ?

Prevention

The incubation period, or a time that elapses between the bite and the first symptoms, is usually between one and three months. This gives a chance to interrupt the disease otherwise the process of infection is inevitable. So the principle of prevention is to neutralise the virus at the site and near the site as far as possible. In addition, neutralisation of virus if it has entered in, by antibodies production through vaccine.

1. First aid treatment :

(a) Local treatment of wound is the first priority. It consists of the prompt washing of bite wounds with thick soap water eliminates the causative 'virus and saliva from the wound.' Couterisation of the wound with a swab of *tincture of iodine* or *carbolic acid* kills the residual virus.

(b) Ordinary antiseptic, antibodies and antitetanic procedures are often indicated and should follow local treatment.

(c) Bite wounds should not be sutured.

(d) *High titre antirabies serum* and its globulin fractions in liquid or powder form used tropically are highly affective in preventing rabies. But before any decision, regarding the treatment of the exposed person, information must be gathered about the biting animal. If traceable, confinement and observation of the biting animal should be done for 10 days. In case the animal is not traceable or even when the animal is under observation and bites are multiple and on hand and neck or if the animal dies, treatment should be started immediately. Where it is possible the animal should be subjected to a laboratory diagnosis for rabies, but treatment should not be withheld for the same. Because the long incubation period gives a better chance for vaccination, if once the disease has developed, vaccination is useless.

•IDENTIFICATION KEY

[Generally post exposure quiaries and prophylactic decision are made by the following observations]

Rabies prophylaxis

I. Was person bitten or licked on an open wound or mucous membranes by a possibly rabid animal? **No** ⟶ None

↓ **Yes**

II. Is rabies known or suspected to be present in the species and area? **No** ⟶ None

↓ **Yes**

III. Was animal captured? **No** ⟶ RIG* and vaccine

Yes
↓

IV. Was the animal a normally behaving vaccinated dog or cat?   V. Does animal become ill under observation durring next 10 days?
  Yes

↓ **No**   **Yes**   ↓ **No**
                    ↓
V. Does laboratory examination ⟵ None
of brain by fluorescent anti- ⟶ **No** ⟶ None
body confirm rabies?

↓ **Yes**

RIG and vaccine

* RIG- Rabies Immune Globulin.

Antirabic treatment : *Generally antirabies serum globulin of human or equine antirabies serum* (derived from immunized horse blood) is used as prophylaxis.

14 injections of antirabic vaccine are to be given i.e. one injection a day for continous 14 days.

The recommended treatment by I.C.M.R. is as follows :

(a) For licking by a rabid dog. 7 injections of 2 cc. each is given irrespective of age.

(b) For several bites or bite on the head, neck or face, give 14 injections of 10 cc. each to adult and 14 injections of 5 cc. each to children.

(c) For other bites and scratches give 14 injections of 5 cc. each to adult and 3 cc. each to children.

If the dog can be kept under observation then give 3 injections. If the dog does not develop paralysis, then no further injections are necessary, as the dog was not a rabid dog, if the dog has run away and nothing is known about the dog then give 14 injections.

Recently *Human Di oid-cell Rabies Vaccine* (HDCV) is given immediately and also three, seven, 14 and 28 days later. This vaccine is more effective than previous. The dangerous side effects seen in association with the older vaccines have not been problem with the use of HDCV (5 cc. is used and injection is given over the abdomen for 14 consecutive days).

2. General measures and control of rabies amongst dogs :

The ultimate solution to the rabies problem is predicated on the control and eventual elimination of the disease from animal population. This may be accomplished by the setting up to transmission barriers, e.g. by animal vaccination, elimination of stray dogs and the reduction of excessive number of wild life vectors.

Extensive laboratory research and field projects have proved that these techniques may be applied successfully to eradicate the disease from a given area, if integrated into carefully planned and well executed programme.

COMMUNICABLE DISEASES 379

1. General measures :

(a) Mass Vaccination of all the pet dogs at 3 months of age and report after every 3 year with L.E.P. Flury vaccine.

(b) Elimination of stray dogs. All the ownerless dogs should be caught and killed, and all the pet dogs should be licensed, and collared.

(c) Reduction of excess number of wild life vectors.

(d) Management of known exposed animals. All dogs and cats bitten by a known rabid animal should be :

    i) destroyed immediately.

    ii) if the owner is unwilling to destroy the exposed animal, it should be placed in strict isolation in a kennel for 6 months.

    iii) if the animal has been vaccinated previously within one year with nervous tissue vaccine or 3 years with chicken embryo vaccine, revaccinate and keep restraint for 30 days.

(e) *Education of the public*—is the necessity of complying with restrictions and vaccinating dogs, of seeking immediate medical attention if bitten by a dog, of confirming and observing animals that have inflicted bites, or manifest strange behaviour (dogs may become furious or quite depending on the type of disease).

(f) *International level*—Either the valid certificate of vaccination or quarantine for 6 moths is required for dogs.

XVII. LEPROSY

Introduction :- *Leprosy, or Hansen's disease* is one of the dread diseases, a dread that stretches back into antiquity, the leper has always been regarded as "unclean". It is also a contageous disease and intimate family contact is needed for its spread from one person to another. It is a disease of human beings. It does not occur in animals. The disease is due to an Acid Fast Bacillus-*Mycobacterium Leprae*. In India there are about 25 lakhs of lepers and 5 lakhs are of infective type. Leprosy is more common in males. Children are more susceptible. Infection enters the skin after prolonged contact, though infection may spread by flies droplets or fomite.

Q. 13.57. What are the suspicious symptoms of leprosy ?

Onset of Leprosy is insidious, the earliest symptoms includes :

(a) appearance of one or more hypopigmented or erythromatous patches in the skin.

(b) slight changes in the texture of colour or symptoms due to involvement of peripheral nerve e.g. formication, tingling, numbness in hands and feet usually localised in one part of the body.

The main suspicious symptoms are :

(i) Numbness, burning or tingling sensation or pain in the distribution of nerves.

ii) Impairment of pain sensation in any part of the body or feeling of heaviness.

iii) Coldness or feeling of heaviness in a limb without sweating.

iv) Partial loss of pigment of the skin.

(v) Inability to perform some movements like fastening of buttons, lacing shoes, writing, playing musical instruments, or a tendency to foot drop.

(vi) Deformities e.g. of finger.

(vii) Wasting of muscles of hands and feet.

(viii) Painless blisters and ulcers.

(ix) Thickened nerves, loss of sweating, and diffuse thickening of skin.

(x) Keratosis and ichthyosis.

COMMUNICABLE DISEASES

(N.B. : A patient may have more than one disease, e.g. leprosy and tinea versicolor or ringworm or scabies, leprosy and syphilides, leprosy and dermal leishmaniasis.)

Q. 13.58. How leprosy is transmitted ?

Generally the bacilli are discharged through nasal secretions and broken down nodules of the patient. The exact mode of transmission is not yet definitely known but possibly the following are the modes of its transmission :

1. Contact :

The commonly accepted view is that leprosy is transmitted by direct or indirect. Contact between an infectious agent and a healthy person who is otherwise susceptible. This contact should be close and of a long duration. So the bacillus probably gains its entrance through the skin.

2. Other possibilities :

The possibility of transmission other than contact are :

(a) through respiratory tract, or (b) by the insects, or (c) through breast milk.

But the factors that favours transmission are : (i) early age, (ii) closeness of contact, and (iii) massiveness of infection.

Q. 13.59. What are the various types of leprosy are seen in clinical forms ?

The various types of leprosy with their characteristic lesions mainly grouped into 6 types under 3 broad divisions :

1. Neural or Non-lepromatous type :

Sub-types :

(a) *Maculo-anaesthetic*—Cases show hypo-pigmented usually anaesthetic macules of varying sizes and number without raised margin, sebaceous function and other growths, asymmetrical in distribution and more commonly found in the face, lateral aspects of extremities and buttocks.

(b) *Tuberculoid*—Cases show markedly thickened anaesthetic patches on the skin accompained by sensory and motor changes. It has minor, major and reactional varieties.

(c) *Poly-neuretic*—Loss of cutaneous sensibility and sweating, paresis and trophic lesions.

2. Intermediate type :

Sub types :

(d) *Indeterminate*—Characterised by slightly hypopigmented flat patches with margins not well defined, no loss of sensation and not thickening of cutaneous nerves, smears are usually negative.

(e) *Borderline*—A large majority of lesions in leprosy in leprosy in skin belong to one or the other of the above 4 or lepromatus type. A minority shows both tuberculoid and lepromatous lesions.

3. Lepromatous type :

(f) *Nodulor or lepromatous*—This is the type with poor resistance and consequent generalisation of infection. Smears are invariably positive. Skin, nerves, mcous membranes, lymphatic glands, testes and internal organs are affected and cause ugly appearance. The lesions are diffuse infiltration, macules or nodules or non-infectious to infectious type. The proportion of neural to lepromatous type is more or less 75 : 25.

Q.13.60. How can we get it? and What happens after infection?

How it gets into the body is not clearly known. The bacillus discharged in enormous quantities from the nose of patients with one from leprosy but also from broken-down skin sores, it may, therefore, be inhaled by contacts of the patients or be spread from skin to skin. The first reaction to its presence takes place in the deep layers of the skin, and the reaction may be one of two kinds. *In one form* there is a sharp reaction to its presence body cells crowd into the area in an attempt to seal off the invader, and in these areas very few bacilli can be found. The intense cellular reaction involves all of the thickness of the skin and the tissues under it. the sweat glands, the hair follicles, and the nerve fibrile that end in the skin. This shows on the patient's skin as a firm, dry spot in which there is no sense of heat, cold or touch. The cellular reaction continues to spread into main trunk of the nerve, tending to strangle it so that impulses cannot get up or down. This causes a loss of power in the muscles of the area, loss of sense of pain, and loss of circulation in the part affected. This is most commonly seen in the fore-arm or lower leg, and it lead to claw hand and gross deformity of the foot, but paralysis of muscles of the face, eye, and neck may also occur. Because the person cannot feel-pain, minor injuries pass unnoticed, and the large croding ulcers can form, causing loss of fingers and toes; sometimes the condition of the limb may be so bad that amputation is the only remedy. This form of leprosy is known as *tuberculoid leprosy* because of the hard nodules, or tubercles, in the skin. It is ironical that it occurs in patients whose tissues resist the disease, for intense cellular response is a reaction of resistance, successful in so far as it prevents local multiplication of the leprosy bacillus and spread through the body but unsuccessful in that it grips and destroys the vital tissues in the invaded areas.

The *second from* the disease is *lapromatious, or cutaneous leprosy*. In this there is very little cellular response, and the bacillus can multiply freely. It can always be found in enormous numbers in the deep layers of the affected skin, and it spreads wide by the skin's lymphatic channels. It spreads up the nerves but does not grip them as in the tuberculoid form. It very often spreads to the skin of the face, where it causes thickening and corrugation of the skin and a typical leonine appearance. Soft nodules appear on the ears, nose, and cheeks and sometimes break down into discharging sores. The nose is often teeming with bacilli, and this sometimes leads to destruction of the sputum of the nose and the palate.

But the progress of leprosy is slow, it may be years before a child infected by a parent shows the first sign of the skin. Years may pass before any change is noticed, and the child has often grown to an adult before he is recognised as a leper. Patients suffer occasionally from bouts of fever, but the course of the disease in mainly one of increasing disability and disfiguration. Lepers do not often die of their leprosy; they can live a normal span of years and, with proper medical and rehabilitative care; can live in some measure of comfort.

Q. 13.61. What is leprosy (Hanse's disease) ?

It is an infectious disease caused by *Mycobactorium leprae* characterised by dip pigmentary changes in the skin, involvement of peripheral nerves with consequent para-aesthesis, anaesthesia, muscle weakness and paralysis, and trophic changes in skin, muscle and bone (neural, maculo anesthetic or tuberculoid leprosy), and in certain other instances by various types of skin lesion- infiltration macules, papules and nodules (Nodular or lepromatus leprosy). The degeneration of tissues and bones lead to ulceration, progressive constrication, and mutilation of extremities causing deformities. After a long course it usually ends in fatality.

Q. 13.62. How we can prevent the disease leprosy ?

Leprosy is an infective and preventable disease. So general principles of prevention for other disease should be apply to this case also. However, because of certain difficulties, some of the important measures available for the control of their infective diseases are not applicable to the control of leprosy. These difficulties are mainly for :

(i) Non-availabity of a culture of the causative organism, so immunisation of the healthy persons at risk is not possible.

COMMUNICABLE DISEASES

(ii) Very prolonged and marked by variable incubation period—a measure like quarantine is unthinkable.

(iii) Very prolonged course of the disease and the large number of patients :

Isolation of all infective cases are impracticable.

(iv) Lack of a quick acting remedy also makes it difficult to render infective cases to non-infective in a short period.

So taking into consideration the above limitations the main measures for leprosy control and prevention are :

1. Prevention

(a) Raising of the economic, social and sanitary conditions of the general population—better diet, housing and sanitary facilities as a part of the National Development Programme.

(b) Health education of the public for stressing greater rick of leprosy in early life and in contacts and for removal superstitions, false beliefs and social ostracism by asserting that neither God or sin or not any unnatural phenomena are involved in the causation of the disease nor it is hereditary. Above all, it is necessary to stress to all concerned that leprosy is curable.

(c) Establishment of mobile units of mass survey and treatment.

2. Control of Patients, Contacts and the Surroundings

(a) Reporting of cases to the nearest health authority.

(b) Selective isolation of infective patients at home if possible or in any hospital till the patients become bacteriologically negative for atleast 4 months. Also separation of infants from the leprous mothers.

(c) Mass scale treatment of all leprosy patients with D.D.S. (Diamino Diphenyl Sulphone) or with other available effective drugs. the treatment is to be continued generally for 3 or more years.

- (d) For protection of children, a part from removing them from contact, chemoprophylaxis treatment with doses of sulphones (Dapsone or DDS) or by immunoprophylaxis with BCG vaccination may be tried.
- (e) Sterilization of leprous patients helps to reduce the susceptible population and contacts.
- (f) Investigation of contacts and their periodic check up.

3. Epidemic Measures

In areas of high endemicity and in uncommon situations the programme of control should have the following facilities : *laboratory, diagnosis, treatment of clinic, case finding programme, isolation of infectious patient etc.*

4. International Measures

- (a) Refusal or entry of immigrants with active or suspected leprosy infection.
- (b) Reciprocal measures between governments at authorized points to prevent introduction of spread of the disease by immigrants.

5. Rehabilitation of Leprosy Patients

With the improvement of treatment much of the deformities and defects can be prevented by early treatment, but for those who have been cured with deformity surgical as well as economic rehabilitation should be undertaken by the Government or the appropriate social organisations.

6. Training and Research

To carry out various antileprosy treatment service and campaigns a large contigents of doctors, social workers and para medical personnel need to be trained. Besides knowledge on the disease and its causative organism being largely deficient a continous research work should be organised.

7. Leprosaria or Leprosy Colony

For both segregation and rehabilitation of leprosy patient at least one leprosaria or leprosy colony is to be maintained by the governments of the affected states. In this colony there should be proper arrangement for treatment as well as for vocational training and remuneration or productive work according to the capacity of the individual e.g. agriculture, poultry keeping, weaving, basket and toy making etc. Early case can, however, be best isolated at his own home for both socio-economic and psycological reasons.

8. Leprosy Hospital

Instead of a hospital exclusively by for leprosy patients it would be better to allot a special wing for such cases in general or infective disease hospital where highly infectious or much more dangerous are admitted without any public objection. It is, however, essential to maintain a hospital for the treatment of severe and main patients.

But to put into practice the principles lined as above, the antileprosy campaign a comprehensive one. The various steps needed in an antileprosy campaign are :

(1) A case finding programme.
(2) Treatment of all patients.
(3) Selective isolation of infective patients.
(4) Health education of the public.
(5) Protection of children.
(6) Welfare services for patients and dependents.
(7) Training of personnel.
(8) Legal measures to be used under special circumstances.

So for the successful implementation of these measures there is need for a well organised antileprosy campaign with multisided activities. Fortunatelly the Govt. of India with collaboration of the State governments, has launched a National Leprosy Control Programme to which various voluntary organisations in the field also contributing to some extent.

Q. 13.63. What are the barriers present before the success of leprosy eradication programmes in India.

1. Social Stigma—Untouchability and Leprosy

The social stigma attached to leprosy is still a major obstacle to the eradication of the disease.

For hundreds of years the society has been shunning leprosy and its sufferers. This has resulted in patients hiding the disease and neglecting treatment till, due to advanced stages of the disease, it is no longer possible to hide the disease. This leads to a continuous and an increased spread of infection in the community. Deformities lead to handicap, unemployment and economic disaster to the person and his family. Further, because of the society's attitude towards the disease, not many doctors, scientists or people from other works of life are attracted to work in this field. Research is also severely affected. All these factors further lead to aggravation of the disease in the community, thus bringing about more apprehension and hatred.

As it is an infective and a contagious, disease, spread by constant touch with an infective patient was also one of the major reasons that induced fear in the minds of the people that leprosy will occur if they touch. So leprosy patients were considered untouchable and become a site for hatred. For centuries people hand no scientific knowledge about the disease and hence leprosy and untouchability become more or less synonymous.

So the vicious cycle can be interrupted not only by compassion but by the right scientific attitude of the society towards leprosy and it suffers with personal hygiene.

2. No Availabity of Proper Drugs

Drugs do help to arrest the disease and make the patient non-infectious, but none that acts quickly is yet available. DAPSONE is one of the more effective, but in the early 1980s a world wide increase in resistan to dapsone lead health officials predict renewed increase in of the disease.

One of the difficulties is that so far no one has been able to grow the leprosy beacillus in laboratory plates, and only since 1960 has it been possible to grow it in a laboratory animal. The foot pad of a mouse can be infected, and the disease in the mouse resembles the disease in humans, so that the progress of the disease can be studied and the effect of new drugs tried first on the infected mouse.

3. Other Causes

Apart from the use of drugs, the management of the disease is a vast problem. The leper must be helped in his disfigurement and his paralyses. The greatest problem is the prevention of infection. A baby born to a leprous mother has little chance of escape unless it is separated from her. A father is almost bound to infect some members of his family unless taken away from them. The fear of separation makes the family conceal the disease and so increases the danger of spread. The ideal must be not a colony for lepers only but, rather, village or the community groups in which whole families can live in good conditions and the leper can be given the treatment he needs and encourged and enabled to work within his limitations.

XVIII. ENDEMIC GOITRE

Q. 13.64. Endemic goitre. What is meant by endemic goitre ? How we can prevent it ?

Goitre is an enlargement of the Thyroid gland presumably due to insufficient Thyroid hormone production. But if the deficiency is caused by inadequate dietary intake of iodine and occurs in a significant number of people in a defined geographic area, it is called *endemic (colloid) goitre*.

In India about 10 million people suffer from goitre and it is prevalent in the southern slops of the Himalayas, northern part of Kashmire, Punjab, Himachal Pradesh, Uttar Pradesh, Bihar, Assam, NEFA and Manipur.

In normal condition, when iodine is taken through food, it is absorbed in the body and circulates in the blood in organic form. The alveolar cells of the thyroid takes up iodine, where it is trapped and stored in the thyroid gland as thyroglobulin, in the following manner :

Tyrosine + Iodine = Di-iodo Tyrosine. Two molecules of Di-iodo Tyrosine = Thyroxine. Thyroxine + Protein globulin = Thyroglobulin.

So it is seen that iodine is the universal accepted materials for thyroxine production and lack of iodine produces endemic goitre. The daily requirement of iodine are about

75 micrograms and intake of 100 ug-150 ug is the recommended levels.

Signs and symptoms, and diagnosis :

In the early stages, diagnosis depends on the presence of a soft, symmetric, smooth goitre. There may be a history of low iodine intake or ingestion of goitrogens. Thyroidal radio-iodine intake may be normal or high, with a normal thyroid scan. The serum T(4) and T (3) resin uptake are usually normal. Later multiple nodules and cysts may appear. Endemic goitre is considered to be of public health importance when 4% or more of girls aged 12 to 14 years show grade I enlargement of the thyroid gland.

Prevention

The principle of prevention of goitre is to prevent deficiency of iodine, and to avoid goitrogenic food e.g. cabbages, mustard leaves, green stalk of onion etc.

Far endemic goitre iodized salt or bread has been practised in different parts of world since 1929. In India considering the severity of the problem iodized salt has also been introduced inendemic zones of our country and number of salt-iodization plants have been set up. Here potassium iodate, which is more stable compound than 'iodide' is mixed with common salt,at a level of 1:100,000 to 1:20,000 are used.

(a) Iodized salt

Common salt fortified with small quantities of sodium or potassium iodate has been widely used in reducing the the prevalance of goitre. The level of iodization varies from country to country. In India, it is 1 in 40,000, iodization of salt is the most economical, convenient and effective means of mass prophylazis in enedemic areas. Under the normal Goitre Control Programme in India iodized salt is made available for public consumption in goitre endemic areas

(b) Iodized oil

In the areas where salt iodization cannot be employed. Intro-muscular injection of iodized oil has been used for preventing endemic goitre. It is cheap, long lasting and relatively free from side effects. Iodized poppy seed oil containing 37% iodine has been successfully used. The dose recommended is 1 to 2 ml for adults and smaller doses for infants and children to be given once in every three years.

(c) Marine fish—a prophylactice against goiter

Marine foods-seafish and shelfish are by far the richest sources of iodine in ordinary human diet. Fresh water fish contain the least (30 ug/kg); anadromous fish, which spend part of their life at sea and part in fresh water, have 11 times as much (330 ug/kg) and at the top of the scale come the true marine fish with an average content nearly thirty times that of fresh water fish. So inclusion of marine fish in diet once daily provides an abundant iodine intake and acts as a prophylactic. As seen that populations near the sea are without goiter that those father inland.

XIX. BERI-BERI

Q. 13.65. What is meant by beri-beri or thiamin deficiency disease?

Beri-beri is a disorder characterized by peripheral neuropathy, myocardial weakness and frequently oedema, due to consumption of milled rice, deficient in vitamin B1 (thiamin).

Clinical features :

Generally this disease is manifested by one of the following types :

(i) *Mild Type*—It is characterised by numbness or weakness of less and diminished knee-jerk.
(ii) *Dry Beri-beri*—The muscles such as calf, become wasted and tender on pressure. There is loss of breath on exertion and loss of knee-jerk. There may be wrist, or foot drop.
(iii) *Wet Beri-beri*—There is oedema, first at the feet, which extends upwards to trunk, arms, and face.
(iv) *Acute Cardiae*—There is dilatation of heart, associated with congestive failure.

Causes : The pathological changes in Beri-beries are due to the toxic effect on pyruvic acid which accumulated in thiamin deficiency. Deficiency of thiamine in pregnant mother may lead to the birth of a baby without any storage from the mother. Such a baby may suffer from 'Infantile Beri-beri' within the first six months of life if the infant's diet is not supplemented with the vitamin. In india, cases of beri-beri are frequently reported due to the consumption of raw and highly polished and milled rice and to the throwing away of the water after boiling the rice whereby the thiamine which is concentrated mainly in the scutellum and aleurone layer of the rice grain is lost. This can be prevented by using 'parboiled' rice.

Prevention

Avoid over milled rice in the diet. Use homepounded. Health education to the public regarding use of food rich in Vitamin B_1, such as yeast, ground-nuts, tomatoes, green leaves, etc. is also helpful.

XX. PELLAGRA

Q. 13.66. What is meant by pellagra or niacin deficiency disease or nicotinic acid deficiency disease ?

Pellagra is a disease caused by consumption of food poor in Nicotinic Acid or Niacin. Generally the deficiency of niacin produces the classical picture of pellagra. Pellagra is known to occur among the maiz-eaters. It is believed that niacin in maize is present in a bound form and not much of it is available to the body. Moreover, the maize protein being deficient in tryptophan (an essential amino acid) the conversion of tryptophan to niacin with in the body is not adequate (60 mg of tryptophan = 1 mg. of niacin).

It has been also suggested that the disease may be associated with (i) some protein produced in the maize, (ii) relative lack of high class proteins in diet, (iii) deficiency in nicotinic acid and (iv) lowered vitality of the affected person.

COMMUNICABLE DISEASES

Clinical Features

In India, pellagra is endemic in the Deccan plateau affecting the poor agricultural people of the area, who are predominant by 'Jowar' eater. It has been found that Jowar contains an excess of the amino-acid-leucine, which is responsible for the deficiency of niacin. Generally the deficiency disease of nacin(pellagra) is characterized by lassitude, loss of weight, gastro-intestinal disturbances, soreness of tongue, diarrhoea, dermatitis and mental disorder. The characteristic skin lesions may be noted on the back of the hands and malar eminences, etc., which are most exposed to sun. Tongue is scarlet red. There are also tremors of the tongue and face muscles, fleeting pains in the body, numbness, anxiety neurosis, toxic symptoms etc.

Prevention

Health education about the cause of pellagra. Introduction of fresh meat, pork, liver, green leafy vegetables, whole cereals specially in the pelagra affected community, to increase protein and Nicotinic acid contents in their diet.

PART IV

Health for All by 2000—A.D.

CHAPTER-XIV

IMMUNITY-IMMUNOLOGY PROPHYLAXIS

DISCUSSION FOR LEARNING

I. Immunity and its various types.
II. Natural and artificial immunity.
III. Immunization active and passive.
IV. Prophylaxis (Allopathy and Homoeopathy views).
V. Routine Immunization Procedure and Recommended Immunization Schedule.

(INTRODUCTION)

I. IMMUNITY AND IMMUNIZATION

Immunity may be defined as the ability of the individual to resist or overcome infection; it may be innate or acquired. For many infectious diseases, immunity is acquired during recovery from an infection or induced by the administration of vaccines prepared from inactivated or live microorganisms of modified disease producing potential, or from specific antigens derived from these organisms. The purpose of immunization, therefore, is to provoke a specific immunological response to a selected microbial agent or its antigens with the expectation that this will result in humoral, and/or secretory, and/or cell-mediated immunity. While this protection may diminished over time, future exposures to the same stimulus will result in a rapid return of the immune response because of heightened reactivity of antibody forming, phagocytic, and other cells that mediate immune mechanisms.

Q. 14.1 What are the different types of immunity?

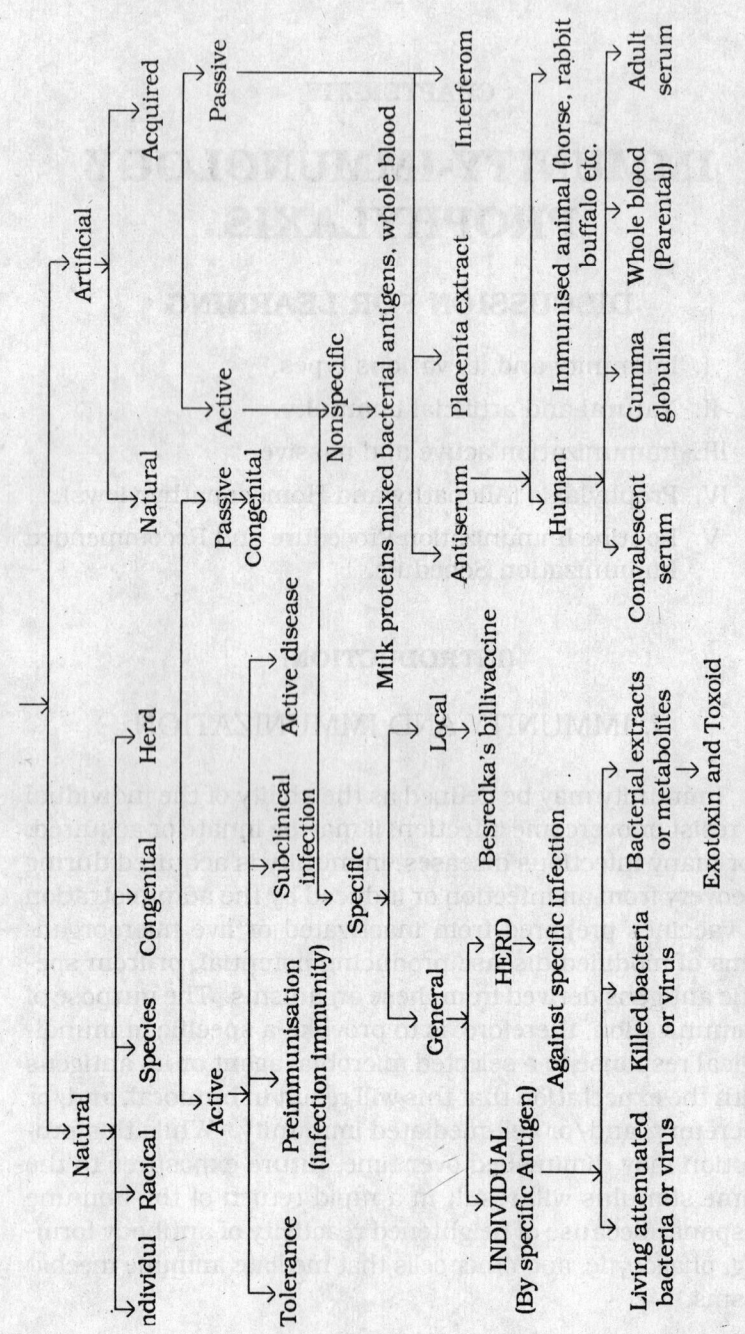

Q. 14.2. What is meant by Immunity ?

Immunity means non-susceptability to a disease or an organism either under natural conditions or under conditions experimentally produced. It also may be defined as the ability of the living individual to resist or overcome infection. The state of resistance is indicated either by the failure of the individual to develop the disease upon exposure, or in some cases by the demonstration of specific immuned bodies (antibodies) in the blood which are considered effective against the invading organisms.

So the term *immunity implies resistance or non-susceptability to a disease or any organisms naturally or artificially acquired.* It may be against the organisms (antibacterial or antiviral) or the toxin liberated by them (antitoxic). Immunity may be :

(a) **Congenital** i.e. from birth.
(b) **Acquired**—*(i) Active-by* suffering from disease or by vaccination
   (ii) Passive—by serum.

Q.14.3. What are the significance of immunity in homoeopathy ?

Immunity means the resisting power of the body against the foreign inimical influences, and vital force of the body resists the invading disease force. If it is weaker than the disease force; on in other words if the body is not immuned, the disease gets a foothold in the body; but on the other hand, if the vital force is stronger or if the body has got immunity the disease will not develop and it will die of itself.

Secondly, Homoeopathy is based on the principle that in order to cure we produce a similar and stronger disease in the body on the presumption that, out of the similar diseases the stronger one will repel the weaker one. In the same way, on the basis of genus epidemicus in order to prevent the occurrence of the disease, with the help of drugs, we produce the artificial disease in the body which is similar and stronger than the one prevailing in the form of epidemic. According to the above principle, the drug disease is stronger than the natural disease, it will repel the natural disease and they will not allow it to develop. Here also we see that the creation of the drug disease is nothing, but immunity, that helps to keep the body free from the natural disease.

So, keeping the above in view, we can safely say that *immunity* and *vital force* are two identical terms; that is to say *immunity is a physical name of the Vital Force.*

Further, immunity is created by the introduction of the morbid products into the system which in turn produce the hypersensitive and allergic states in the body. Hahnemann's ideas regarding the theory and nature of chronic diseases have been corroborated by the modern investigators in the field of Allergy and Immunity. Generally the immunity type of the response may be considered as analogous to the effect of the *isopathic* or *homoeopathic* remedy which is supposed to raise the body resistance to infection by vital stimulation. So the following homoeopathic drugs can produce immunity *Variolinum, Morbilinum, Typhoidinum, Diphtherinum, Pertussin, Hydrophobinum* etc.

II. NATURAL AND ARTIFICIAL IMMUNITY

Q. 14.4. What is meant by Natural Immunity ?

or

What is meant by congenial, genetical or inherited immunity ?

Natural Immunity—This is a type of Immunity with which an individual is born.

In this case the resistance is offered by the body under the normal conditions without any external stimulation of previous infections. In this the immunity to a given infectious agent is conditioned by innate factors which are transmitted according to the laws of heredity from one individual or generation to the next and which consists in functioning of stimuli arising from contact with the environment.

So this immunity is possessed by a person either from birth or acquired during growth. It is of *following types* :

(a) *Species*—This type of immunity bears some definite character according to the different species of life. Immunity relating to species are *Rats to diptheria, Fowl to tetanus, and Goat, Horse to tuberculosis.*

(b) *Racial*—This type of immunity develops in some particular races. e.g. Negros to yellow fever, Jews to tuberculosis.

(c) *Individual*—This type of immunity develops according to constitution of individual. Gastric juice, Lysozyme and some other internal and outward secretion of our body having power to protect of different organism. As seen in case of epidemic where certain persons remain immune and are not affected by influenza, smallpox etc.

(d) *Congenital*—This is found in the newborn due to the passive transfer of antibodies from the mother to the child through placenta. Thus on infant in the first year of life is resistant to *diptheria* and *scarlet fever.*

Q. 14.5. What is meant by Herd Immunity ?

By the term *herd immunity* is meant the level of immunity in a *group* or *community* exposed to an infection. During an epidemic prevalence a large number of people gets infected and acquires immunity either subclinically or by active disease and a part of the community remains susceptible. A herd immunity may be achieved through natural selection i.e. by weading out of susceptibles in successive generations by disease and death. In the post epidemic or inter-epidemic stage the estimated level of immunity in such a community is defined by the term *herd immunity*, which if high can avert an epidemic and if low may result in an epidemic. Thus herd immunity can be raised in a community by artifically immunising 70-80 percent of the population. In tuberculosis the civilized nations have achieved herd immunity while the hill tribes have remained highly susceptible.

Q. 14.6. What is meant by Acquired Immunity ? What are its various types ?

Acquired Immunity means the immunity which is developed by the individual during his life time after an attack of a disease or by artificial means.

From the point of view of Preventive Medicine, acquired immunity is the most important. Generally acquired immunity is of two main types e.g. *Natural* and *Artificial.*

(A). The various forms of *naturally acquired immunity* are :

    (a) *active*—i) tolerance, ii) infection immunity or premunition, ii) sub-clinical infection, iii) clinical disease.

    (b) *passive*—congenital.

(B). The *artificial acquired immunity* may be :

    (a) *active*—i) *Specific*-general and local, and ii) *non-specific.*

    (b) *Passive*—from animal, man and bacterial agent.

A. Natural acquired immunity :

(a) *Active*: *i.e. when the tissues of an individual take active part in raising the mechanism of resistance.*

It is of following types

    i) *Tolerance*—means limited : resistance developed as a result of continued infection or reinfection e.g. against malaria, hookworm etc.,

    ii) *Premunition or Infection immunity*—It is developed by harbouring the parasite in the body in small numbers e.g. in tuberculosis, viral infection, the immunity disappearing with the disapperance of the organism from the body.

    iii) *Sub-clinical infection*—In an endemic situation many individuals, particularly in the early stage of life, get infected with various organisms but immunity develops before such infection leads to clinical symptoms e.g. diphtheria, meningitis, poliomyelitis, infective hepatitis.

    iv) *Clinical disease*—By actual suffering from a disease a high and long standing immunity against second attack is developed in the survivals e.g. second attack of smallpox, chicken pox, mumps, measles, etc. are rare.

IMMUNITY-IMMUNOLOGY PROPHYLAXIS

(b) *Passive* : i.e. *when the resistance is obtained for a short duration by introduction of performed antibodies or protective substances from man or animal into the body of an individual.*

e.g.: Congenital—The offspring of a mother who has been previously immunised and carries antibodies against a specific infection obtains at birth passive immunity from the circulating mother's blood (serum) and also partially through colostrum and milk. So a baby becomes immune to diphtheria or tetanus.

B. **Artificially acquired immunity :**

(a) **Active**

(i) *Specific*—When any material containing antigenic substances (antigen) which include bacteria, viruses, toxins, or any protein introduced into a body intramurally, subcutaneous or orally it induces the production of a particular kind of serum protein of the nature of globulin called antibody and the process is called artifically acquired immunity. So inoculation of certain materials containing antigen substances derived from bacteria or viruses to give rises the protection against potential future exposure to infection of an individual is known as *active specific artifically acquired immunity*. It is generally done by (i) cutaneous vaccination, (ii) injection of toxin, (iii) injection of bacteria or by orally (e.g. Bilivaccine) and the vaccines including toxoids are :

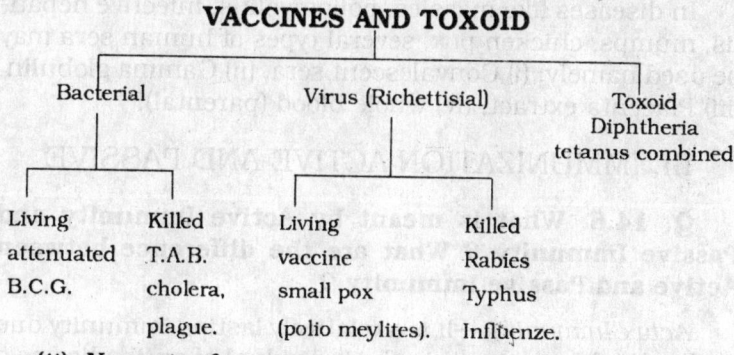

(ii) *Non-specific :*

In persons suffering from subacute long drawn septic conditions such as salpingitis or other infections leading to leucopenia, the resistance can be enhanced by injecting non-specific antigen in the form of milk protein, mixed bacterial antigens or whole blood.

(b) Artificially Passive Acquired Immunity

Artificially acquired passive immunity means giving ready-made immunity. Usually, a horse or buffalo, rabbits etc. are immunized by injecting the toxins of diphtheria, tetanus, snake venom etc. in increasing doses. The blood of the animal gets super immunized. The immunity is in the gamma-globulin part of the blood serum. The gamma-globulin is separated, and from this, serum is prepared. The serum when injected in a person suffering from tetanus, diphtheria etc. will destroy the exotoxins in the patient's blood. So the immunity that is conferred by this procedure is called artifically passive acquired immunity. It is short lived but is of particular value to tide over the crisis when antibodies are lacking in the blood of the patient. This kind of antiserum has also been used as a prophylaxis e.g. in diphtheria and tetanus but its value is being doubted now.

The application of these *antibacterial and antitoxic sera have certain risks of producing (i) anaphylactic shock, (ii) serum sickness and (iii) fall in protective value* after the second or subsequent injections. Generally the above reactions follow a previous serum injection so necessary precautions and history should, therefore, be taken before using these sera either prophylactically or therapeutically.

In diseases like measles, poliomyelitis, infective hepatitis, mumps, chicken pox, several types of human sera may be used namely: (i) Convalescent sera, (ii) Gamma globulin, (iii) Placenta extract, (iv) whole blood (parental).

III. IMMUNIZATION ACTIVE AND PASSIVE

Q. 14.6. What is meant by Active Immunity and Passive Immunity ? What are the difference between Active and Passive Immunity ?

Active Immunity :—It is a relatively lasting immunity due to the development within the individual of antibodies as a result of contract with the micro-organism or their products.

Passive Immunity :—This is acquired immunity which is temporary in which antibodies are produced in another animal, whose blood serum is injected into the person.

DIFFERENCES

Active Immunity	Passive Immunity
1. It is produced by cellular activity of individual. It is not borrowed or performed.	1. It is always performed or borrowed and not related to celluler activity or a person.
2. *Produced by* : (i) suffering from the disease, (ii) using vaccine, (iii) by repeated sub-clinical infection.	2. (i) Inherited. (ii) Produced by serum therapy.
3. Takes 8 to 10 days to develop.	3. No time is lost. Immunity develops as soon as serum therapy is instituted.
4. During first 8-10 days the person is more susceptible and has no antibody.	4. No such negative phase as the effect is immediate.
5. It is long lasting.	5. Duration is very short.
6. Reaction is severe and it may be local or general.	6. Reaction negligible except that due to protein shock.
7. Main use in prophylactic.	7. Main use in therapeutic.
8. Cannot be inherited.	8. Can be inherited from mother.

Q. 14.7(a). What are the factors responsible for producing immunity in a man ?

A. For Individual Immunity :

The defensive forces of the body vary from one person to other. For the *following facts the immunity produce in a man* :

1. **Physical factors** (Reflex action) :
   (i) Integrity of skin and living epithelium of skin and stratified squamous epithelium.
   (ii) The lining epithelium of respiratory and alimentary tract secreates thick tenecious mucus which provides a protective coating, so that bacteria can penetrate with difficulty. The ciliated epithelium of respiratory tract by their ciliary movement helps to expel out foreign bodies, bacteria get entangled due to its stickiness and they are expelled out. This is way lowering of muco-ciliary resistance of respiratory tract due to any factor will predispose to bacterial infection.
   (iii) The acid sweat liberated by skin helps to keep the skin free from infection. In other words the sweat acts as auto-sterilising agents.

2. **Chemical factors** :
   (i) *Gastric juice*—HCL content of stomach has a high bacteriocidal action and it protects against infection of alimentary canal.
   (ii) *Lysozyme*—It has a bacteriocidal action and present in all secretion and excretion of the body except urine, sweat and C.S.F. It is present in maximum concentrativa in lacrimal secretion and cartilages. The conjunctive is normally kept free from bacterial infection as it is bathed in lysozyme.

3. **Cellulo-humoral mechanisms** :
   Cellular Mechanism—The various phagocytic cells of the system help, in the process of phagocytosis of bacteria and latter on undergoes intracellular lysis. The following are the phagocytic cells :
   (a) Cells of circulating blood—Polymorphous and monocytes.
   (b) Cells in the tissues—These tissue cells concerned in phagocytosis may be of two types—viz :
   i) *Fixt* celled cells of particular organs :
   (1) *Kuffer's* cells of the liver.
   (2) *Endothelial cells* of the bone marrow.
   (3) Cells living in the sinus of the lymph gland.

IMMUNITY-IMMUNOLOGY PROPHYLAXIS

ii) *Wandering cells*—are also histocytes tissue and they are mono-nuclear cells.

***Action of *cellulor components which help in immunity* are :

i) the cells elaborate proteolytic enzyme which produce healing and immunity against infection.

ii) The cells also concerned with the formation of complement *Opsonin*—which add to defensive force.

(2) Humoral Mechanism :

i) *Bacterial element in blood*—There are some bacteriocidal substances present normally in serum e.g. L-lysin, Lukin, plakin etc.

ii) *Antibodies like*—Agglutinin, Bacteriotropin etc. are produced in the serum, which defensive against infection.

iii) *Aritificial Immunity :*

This immunity results by artificial means. It is of 2 types, viz. :

(a) *active* and (b) *passive*.

(a) Active Artificial Means :

This immunity results form a course of *specific vaccination or by infection* e.g. T.A.B.C. vaccine, Plague, Autovaccine etc.

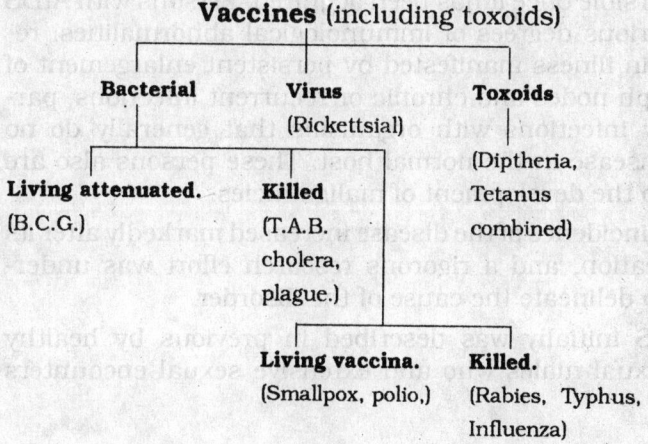

Vaccines (including toxoids)

Bacterial
- **Living attenuated.** (B.C.G.)

Virus (Rickettsial)
- **Killed** (T.A.B. cholera, plague.)
- **Living vaccina.** (Smallpox, polio,)

Toxoids (Diptheria, Tetanus combined)
- **Killed.** (Rabies, Typhus, Influenza)

(b) Passive Artificial Means :

(a) **Serum Therapy**—Readymade antibodies are supplied to the person through the serum. The serum used for passive immunity may be either of the following types :

(i) *Autoxic serum*, against Diphtheria, Tetanus, Gas gangrene. Acts by neutralisation of exotoxin elaborated by bacteria in the body.

(ii) *Antibacterial serum*, against pneumonia and meningo coccal infections. Acts by destruction of bacteria and thereby preventing increase by endotoxin.

(iii *Convalcent or antiviral serum*, measles, actue antpoliomyelitis, serum obtained from an individual recently recorded form of infections.

(b) **Bacteriophase Therapy** : Recently passive immunity also be induced by bacteriophase therapy.

N.B.

**[Q. *What do you mean by artificial immunity? Describe the various methods by which it can produce in a man.)*

Q. 14.8. What is meant by AIDS (Acquired Immune Deficiency Syndrome)?

In *Acquired Immune Deficiency Syndrome* (AIDS) the cellmediated (T-cell) immune regulation and surveillance system of the human body is affected. First recognized in 1979 in the United States, AIDS appears to be a defect that is irreversible once it has been acquired. Persons with AIDS have various degrees of immunological abnormalities, resulting in illness manifested by persistent enlargement of the lymph nodes and chronic or recurrent infections, particularly infections with organisms that generally do no cause disease in the normal host. These persons also are prone to the development of malignancies.

The incidence of the disease increased markedly after its identification, and a rigorous research effort was undertaken to delineate the cause of the disorder.

AIDS initially was described in previous by healthy homosexual males who and extensive sexual encounters with a variety of partners. It has come to be known, however, that this disorder also occurs with increase frequently in persons who abuse drugs intrafusions, as well as in a disproportionate number of people who live in or have immigrated from Haiti or who are of Haitian descent. A heterosexual female whose male partner has AIDS also may be afflicted, as may infants born to mothers who are drug abusers or who are of Haitian descent.

*The *mechanism* by which the disease is transmitted from one individual to another is not known. It appears, however, that the transfer of blood or blood products may be an important vehicle for transmission.

**The *etiology* of AIDS also is not known, but it is presumed to be caused by an infectious agent. Viruses that have been found with great frequency in individuals with AIDS and that have been postulated as playing a causative role in the syndrome include cytomegalovirus, Epstein Barr virus (the cause of infectious mononucleosis, hepatitis B virus, or a 'new' virus that has the potential for causing malignant change. It also seems likely that both genetc and environmental factors are important since there are variations in the expression of the syndrome.

The *incubation period* for AIDS appear to vary from six months to two years. During this time there is a gradual deterioration of the immune system, resulting in impaired T-cell regulation and surveillance mechanisms. Those who are afflicted develop recurrent or chronic infections with organisms that are otherwise well tolerated in normal individuals. In patients with AIDS, however, these organisms produce life threatening disease and frequently cause death.

Many persons with AIDS are at increased risk for malignancies, particularly kaposi's sarcoma, a cutaneous disorder, with dark blue or purple-brown plaques or nodules on the extremities, which progresses at a more rapid rate than normally seen in individuals who do not have the syndrome. Other malignancies noted with increased frequency in persons with AIDS include lymphomas and squamous—cell carninomas.

Some perons with AIDS have chronic and recurrent

fever, night sweats, weight loss, mal-absorption of food from gestro-intestinal tract, and generalised enlargement of the lymph nodes. These symptoms may persist for variable periods of time before malignancies become apparent or before overwhelming infection with an otherwise innocuous organism has been documented.

The *diagnosis* of AIDS should be considered in persons whose symptoms include recurrent or unusual infections (Pneumocystis carinii, Cytomegalo virus, or Cryptococcal disease), weight loss, persistent fever, and lymph adenopathy, particulaly if they belong to one of groups known to be at risk.

Antibiotics used to treat specific infections, are the only treatment that ameliorates the symptoms of AIDS.

The death rate is as high as 50 percent and usually results from infection that either no longer responds to antibiotics or for which no therapy is available.

Q. 14.9. (a) What is meant by Immunization (or Sensitization) ?

The terms *immunization means the process of stimulatng an immunological response in an animal by the administration of antigen.* When an antigen is reintroduced into an organism several weeks after the first introduction, the immunological response is usually greater and occurs more rapidly that did the initial response, the phenomenon is commonly known as *immunological memory.* An animal that fails to make the expected immunological responses to an antigen is described as *immunological tolerant.* The ability of an animal species to make immunological response to own constituents, although many of them would act an antigens in another-animal species, is termed *self tolerance.*

Q. 14.9. (b) Discuss Antigen is for immunization.

Proteins generally are potent antigens, as are certain carbohydrates. Lipids are sometimes able to elicit immunological responses but do not do so readily, probably because they are broken down rapidly in the body and have few destinctly foreign molecular patterns. Nucleic acids are composed of a limited number of building blocks (the nucleotides, and are not antigenic unless modified chemically. Antibodies react only with altered or denatured nucleic acids ; this means that antibodies are not normally formed against a body's own gentic material or against the genetic material of invading microbes.

The early 20th century discovery that minor alternations in the structures of antigens, such as bacterial toxins, destroy poisonous properties without affecting the capacity to stimulate the formation of antibodies capable of reacting with untreated toxins was an extremely important one; minor structural alternations convert toxins to toxoids and provide the basis for proplylactic (protective) immunization against the toxic products of various diseases eg., diphtheria, tetanus. In a similar manner, microbes killed by various means retain their surface antigens and they are able to stimulate the formation of antibodies against living bacteria of the same species; this method is used in immunization against disease such as typhoid, typhus, and plague. It is important and often difficult, however, to ensure that antigens produced by bacteria after they invade the body are also found in the vaccines produced by these organisms when grown outside the body.

Whenever possible, immunization against a virus is achieved by the administration of an attenuated form ; i.e. the virus can multiply to a limited extent in the body without causing manifestions of disease and thus provides a strong antigenic stimulus. Attenuated stain of virus are obtained by careful selection of variants that have been grown in abnormal hosts or under abnormal conditions. Attenuated stains must be able to stimulate immunity against the antigens of fully virulent strains and should not revert to virulent forms. Attenuated strain of microbes have been used to immunize man against smallpox since 1978, tuberculosis 1927, and the 17 D stain of yellow fever since about 1938.

Q. 14.10. What is Antigen ?

The term *antigen* is used to describe any material,

usually of a complex nature, that stimulates a specific bodily immunity because the body recognizes it as foreign. More than one component of the structural pattern of an antigen can be recognized by the immunological system as foreign; each component so recognized is known as an *antigenic determinate*. An antigen can be modified by the addtion of a simple chemical group, which acts as an antigenic determinant and is called a hapten (Greek Haptain, "to grasp").

Q. 14.11. What is Antibody ?

An *antibody* is a specialized protein (called an immunglobulin) that is able to combine especially with an antigen. After antibodies are released from the cells in which they are synthesized, they enter body fluids and are responsible for specifc protective properties, sometimes called *humoral immunity*, that are present, especially in blood. Antibodies also cause certain forms of hyper-reactivity or hyper-sensitivity to antigen. Other hyper-sensitivity reactions are caused by the mechanisms of cell-mediated immunity-i.e. a manifestation of specifc immunity that is not attributable to antibodies circulating in the blood stream but is the result of the action of certain cells (lymphocytes) reacting directly with an antigen and requiring the cooperation of scavenging cells called macrophages to exert some of their effects.

Q. 14.12. What is meant by Immunization ?

The process of stimulating an immunological response in an animal body by the adminstration of antigen is called Immunization. Or *Increasing the resistance of the human body by artificial methods against the communicable disease is known as immunization.* The immunization is either a sole method of controlling disease or is prophylaxis for those persons who are exposed to risk of infection. For smallpox, tetanus, poliomyelitis, diphtheria, whooping cough, immunization is done solely for *control of the disease*, but the *prophylactic immunization* is done for cholera, typhoid, plague, yellow fever etc. However in Homoeopathy, prophylactic immunization is possible for smallpox, tetanus, poliomyelitis, diphtheria, whooping cough etc.

Q. 14.13. What is meant by active immunization and passive immunization ?

(A). Active Immunization means—*immunization of a healthy person*. By immunization, a person can resist infection and the harmful effect of their toxins. *Active immunization is done to healthy person*. The immunity develops in 7 days and lasts for 6 months to about 5 years. Hence if a person is given *vaccination during the incubation period of a disease*, the disease will be prevented, if the disease is occurs, it appears after 7 days of vaccination.

**1) Methods of vaccination are :
   (a) *Oral method*—(i) Oral polio, (ii) Bilivaccine in cho-lera.
   (b) *Intradermal method*—(i) B.C.G., (ii) Cowpox vaccination.
   (c) *Subcutaneous methods are in*—Cholera, typhod, plague etc.

2) Period of immunity varies in different disease :
   (a) *In plague*, cholera and typhoid, the person is immuned for 6 months.
   (b) In *smallpox* and tetanus the person is immuned for about 5 years.
   (c) In *yellow fever* the immunity lasts for about 10 years.

****Mass immunisation* means immunization of a greater population in a affected community during breaking out of an epidemic diseases like plague, cholera, smallpox, typhoid, diphtheria etc. but it is not done in tuberculosis.

Formerly it was thought that by the age of about 10 years every person has active living germs of tuberculosis in his body. Hence active immunization was contra-indicated after 10 years, unless Mantoux test was done and found to be negative. However, at present the Government has advised B.C.G. Vaccination without, doing Mantoux's test upto the age of 19 years.

(B). Passive Immunization is done after the disease has manifested. It is the introduction of ready-made immune bodies i.e. *serum*. Passive immunization is mainly done for diphtheria, tetanus and snake bites.

IV. PROPHYLAXIS

Q. 14.14. Name the various prophylactics used in Alopathy and what are their uses.

(A) Active Immunization in Adults

Type of vaccine	Administration and frequency.		Comments
1. All Adults			
Tetanus and diphtheria.	Adsorbed toxoid.	1M at least every 10 days.	Usually administered together as Td vaccine.
Poliomyelitis.	Live attenuated.	Oral Polio Vaccine (OPV).	Preferred for routine use and during epidemics.
	Formalin-inactivated.	Inactivated Vaccine (IPV).	Selective use in unimmunized adults.
2. Women of Child-Bearing Age			
Rubella vaccine.	Live attenuated.	SC once.	Only to women who are antibody (H,1) negative and if pregnancy can be prevented for 3 months Post-vaccination.
3. Post Pubertal Males			
Mumps.	Live attenuated.	SC once.	Prevention of orchitis in susceptible sero-negative males.
4. Persons at High Risk of Acquiring Disease or Developing Complications of Disease			
Influenza.	Inactivated.	SC yearly.	Directed at reducing morbidity and mortality in those at risk of complications of influenza e.g. chronic heart and lung diseases and those over 65 years.
Pneumococcal polysaccharide vaccine.	Purified tetra-decavalent polysaccharide vaccine.	SC once	Same population as influenza vaccine functional or surgical asplenia, agammaglobulinemia, cirrhosis multiple myeloma, and nephrotic syndrome.

IMMUNITY-IMMUNOLOGY PROPHYLAXIS

Type of vaccine	Administration and frequency.		Comments
Hepatitis B vaccine.	Inactivated sub unit vaccine.	3 doses 1M 0,1, and 3 months	High Risk groups for acquisition of hepatitis B including household contracts of hepatitis B patients, patients requiring a large volume of clotting factors, homosexual men, and selected medical and dental personel.

5. Population Exposed to Localised Outbreaks

Meningococcal vaccine A,C AC.	Purified capsular polysaccharide	SC once	Control of localized epidemics and adjunct to chemoprophylaxis household contacts.
Measles vaccine	Live attenuated	SC once	Control of outbreak usually among adolescents or young adults.
B.C.G. vaccine	Live attenuated	SC or intradermaly once	Used in groups with excessive risk of new infection with individuals persistently exposed to suputum positive tuberculosis.
Adino virus vaccine	Live attenuated bivalent(types 4 and 7)	PO once	Used only for military recruits.
Typhoid vaccine	Inactivated bacilli.	SC in two doses	Household contact of documented Salmonella typhi carrier.
Rubella vaccine	Live attenuated	SC once	Control of outbreak among adolescents and young adults (must screen pubertal females) with HI test prior to vaccination.

6. Travellers to Foreign Countries

Type of vaccine	Administration and frequency		Comments
Small pox	Live vaccinia virus	Intradermally, every 3-5 years.	Not recommended except for travel to countries requiring vaccination certificates.
Yellow fever	Live attenuated	SC once per 10 years	Administered at yellow fever vaccination centers.
Cholera	Phenol inactivated suspension	SC approxi-	Only 50% effective and not effective in decreasing transmission of disease.
Typhoid	Inactivated bacilli	SC in half doses 4 weeks apart.	70-90% efficacy in "normal" exposure.
Typhus	Foamaldehyde -in activated Rickettsia prowazeki.	SC in two doses 4 weeks apart.	Only to persons in close contract to those where disease is indigenous.
Plague	Formaldehyde in activated Yersinia pestis.	SC in three injections of 0.5 ml at least 1 week apart, booster approximately every 2 years.	—
Hepatitis A	Immune serum globulin	1 M every 3 months.	—
Poliomyelitis	Oral or inactivated poliovaccine.	PO	Most adults already immune.

**PO. orally.
SC, subcutaneously;
1M intramuscularly.

(B) Passive Immunization

1. Diphtheria :

Antitoxic serum produced in horses by repeated injections of diphtheria injections of diphtheria toxoid and toxin.

Dose and Methods— For prophylaxis on 1M dose of 500-1000 units. Therapeutic initial dose 10,000-20,000 units.

**Remarks—*For prophylactic purposes combined antitoxin and toxoid injection is used.

2. Tetanus :

Antitoxic serum produced in horses by repeated injections of toxide and toxin.

Dose and Methods— For prophylactic one 1M dose of 1500 units. Therapeutic dose initial 20,000-40,000 units minimum 10,000 units.

*Remarks— For prophylactic purpose combined antitoxin and toxoid injection is used.

Q. 14.15. What are the basis of active and passive immunization?

Antibodies are produced in the body in response to the stimulus either of infection with an organism or the administration of a suspension of an organism, dead or alive by mouth or by injection. When alive, the organisms have been weakened, or attenuated, by some laboratory means so that, whereas they still stimulate antibodies, they do not produce their characteristic disease. However stimulated, the antibodies are produced by the body itself and therefore tend to remain in the body indefinitely. Moreover, the antibody-producing cells of the body remain sensitized to the infectious agent and respond to it again, if it attacks the body, by pouring out more antibody. This is why one attack of a disease often renders a person immune to a second attack and is the theoretical basis of *active immunization* by vaccines.

Antibody can be passed from one person to another, conferring protection on that second person; but in this case the antibody has not been produced in the body of the second person, nor have the antibody—producing cells been stimulated. The antibody is a foreign substance and and is eventually eliminated from the body, so that protection is short lived. The most common example of this form of passive immunity is the transference of antibodies from the mother through the placenta to the inborn child. This is why a disease such a measles is common in babies less than one year old after that age, the infant has lost all of tis maternal antibody and becomes susceptible to the disease, unless protected by active immunization. Sometimes antibody is extracted in the form of gamma globulin from blood taken from immune persons and is infected into susceptible persons to give them protection against a disease for examples, measles or rubella. This *passive immunization gives protection only temporary.*

Q. 14.16. What is meant by Live vaccines ?

Vaccine is a preparation of an antigen for preventive inoculation which when adminstered stimulates specifc antibody formation in the body. The live vaccines are prepared from live attenuated organisms. In general, live vaccines are more potent immunising agents than killed vaccines. The reasons are as follows :

1. The organisms multiply in the host and the resulting antigenic dose is much stroger than what is injected.
2. Live vaccines have all the major and minor antigenic components.
3. They engage certain tissues of the body as for example the intestinal mucosa after adminsitration of oral polio vaccine.

The live vaccines in current use are : 1. B.C.G., 2. *Small pox*, 3. *Oral polio*, 4. *Yellow fever*, 5. *Measles*, 6. *Mumps*. Smallpox vaccine is adminstered subcutaneously, B.C.G. intradermally, yellow fever subcutaneously and polio (Sabin) orally.

V. ROUTINE IMMUNIZATION PROCEDURE, RECOMMANDED SCHEDULE

Q. 14.17. Name the various diseases against which the children should immunised. or Describe the Routine immunization procedures and Recommended Immunization Schedule.

(A) Routine Immunization Procedure :

Infancy and early childhood are the most susceptible periods of human life. They need to be protected against several common infections which affect them namely, *diphtheria, whooping cough, tetanus, smallpox, poliomyelitis, tuberculosis and also enteric infections and cholera* particularly in the tropical countries. It should also be realized that the child should be in fully healthy state to respond to the various antigens which are now recommended for prophylactic use, and that the antibody forming mechanism is not fully developed in very early infant stage. This is why that it should be protected during the first 2 or 3 months by the antibodies passively transferred from mother to the infant. For adequate protections during this period the best course, therefore, is to thoroughly immunise the mother particularly against smallpox and tetanus prior to her undertaking the responsibility of motherhood to take adequate antenatal care to facilitate delivery of a healthy child.

To avoid over crowding of prophylactic injections combined vaccines are often used e.g. *Triple Antigen* containing diphtheria and tetanus toxoids and killed Pertusis bacilli in optimum proportion, is given in three doses with give rise of antibody titre against each. Some countries even prefer to use *Quadruple vaccine* by combining *Polio vaccine* with the *Triple Antigen*. The only risk in triple vaccine reported by some workers is that of provoking polio myelitis following such injection but the risk was found to be negligible, if any. The vaccines should, however, be suitably spaced. An interval of at least *two weeks* should be allowed after triple vaccine or polio vaccine before undertaking vaccination against smallpox and a gap of *three weeks* between smallpox vaccination and other inoculations, between B.C.G. vaccination and smallpox, or yellow fever or polio vaccines either following or preceding it. B.C.G. vaccine may, however, follow *a week* after a killed vaccine or a killed vaccine may follow *four weeks* after B.C.G. vaccine. The arm used for B.C.G. vaccine should be avoided for any other vaccine for a period of three months.

For prophylactic purposes in *diphtheria and tetanus* mass immunization with antitoxin may be followed by one to two days later by toxoid (active) immunization. In tetanus, administration of tetanus antitoxin has beem simultaneously followed by tetanus toxoid adsorbed on aluminium hydroxide instead of formol toxoid, at a different site.

The second dose of absorbed toxoid should be given six weeks after the first dose and the third dose 6—12 months after the second. This will maintain the immunity level for at least five years.

(B) Recommended Immunization Schedule

Age	Immunisation against Diseases
First to 4th week	B.C.G. vaccination (to prevent Tuberculosis) and cowpox vaccine.
3rd month	Smallpox primary vaccination. (if not given during first week of life).
4th month	(1) First dose of Triple Antigen. [Diphtheria, whooping cough-tetanus(DPT)] (2) First dose of oral polio-vaccine (polio).
5th month	Second dose of (1) and (2)
6th month	Third dose of (1) and (2)
8th month	Booster dose of Triple Vaccine.
3rd year	1. T.A.B.C. (Typhoid, para A and para B, cholera). Combind typhoid, Para typhoids, and cholera in two doses subcutaneously at interval of 1-2 weeks. 2. Revaccination against smallpox.
5th year	Revaccination against smallpox.
6th year	Booster dose of combined diphtheria and tetanus toxoids.
8th year	B.C.G. after tuberculin testing.
9th to 10th year	Optimal booster dose of T.A.B.C.
Before school leaving	Revaccination against smallpox.

IMMUNITY-IMMUNOLOGY PROPHYLAXIS

Rest of life
1. Revaccination against smallpox.
2. Booster dose of T.A.B.C. at 5 yearly intervals.
3. Booster dose of tetanus toxiod for those who are exposed to special risk.
4. Other vaccines as needed or in emergency.

N.B.
1. Now the Government has started neonatal vaccination against smallpox. The infant is vaccinated against smallpox together with B.C.G. vaccination, at the maternity home.
2. No immunization is to be done if the person has fever, as the fever may be the manifestation of the same disease.
3. Do not give cowpox vaccination if the child has eczema.
4. Diphtheria and tetanus vaccines are given in 2 doses at interval of 4 to 6 weeks.
5. Cholera, typhoid, plague vaccines are given in 2 doses at interval of one weeks.

Q. 14.18. Can we use Homoeopathic Medicine as a prophylaxis, if so, how and why? Illustrate with examples?

The objective of Preventive Medicine is to intercept or "oppose" the disease process in man or community. This may be done at various levels in the course of the natural history of disease. In this regard, according to Allopathy there are five levels of prevention :

1) *Health promotion*
2) *Specific protection*
3) *Early diagnosis*
4) *Disability limitation, and*
5) *Rehabilitation*

But in the homoeopathy, all these are same, except specific protection by specific immunization. Where it has its own views regarding the principles, use and scope.

The following are the principle methods which are advocated by the different stalwarts of homoeopathy from begining to present era.

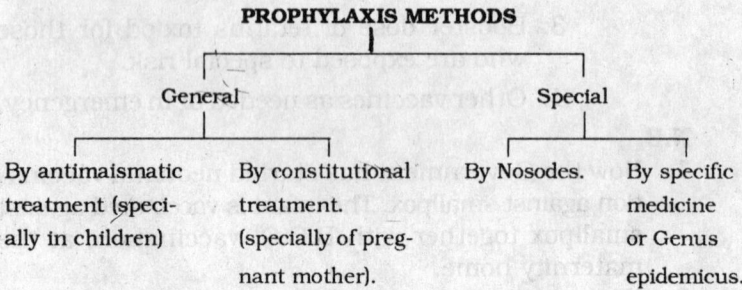

PROPHYLAXIS METHODS — General (By antimaismatic treatment (specially in children); By constitutional treatment (specially of pregnant mother)); Special (By Nosodes; By specific medicine or Genus epidemicus).

(I) General Prophylaxis

(1) By Antimiasmatic treatment :

Dr. Winter, in a essay on prophylaxis, denies the existence of special prophylactics; like—*Vaccininum for Variola, Belladonna for Scarlet fever, Aconite* for measles, but he describes general prophylactics in homoeopathy. He says that those chiefly liable to epidemic, miasmatic and contagious diseases are not in a good relative state of health. There is something wrong with their vegetative system to which these diseases have a particular affinity. He furhter states that if we are able to act on the vegetative system in such a way as to eradicate its faults, we shall put those persons in a condition to resist these disease, or at least to have them very mildly.

In order to effect these changes in the vegetative system, he proposes to give sucessive doses of the 1st, 2nd or 3rd dilution or triturition of *Mercurius* followed by *Sulphur, Calcarea, Lycopodium, Graphites, Arsenic* etc.

A similar idea seems to have occurred to Dr. Gastier of *Thoissery*, who wrote a special work on the subject of prophylaxis. His object is chiefly to prevent chronic diseases.

As regards *chronic diseases* he starts the idea that they originate from the *Psoric Miasm*, in most cases transmitted by the parent to the offspring. When there is reason to suspect such a hereditary psoric constitution in as infant, which in later life would become developed into different dyscrasias recommends that the child be subjected to an antipsoric prophylactic treatment consisting of a succession of the so-called antipsoric remedies. The recommended for these courses are :

1. Sulphur
2. Sepia
3. Carbo vegetabilis
4. Arsenicum
5. Belladonna
6. Lachesis
7. Nitric Acid
8. Silica
9. Thuja occidentalis.
10. Lycopodium.
11. Graphites
12. Calcarea carb.
13. Phosphorus.

Mode of administration:

A dose of each of these medicines consisting of one globule of the 30th dilution, is to be administered to the child every 5th day until the course is finished, unless there should occur after any of them an erruption on the skin in which case the course is to be interrupted until this artificial erruption has gone off. If no erruption takes place, the preservation is, says *Gastier equally certain*. But, in order to make assurance doubly sure, he recommends that the course is to be repeated every year. This medicine in the above course may, Dr. Gastier remarks, be given either by the mouth or by olfaction.

Criticism : But there is great doubt regarding the efficacy of the courses of medicine advised to be given to infants by Dr. Winter and Gastier. Regarding this Dr. R.E. Dudgeon is in the opinion that the best plan to adopt with infants is to place them in the best hygienic conditions and not to resort to medicinal interference until we see something to treat. It will often happen that we may obtain a correct knowledge of the peculiar diathesis of a child from very trivial signs during the first weeks or months of its life and be enabled by the administration of the appropriate remedies, to check such diathesis in the bud. Moreover to fix on a certain definite course of medicine that is to be crammed down every suspected infant's throat is a very senseless and illogical procedure.

2. General Prophylaxis by constitutional treatment:

Dr. Fearson also advocated general prophylaxis by constitutional treatment especially of pregnant mother. He has favoured a course of preventive treatment in cases of suspected constitutional tendency to disease, not only in the very earliest infancy but also from the very moment of conception when that can be ascertained. The constitutional treatment of the foetus shall be through the system of mother. He does not enter into any detail respecting the constitutional preventive treatment to be adopted like Dr. Winter and Gastier. However, if the mother is unhealthy during the gestation, we should devote great attention to her treatment, as by rendering her healthier we may greatly influence the constitutions of the foetus that dervies sole nutrition from her.

(II) Special Prophylaxis

1. By Nosodes :

The prevention of illness by using the agent which may cause or transmit the disease has been known for centuries, and some of the earliest examples of this were to protect against virus infections. The *Chinese* used to give protection against smallpox by compulsory wearing of the garments of a patient in full suppuration, or by the introduction of a one-year-old dried pustule into the nostrils, and during the 17th and 18th centuries in Europe vaccination against using inoculation with variolic pus was carried out. Hippocrates recommended the slimy saliva from under the tongue of a rabid dog, taken as a drink, as a protection against rabies.

These are examples of *Isopathy*, a form of therapy based on the principle of treating with the same agent that may cause or transmit the disease, as compared with *homoeopathy* which is based on the *law of similars*. We wonder how many antagonists of homoeopathy realise that the work of Edward Jenner, who confirmed the belief that infection with cowpox would protect a person against smallpox and so laid the foundation of mordern immunization, is in fact a clear illustration of the homoeopathic principle.

Every immunization procedure carries some risk of adverse reactions when material amounts of disease agents are used, be it an actual infection of else an immunological reaction, and these risks may deter both doctor and patient from using them in individual cases. Here homoeopathic preparations of disease products in potency, known as *nosodes*, can be used, and as a result of many years of clinical use there seem to be good grounds for recommending their efficacy and safety. Though the efficacy of all homoeopathic prophylactic remedies for various conditions have not been proved by controlled studies and statistical records, yet generations of homoeopaths have used these remedies to prevent the disease conditions and claim to have done successfully. So their efficacy may be accepted on the basis of experience even if it is not proved experimentally.

Recent Research on Nosodes: Little research has been carried on the immunological effects of nosodes in the body, although *Diptherinum*, a homoeopathic preparation of diphtheritic membrane, has been shown to induce a positive Shick-test 2 to 9 weeks after giving the 200 potency.

Meningococcin, the homoeopathic preparation of Neissaria meningitiis, in 1974; there was on epidemic of *cerebro spinal fever* in the Sao Paulo region of Brazil, and about 18,000 people were immunized with a single drop of *Meningococcin*-10M on tongue, and only four of these developed meningitis during epidemic. Compared with the incidence in the non-immunized group, the results were statistically highly significant.

We have also found similar results using *Pertussin* in the prevention of whooping cough syndrome. *Pertussin* is prepared from the sticky mucus in the throat of a patient suffering from whooping cough, and has been used in the treatment and prevention of this illness for about 80 years, usually in the 30 potency. It appears to be helpful in both true *Bordetella pertussis* infection, and the similar symptom picture casused by several different viruses. It is safe to immunize the child with pertussin at any age, even the neonatal period, and addvisable to give booster doses either annually, or when there is risk of future contact. A single dose, or a split dose of the 30 potency, does not enough to prevent an infection that is already being incubated, and in such cases *pertussin* 30 is need for seven days twice daily with great success.

Morbillinum is prepared from the exudate taken from the mouth and pharynx of a patient with measles, and has been prophylactically in the 30th potency given at weekly intervals during the incubation period. Alternatively, homoeopathic remedies which have a similar symptoms picture to that caused by the infection can give prophylaxis.

In the case of *Measles*, *Morbillinum* has been used as a preventive, given in the 30th or 200 potency daily during the incubation period until the danger of infection is past.

Various *influenza* nosodes have been used over the years and *Influenzinum* appears to be a safe and effective alternative to the orthodox vaccine, given each winter in the 30th potency. Different types of influenza nosode are also available e.g. A,B, AB, A_2 (Hongkong 1968), B (Hongkong 1972), etc. concerning the prevention of recurrent respiratory infections in general, the tubercular nosodes *Tuberculinum bovinum* and *Bacillinum* have been found effective, especially in children.

Oscillococcinum is nosode used especially in France to prevent and treat respiratory tract infections. It is prepared from autolyzed duck heart and liver, and is so named because the germs observed in the original culture, exhibited an oscillating movement. It is most often used in the 200th potency at regular intervals through the winter months as a preventive for influenza and other respiratory infections.

Other nosodes that have been used to give prophylaxis are *Rubella nosode*, *Lyssin* prepared from the saliva of a rabid dog, *Variolinum*, prepared from the discharge from a smallpox pustule, and Malandrinum, prepared from the serous discharge of a horse with *malandra or "grease"* a weeping eczema in the hollow of the fold of the knee, believed to be cause by the same virus as causes cowpox.

2. By Specific Medicine or Genus Epidemicus :

Medicine which is indicated in majority of patients affected from an epidemic disease is termed as *Genus Epidemicus*. It can only be obtained after the break out of an epidemic disease in the community (by the homoeopathic method) and when the *Genus epidemicus* is applied to healthy persons of that particular locality, it acts as a preventive medicine and escapes those persons from that particular disease. Homoeopathic law provides specific remedies for specific disease condition during epidemics such as *Belladonna* for scarlet fever, *Diphtherinum* and *Merc cyanide* for diphtheria, *Carbo veg.* and *Cuprum met.* for whooping cough, *Lathyrus sative* and *Gelsemium* for poliomyelitis, *Veriolinum* for smallpox etc. They have also a much higher degree of efficiency when the remedies are given for protection.

As the law of similars excels in the power to cure, it excels more forcibly and certainly in the art of disease prevention. But they never causes *anaphylaxis of shock, never results in secondary infection, never leaves in its wake serum or vaccine disease or any other severe reaction; it simply protects surely and gently.*

An epidemic of *Scarlet fever* may have more cases with a rough or a purplish rash than those having the typical smooth, shinning, red rash which *Belladonna* is specific where the typical rough, darker rash prevails remedies like *Ailanthus* and *Phytolacca* and *Sulphur* will give more certain protection, but after the single epidemic remedy is found it brings the highest protection of any other. (Hahnemann).

In *diphtheria* protection, the remedy *Diphtherinum* is the leading prophylactic but in some severe epidemics of the past *Merc cyanide* has proved to be very effective as well as curative in this disease.

In whooping cough, *Carbo veg.* has been a reliable protection in hundreds of cases of young children an infants. But some epidemic require like *Drosera* and *Cuprum metal licum* and then they afford the most certain protection.

The remedy *Lathyrus sativa* gives the most certain protection in thousands of cases exposed to polio through many epidemics over the last forty years. It easily heads the list of homoeopathic remedies for protection against that dread disease. This remedy has the same affinity to the same centres in the spinal cord and brain as the polio virus and acts as the most perfect antidote both for protection and cure. This single instrument in Homoeopathy's citadel of power should command world-wide recognisation both from the medical profession and the laity at large.

Against smallpox, *Variolinum* is effective weapon, but we have others that have proved curative and effective prophylactic agents in many epidemics of the past, such as *Sarracenia purpurea, Antim tart, Vaccininum,* and *Malandrinum. Ant tart* in the third trituration rubbed on an abrasion of the skin produces a typical vaccination scar.

Malandrinum is the most potent antidote to the dangerous septicemia sometimes following *vaccination* and *Thuja* is the best antidote.

Conclusion :

So it is strange, so little has been said by homoeopathic doctors familiar with the wide spread possibilities of homoeopathic prophylaxis, especially in the face of the so many harmful and even deadly accidents that have followed the application of the prevailing methods of protection against acute epidemic diseases.

As true healers and educaters in progressive medicine it is our duty to give to the world this knowledge for its protection and well being.

It is also duty to invite physicians of all schools of healing to test fully the homoeopathic art of protection against epidemic diseases. If such tests are honestly done by sincere men of all schools of healing, Homoeopathy would reach its place in the sun.

Recently it is known that the vast majority of *respiratory infections* are of viral origin and for the most part allopathic medicine has little to offer other than symptomatic palliation, which may indeed be detrimental through suppressing what could be regarded as one of the body's emergency excretion routes *catarrhal discharge* only in the relatively few cases of septic tonsillitis, diphtheria, epiglottitis and bacterial pueumonia are antibiotics of benefit. But being able to prescribe homoeopathic remedies with confidence is one way in which the honest general physician can overcome the almost superstitions demand for an antibiotic by the anxious parents of children whose respiratory infections comprise a major part of the work load in general practice in this country.

Anti-viral chamotherapy is still very much in its infancy, and, therfore, homoeopathic treatment can play a leading part in the prevention of management of acute virus infections. If in such cases where there is no effective alternative, doctors would prescribe homoeopathic remedies in accordance with the law of similars. I believe that they would be pleasantly surprised and encouraged to go on further with homoeopathy.

Q. 14.19. Whether the potentised homoeopathic medicine can produce immunity or not?

Yes, it can do. Homoeopathic physicians are curing plenty of cases of diphtheria, whoopoing cough, typhoid etc. by homoeopathic medicines and this is possible because antibodies are formed against the antigens of these diseases which counteract the antigens and the action of their toxins, unless it can never cure diseases. But until we can prove this in the laboratory or we can give some scientific explanation, it may not be accepted by the scientific world and the public may not understand.

Explaination :

When a Homoeopathic medicine is applied in potentised form it excites the vital force. The supreme commander on its part immediately directs its subordinate forces (resisting force, chemical defence substances of the blood etc.) to organise such groups of army as would be able to fight out the ensuing drug action. Any medicine in its crude form creates a disease in this economy, but the peculiarity of the potentised medicine when applied on a healthy person is this; that the potentised medicine does not create a disease in the body; but excites the vital force to be prepared for combating with such disease as can be produced by the potentised drug in its crude form. A potentised medicine creates similar symptoms as those of its crude form without manifesting the disease on the body. It only excites the vital force for getting ready to fight out such symptoms.

In this process when preventive drugs are applied on healthy persons and repeated twice or thrice considering the action of the drug, the vital force is enriched with groups of fighting forces (antibodies) for that particular disease. Thus the body becoming immune from that disease. In this process we can immunise the mass against such epidemic diseases after selecting the appropriate remedy for particular epidemic (Genus Epidemicus).

Homoeopathic Therapeutic Law of Nature can also be explained by immunological phenomenon as that homoeopathic medicine acts through the vital force on the endogenous protein to act as antigen and during this phase, a similar but stronger disease tends to be produced in the system; but meanwhile antibodies start forming against *medicine stimulation*, and the medicinal antibodies jointly with the antigenic antibodies counteract the disease antigen and the patient gets cured. There is not actually stronger permanent disease being produced in the system but a tendency or threatening for the same. But if the doses are repeated for a long time unnecessarily then the patient instead of being cured, suffers terribly from the drug action and may even lead to a drug disease.

Recently with the help of latest laboratory techniques like fluoroscent antibody lebelled test, complement fixing antibody test, radio active iodine test radio-immuno assay etc. We can easily prove that homoeopathic medicine can produce immunity in a body. Generally this can be done by the use of homoeopathic nosodes as well as medicines in a group of persons and it is seen as soon as some reactions start in the form of symptoms.

IMMUNITY-IMMUNOLOGY PROPHYLAXIS 429

Q. 14.23. How to test whether a man immune or susceptible to a particular type of epidemic?

This can be tested by giving few doses of a potentised medicine similar to the epidemic in quick succession. If the person reacts soon after the first, second or third doses, it may be presumed that he hypersusceptible to that medicine and consequiently to that type of disease having similar symptoms. But if he does not manifest any reaction even after 8, 10 or 12 such doses, it may be presumed that the person is more or less immune, of course this requires experiment and verification.

Q. 14.24. What medicines are best for the purpose of homoeopathic immunization ?

Nosodes prepared from the respective disease products are best for immunization purpose. Because they contain the "simple substance" or the dynamis of the organisms responsible for specific diseases and as such they excite both the cellurar and humoral antibodies. There are many nosodes in homoeopathy, e.g. Morbillinum for measles, Diphtherinum for diphtheria, Pertussin for whooping cough, Parotidinum for mumps, Typhodinum for typhiod, Veriolinum, Vaccininum and Malandrinum for smallpox, Pyrogen for sepsis, *Tuberculinum* and *Bacillinum* for tuberculosis, *Medorrhinum* for gonorrhoea, *Syphilinum* for syphilis, *Psorinum* for psora, *Lysin* for hydrophobia and so on.

But for diseases where the respective nosodes are not available, any homoeopathic medicine capable of producing similar symptoms to that of the disease intended to be prevented, may be give safely. Because any medicine having similar symptoms will produce similar antibodies in the system which undoubtedly will prevent the advent or action of similar weaker antigen (disease) curing later according to the phenomena observed and stated by Dr. Hahnemann in his *Organon* when two similar diseases meet together in the living human organism at the same time. This is also true in even cases where nosodes are inavailable, e.g. we can prevent smallpox by *Thuja occidentalis*, (instead of Malandinum, and Vaccininum), Measles by *Pulsatilla* (instead of Parotidium), Whooping cough by *Drosera*. Diphtheria by Apis mel etc. and also shown by many renouned homoeopaths of the world.

Q. 14.25. What are the Homoeopathic Medicines ? Are they prophylaxis of the following diseases ?

Name of the Diseases	Homoeopathic Medicines are used
1. Tuberculosis	*Tuberculinum.* (Kent)
2. Cholera	*Ars alb, Cup ars, Verat alb. Sulph.* (Farrington)
3. Diphtheria	*Apis mel, Diptherinum, Merc cyanide.*
4. Influenza	*Influenzinum.*
5. Smallpox	*Variolinum, Vaccinanum, Malandrinum, Ant tart, Hydrastis, Thuja.*
6. Measles	*Pulsatilla, Morbillinum.*
7. Mumps	*Pilocarpus, Parotidinum, Trifolium repens*
8. Yellow fever	*Carbo veg.*
9. Hayfever	*Ars alb, Psorinum.*
10. Whooping cough	*Drosera, Pertussin.*
11. Hydrophobia	*Bell, Canth, Cuprum met, Hydrophobinum, Lysin*
12. Erysipalas	*Graphites.*
13. Intermittent fever	*China, Arsenic alb, Malaria officinalis. Nat mur.*
14. Scarlet fever	*Bell, Eucalyptus.*
15. Haemophilia	*Sanguinaria, Phoshphorus.*
16. Quinsy	*Baryta carb.*
17. Poliomyelitis	*Gelsemium, Lathyrus Sativa.*
18. Respiratory tract infections	*Occillococcinum.*

*All the disease should be treated by the homoeopathic medicine after symptomatic consideration.

CHAPTER-XV

DEMOGRAPHY AND FAMILY PLANNING

DISCUSSION FOR LEARNING

I. Demography.
II. Population growth in India with different Demographic Data.
III. Various Demographic features.
IV. Importance of population projections.
V. Family planning—its definition and needs.
VI. Contraception, and contraceptive methods.
VII. Contraceptives, M.T.P. and Sterilization.
(Vesectomy, Tubectomy and Laparoscopy)
VIII. Advantages of Family Planning.
IX. National Family Planning Programmes and its organisational set up.
X. Present attitude towards Family Planning.

I. DEMOGRAPHY

Q. 15.1. What is meant by Demography?

The word *'Demography'* is derived from two Greek words, *demos* means people and *graphein* means to write, thus demography is the scientific study of human population, through the following demographic process, namely—*fertility, mortality, mairrage, migration* and *social mobidity*, focusing readily obserable human phenomena like :

(i) *changes in population size* (growth and decline);
(ii) *the composition of the population*;
(iii) *the distribution of the population in space.*

Q. 15.2. What are the sources of Demographic information?

Sources of Demographic information are :
1. *Census.*
2. *Vital ragistration.*

3. *Institutional records.*
4. *Adhoc survey reports.*

Apart from these sources, which can give information for any country, organisations like UN and WHO's periodical reports e.g. Demographic Year Book, World Health Situation, Epidemological and Vital Statistical Reports etc.

II. POPULATION GROWTH & DEMOGRAPHIC DATA

Q. 15.3. Describe the population growth of India with the various demographic features affecting the population growth.

Growth of World Population

Our knowledge is very limited about the growth of the human race during the early preleolithic age. It is evident from archaeological discoveries that men using tools living were on the earth about 100,000 years ago. At that stage they were always moving about in small groups in search of food and shelter. Their number increased or decreased depending on the availability of edible seeds, fruits and roots they could obtain and flesh of animals they could kill. Many of them died of hunger and exposure to extremes of weather, attack of wild animals and tribal wars. After the discovery of shardedged stone weapons, men could kill animals more easily for food and also protect themselves better. After 6000 B.C., men discovered agriculture and fire and such discoveries brough a revolution in their way of life. Thus their number began to increase slowly as the limiting factors were still severe, in the forms of disease, epidemics and war between different tribes.

But the world population showed increase in the three successive stages. The *1st stage* was when human society developed primitive agriculture, reared domestic animals, developed poultry, used flint and fire.

The *2nd stage* of growth began with the development of towns and cities, use of minerals and machinery. The *3rd stage* was heralded by extensive use of natural resources, electricty, transport, complex machineries and life-saving drugs.

Population Growth in India

Some workers have estimated that India's population was almost stationary at 100 millions during the long period from 300 B.C. to 1600 A.D. The first census in India was taken in 1871 and thereafter every 10 years, the last in 1981. It is believed that at first three censuses population was under recorded. Even so, it increased at slow rate upto 1921, which may be termed a year of transition. During this period the growth was irregular and sometimes negative. The rate of growth showed an upward trend after 1921 and 1981 it was recorded maximum (2.16 per cent per year). Now India, the second most populous country of the world next to China, is multiplying her population. By adding one prospective citizen every one and half second, she has already over stressed her resources in respect of *food supply, housing, clothing, education and employment.*

Through only about half of Australia in size (*Australia is 2.5 times the size of India, 14.8 million entire people*), India is adding about 13.6 million people to her present census (685 million 1981, 711 million in mid 1982, and 720 million in 1985), every year, which is more than the total population of the island continent. This continent of Asia has 15.6 per cent of world's land with 53.0 per cent of the world population. Compare to this 2.4 per cent of world's land are India supports 15.5% of the world population.

Following independence and partitioning of the country 1947, India had to face an unprecedented inflow of displaced persons from both wings of Pakistan of a magnitude which had no parallel in history. Though some people from India migrated to Pakistan, the immigrants vastly out numbered the emigrants. Moreover India had also to take back many people of Indian origin from Burma, Sri Lanka and some East African countries, who were dislodged after independence of these countries. According to the report of the Refugee Relief and Rehabilitation Department of Government of West Bengal, 21,52,185 people (registered East Pakistan) between 1950 and 1970. According to the census taken in 1901 the population of India was 238.3 million; it increased to 252.0 million in 1911 but declined slightly to 251.2 million in 1921. From 1921 onward the population recorded gradual increases to 279.0 million in 1931, 318.5 million in 1941, 360.9 million in 1951, 439.0 million in 1961, 547.9 million in 1971 and about 685.0 million in 1981, and at present it is about 711 million.

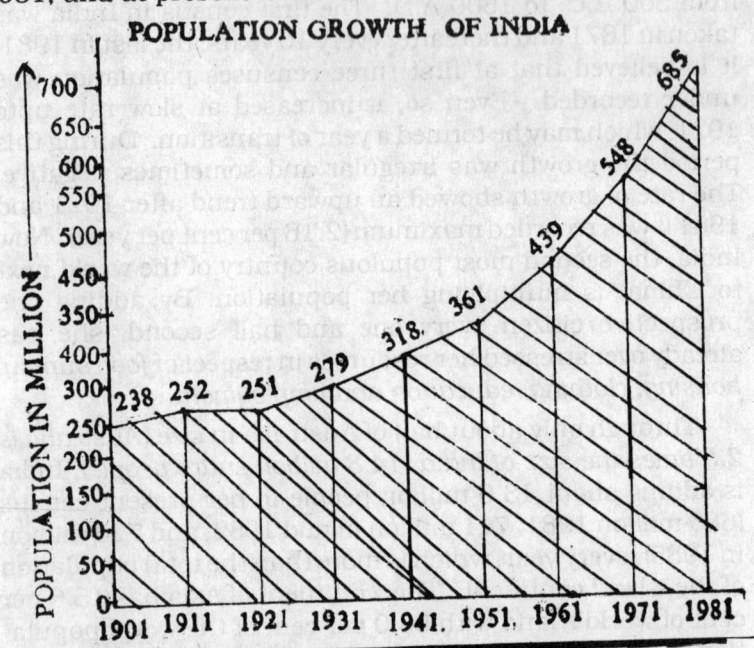

The 1981 census also showed that India's population grow by 137 million between 1971 and 1981, as against 109 during the previous decade. So it showed that after 37 years of Independence the population of India has been doubled (it was 340 million in 1947), i.e. a second India has been added.

Different Demographic Data of India

1. *Area :* 3268090 Sq. Km. or 2.4 percent of world land area.
2. *Population (1981)* - 685. 148. 692—(685.1) crores.
3. *Decinnial growth rate (1971—1981)*—25.00 percent.
4. *Density of population (1981)*—221 per Sq. Km. (West Bengal have the highest densities 614 per Sq. Km, Bihar-402, UP-377, Tamil Nadu-371 and Panjab-331. India ranks 7th among major countries of the world).

5. *Ages and Sex ratio of population (1981)* :
   Females—1000, males—935.
   0-14   years=42%
   15-64   years=55.4%
   over 64 years=2.6%
6. *Percentage of Urban and Rural population (1981)* :
   Urban population—20 percent.
   Rural population—80 percent.
7. *Literacy Rate (1981)—36.17%*
   Males—46.74%
   Females—24.88%
   Kerala has the highest literacy rate (69.17) and at the bottom Bihar (26.01) and Rajasthan (24.05).
8. *Birth Rate and Death Rate (1971 to 1980)* :
   Birth rate—37.1%
   Death rate—14.8%
9. *Infant mortality rate*—110 per 1000 live birth :

N.B. :

So from the Data it is seen that the high birth rate with low death rate is the main causes of population explosion in India.

(i) On the basis of the caste and religion it has been observed that the fertility rate is higher amongst the Muslims and the so-called lower castes in Hindus.
(ii) The custom of early child marriage in India is another contributory factor towards this end.
(iii) High dependency ratio and heavy burden on the younger wage earner groups creating unrest of the society and nullified all the programmes of the Governments for the progress of life and the society.

III. DEMOGRAPHIC FEATURES AFFECTING

Q. 15.4. What are the various demographic features or stages present in the world population and also in India?

Different demographic stages of world as well as India are characterised by :

1. *High stationary* : i.e. high birth rate and high death rate; which balance each other in the past, so that the population of India remained stationary up to 1921.

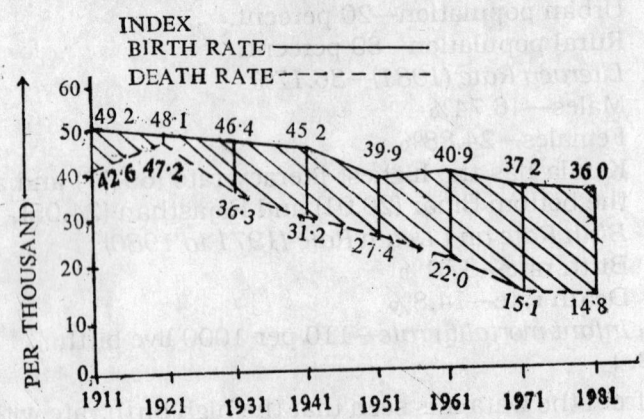

2. *Early expanding* i.e. high birth rate and falling of death rate : It is now seen in India (also other developing countries of Asia, Africa and Latin America), where the population is increasing due to imbalance between births and deaths. It is possibly due to the improved health conditions and shortening the period of breast feeding.

3. *Late expanding* i.e. low birth rate and low death rate : as attended by most of the developed countries of Europe and America, where the population increase has been checked due to balance in births and deaths.

India has now entered this place. China and Singapore also decline death rate still further, but birth rate tends to fall.

4. *Zero population growth* i.e. Very low birth rate and low death rate : Causing the population stationary. It is seen in Sweden, Germany in 1982 (Growth rate 0.1 have been recorded in Switzerland and Belgium in 1982).

5. *Declining* i.e birth rate is lower than the death rate : as seen in some European countries like Germany F.R and Luembourg (growth rate and death rate ratio = 0.3 : 0.1).

IV. IMPORTANCE POPULATION PROJECTIONS

Q. 15.5. What are the importance of population projections ?

Under existing conditions it is of utmost importance for planners in Government and outside, to know the future projection of population growth in the country, for realistic and effective planning. *Population projections* are, at best conjectural and depend upon the pattern of birth and death rates in country. Since serious attempts being made to curb the birth rate, population projections have made on the basis of three variants, namely *high, medium and low decline of birth rate*. It has been calculated that if the birth rate is reduced at a slow pace we could expect the population of India to reach about 750 *million* in 1985 and 1122 *million* in the year 2000. At a medium rate of reduction of birth rate the corresponding figures will be 682 and 981 million and at a high rate of reduction birth rate two population will be 661.5 or 908 million in the year 1980 & 2000 A.D. respectively. There calculations assume a static crude death rate. If the decline in death rate is also accepted as a variable then the projections have to be altered.

V. FAMILY PLANNING

Q. 15.6. What is Family planning?

There are several definitions of family planning. In 1971 *An Expert Committee of the WHO defined* :

"Family planning is a way of thinking and living that is adopted voluntarily, upon the basis of knowledge, attitudes and responsible decisions by individuals and couples, inorder to promote health and welfare of the family group and thus contribute effectively to the social development of a country."

(*WHO 1971*, Tech. Rep. Ser. No 483)

Another Expert Committee defined and described :

Family planning refers to practices, that help individudals or couples to attain the following objectives :

(i) to avoid unwanted births,
  (ii) to bring about unwanted births,
  (iii) to regulate the intervals between pregnancies,
  (iv) to control the time at which births occure in relation to the ages of the parent; and
  (v) to determine the number of children in the family.

Q. 15.7. What is meant by Family welfare?

"Children are to be borne because they are desired and not because they can not be prevented". So Family planning means planned parenthood by choice and not by chance, by spacing the birth through the methods of Birth Control by choice not by chance. So as it also includes the following measures to promote the welfare and harmonius growth of family, it is called family welfare.

Various measures :
  (i) *Preparing the young for the responsibility of marriage.*
  (ii) *Eugenics and sex education.*
  (iii) *Marriage guidance and counselling.*
  (iv) *Advice on sterility.*
  (v) *Screening for pathological conditions related to the reproductive system.*
  (vi) *Premarital consultation examination.*
  (vii) *Carry out pregnancy test.*
  (viii) *The preparation of couples for the arrival of their first child.*
  (ix) *Providing services for unmarried mothers.*
  (x) *Teaching home economics nutritions.*
  (xi) *Providing adoption services, which are conductive to health and happiness of the family.*

From the *National point of view*—it is a measure for population control and a means for the improvement of the national economic standard.

Q. 15.8. Why Family planning is needed in India?

Family planning is needed in India for the following causes :

1. Health Benefits :
  (a) Improves population's health and mortality.
  (b) Improves maternal health and mortality as well as infant health and mortality.

(B) Socio-economic Benifits :

(A) HEALTH BENEFITS

1. Control Population

The population of India has grown from 238 million in 1901 to 251 million in 1921, 361 million in 1951, 684 million in 1981. Thus during the 20 years between 1901 to 1921 the total increase was only 13 million, whereas during the next 30 years between 1921 to 1951 it increased to 110 million and lastly (1951 to 1981) it was 323 million. In this way if the population of India increased, the population of India will be 1037 million by 2000 A.D. So such excessive population growth adversely affects the economic growth of the country, lowers the standard of the country, lowers the standard of living, creates housing problem, requires the establishment of a larger number of schools and colleges for education, organisation of medical facilities on an extensive scale, the provision of larger amount of food, safe water and other sanitary facilities. India is already in difficulty about meeting these basic needs, so the family planning is needed to arrange the minimum standard of living.

2. For Food Production

The average land requirement to support an average family of 5 or 6 persons is 3 acres, but it has already reduced to 0.7 acres. Under the present condition of food production it is doubtful whether an individual can get even half of the prescribed balanced diet due to no-availability and high price of all kinds of foodstuff. This lack of food has alreade caused malnutrition and deficiency diseases and will lower the resistance against disease, creat apathy, inertia, fatigue and general reduction of output, ultimately there will be famine, and serious deterioration of health conditions leading to diseases and epidemics. So to meet up adequate balance diet family planning is needed.

3. For the Socio-economic Condition

There is already a serious unemployment in the country to the extent of 30 million. A slum has been created in industries leading to complete or partial closure of many small and even large industries with consequent retrenchment of workers, and increase of proverty, over crowding, starvation, disruption and disorganisation of society, ill-health and deaths. Besides the children born require to be fed, reared, clothed and educated, which entail a serious economic burden for well-neigh 20 years, before they can expected to be gainful employed. So to improve socio-economic condition of a people with employment in gainful occupations are needed family planning.

4. For the Preservation of Health of the Mother and Children

In the context of the existing living and economic conditions danger associated with frequent child bearing increase with the wide prevalance of malnutrition, under-nutrition, incidence of disease and even of deaths in mother as a result of cumulative effect in shattering their health as they go through successive course of the child bearing. At the same time the children that will be borne will get less and less attention and care resulting in malnutrition, illness and premature death. So to preserve the health of mothers ad her children family planning is necessary.

5. For Launched out Successful Planning

One of the most pernicious consequences of this tremendous growth is, even if we double all our resources and existing facilities e.g. schools, colleges, housing, transport facilities, food production, textiles, etc. with in next 28 years, even then, 1999 we will still be living in the same sub-human conditions as we are at present, with the per capita consumption of daily necessitities, among the lowest in the world. This will be mainly for the result of high and relatively stable fertility and decline mortality. The rate of Indian mortality estimated as 48.6 per 1000 population in 1921, come down to 14.8 in 1981, but the birth rate of 49.2 per 1000 population in 1921, stood above or around 36 per 1000 population in 1986. It was seen that due to high rate of population growth the first five yearly plans launched by Government set back to improve the socio-economic conditions and standard of living. So to improve the standard of living and socio-economic condition regulation of Indian's population by size and quality is utmost importance. This is generally done by Family Planning Programme with National Welfare, unless the energy and money spend by Government, or other organisation or any development work will be nulified by the unchecked population.

VI. CONTRACEPTION, CONTRACEPTIVE METHODS

Q. 15.9. What is meant by contraception? and What are its utilities?

Contraception is the practice against conception and is an important primary health care for the population. The basic principle of contraceptions is to prevent or interference of any one of the following condition to fulfil the conception:

1. Sexual union between a man and woman both of whom have reached the age of puberty and are within the reproductive period of lives.
2. To deposit semen containing viable sperms in the vagina.
3. To the passage of the sperm from the vagina, through the cervical canal and uterine cavity to the uterine orifice of the fallopian tube and then towards along the tube to meet the ovum awaiting fertilization. This period is about 4 to 5 days beginning 11th day from the first day of previous menstruration.
4. To enter the unfertilised ovum into the fallopian tube from the peritoneal cavity, where it is discharged by the ovary.
5. To travel the fertilized ovum in the uterine cavity.
6. To receive and accept the fertilized ovum in the endometerium of the uterus.

N.B. : [*Contraception and conceptions :- Prevention of conception by any means or devices is known as contraception. The devices which are used for the purpose of preventing conception are known as contraceptives.*]

Utilities :

1. Contraception can space and limit child births according to the resources of the family and thus a wider concept can stabilize the population with in the resources of the country and the world as a whole. So to improve people's health and lower mortality by improving the living standard and quality of life use of contraceptives are necessary.

2. The women can reduce mostly safely strong healthy intelligent child when she is 20-30 years and child births are at 30 more years interval and two children care born. Women aged beyond 20-30 years and having poorly spaced many child births during the reproductive period increase the risk of maternal death and ill health due to multiparty. These also increase infant mortality and morbidity. So to reduce maternal and infant mortality in the developed country like us spacing and limiting childbirth by contraception and also by raising age of marriage in female beyond 20 years is necessary. Improved health in the family also brings economic benefit and raised standard of living.

Q. 15.10. When contracaptives are indicated ?

1. Socio-economical conditions :

Contraception is accepted by the poor families in India in the National Family Welfare Programme so that they can support a large number of children.

2. Medical conditions :

(a) *Multiparity*—Contraception becomes less risky than that of repeated abortion, pregnancy, deliveries and child bearing in multiparity. One of the reason of high maternal death in India is multiparity.

(b) *Medical disorders*—Women suffering from heart disease, hypertention, renal disease, tuberculosis must be protected by contraception for life safety.

3. Eugenic :

Contraception can prevent perpetuation of seriously harmful genetic disease like Down Syndrome and others.

Q. 15.11. What is meant by effectiveness ?

Theoretically effectiveness means success of the procudure when it is used correctly. Use effectiveness means success of the procedure is actual clinical use where human failure are there. Effectiveness for a Procedure generally means use-effectiveness.

Q. 15.12. What is meant by contraceptive ?

The word *contraceptive* all temporary and permanent measures or devices which are used to prevent pregnancy resulting from coitus.

An *Ideal contraceptive* is one which is :

    (i)   acceptable to both partners,
    (ii) easy to administer and long lasting,
    (iii) quite efficacious and reliable,
    (iv) easily available and cheap,
    (v) does not produce any side effects, and
    (vi) require little or no medical supervision.

Q. 15.13. What are the various methods of contraception?

Methods of contraception :

1. Sexual union can be avoided by *abstinence.*
2. The semen can be prevented from being deposited in the vagina by withdrawing the penis before ejaculation.- *withdrawal or coitus interrupts.*
3. Sexual union can be restricted to only those days when the ovum is not available for fertilisation - *safe period* or *rhythem method.*
4. Semen can also be prevented from depositing in vagina if the male partner wears a protective sheath over his erect penis during coitus. Such a sheath is known as a *Condom* (Nirodh).
5. Barriers can be placed in the path of the sperm so that it does not reach the ovum in the fallopian tube:
    (i) *A Mechanical barrier* in the form of a latex rubber

cap over cervix closes the canal and is then known as a *Diaphragm*.

(ii) *Chemical barriers* in the form of jellies containing spermicidal chemicals may also be use. Attempts are being made to deposit sclerosing chemicals in the internal orifice of the fallopian tube and a plug of plastic material has also been tried for the same purpose. The fallopian tubes can be closed by clips or cut, thereby making the

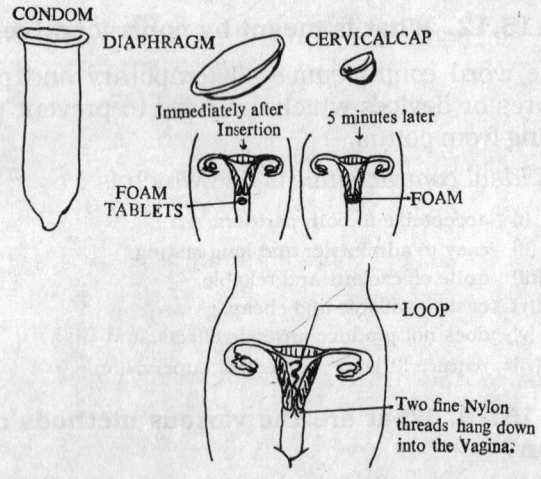

women sterile - A method known as *female sterilization* or *tubectomy*.

6. The embedding of the fertilized ovum in the endometrium can be interfered with either by the mechanical devices known as *Intra Uterine Devices* (IUDs) or by altering the delicate hormonal needed for the preparation of the endometrium through the administration of hormons as pills (Oral contraceptives) or injection. As *pills* and injections alter the hormonal system, they are known as *systemic contraceptives*.

7. The spermatozoa can be prevented from reaching the seminal vesicles by interrupting the vasdeferens. This is known as male *sterilization* or *vasectomy*.

METHOD OF CONTRACEPTIONS

```
                          METHOD OF CONTRACEPTIONS
                                    |
                    ┌───────────────┴────────────────┐
                Temporary                        Permanent**
                    |
        ┌───────────┴───────────┐
  Without any contrivance   With contrivance
            |                     |
        Physiological    ┌────────┼────────┐
                      Mechanical Chemical Drug
```

Physiological
[Those which depends on the voluntary action of the sex partners.]
- a) Abstinence.
- b) Withdrawal or Coitus interruptus
- c) Rhythm method.
- d) Safe period.
- e) Calender method.
- f) Body temperature method.
- g) Cirvical mucous method.

Mechanical
[Those which prevent fertilisation by mechanical contivances.]
- a) Condom.
- b) Diaphragm and cervical cap.
- c) Intra uterine devices (IUD).
- d) Vasectomy (Permanent method in male.)
- e) Salpingectomy or tubectomy (permanent method in female.)
- f) Laparoscopic sterilisation.

Chemical
[Those which act chemically or both chemically and mechanically.]
- a) Sponges and tampoom.
- b) Douches.
- c) Jels, creams and aerosol foam.
- d) Vaginal foam tablets and suppositories.

Drug
[Drugs that counteract the hormons and stimulate ovulation.]
- a) Combined hormonal pill.
- b) Seçomential pill.
- c) Micro pill.
- d) Slow release combinations.

Recent advance —
I. Prostaglandin.
II. Birth Control Vaccine (Immunological method).
N.B.—All are temporary Except—Vasectomy & Tubectomy

** Post conceptional methods.
ABORTION/MR/MTP
(Permature termination and destruction of the Product of conception).

Q. 15.14. What is meant by Oral Contraceptive ?

Oral Contraceptive means drug that prevent ovulation. This drug—an oestrogen progesterone compound, popularly known as the 'pill', is now prescribed under physicians instruction as a simple method of fertility regulation. If it proves effective without complications it will be more acceptable to women as it eliminates the trouble of filling, insertion and special precautions at the time of intercourse.

Is the pill safe ?

The pills are safe except the following causes.
1. It has to be taken regularly for 20 or 22 days beginning from the 5th day of menstruation. Missing even for a day may end in a failure.
2. It is the mose expensive method.
3. There is some apprehension of ill health following prolonged use.
4. Some side effects such as, break through bleeding, spotting, nausea and vomiting, dizziness, headache, dysmenorrhoea, change of flow and weight changes, all simulating symptoms of early pregnancy may arise.

Besides there are certain contra indications, namely :

(i) Liver trouble, (ii) kidney disorders, (iii) hypertension, (iv) history of breast cancer or uterine troubles and blood clots, (v) if the mother is nursing a baby it may interfere with milk production requiring its use to be postponed until the breast feeding is well established.

How it works ?

The oral contraceptive works by mimicking the action of those natural hormones the signal the pituitary to stoop off cell production. The first pill that stood the test was ENOVID followed by ORTHO-NOVIN, OVRAL OVULEN and NOR-INYL-1.

VII. CONTRACEPTIVES, M.T.P. AND STERILIZATION

Q. 15.15. What is meant by M.T.P.? or Premature Termination of the product of conception or pregnancy ?

Termination of pregnancy by destroying the foetus, through induced abortion, is as old as humanity itself. Some cultures permit it under specific circumstances, others tolerate it and still others condem it.

In India recently abortion was illegal, but with the Medical Termination of Pregnancy Act (MTP act., 34 of 1971) which came into effect from 1.4.72 women can take recourse to abortion on three specific grounds-Humanitarian, health and eugenic.

Under humanitarian grounds a women can ask for abortion to get rid of pregnancy resulting from criminal acts i.e. rape, pregnancy can be terminated if it poses a grave danger to the health, physical and mental of the pregnant women. Also in cases, where there may substantial risk for the off-spring, to be born with mental and physical abnormalities the pregnancy can be terminated. There are certain formalities which have to be followed.

A Board of Examiners has to be set up the place where abortions are carried out, has to be registered, and the constitution of the board of experts, examining the pregnant women before deciding whether abortion should be performed or not, depends on, the duration of pregnancy before seeking abortion. Generally the abortion is to be undertaken during the first two months of pregnancy.

Q. 15.16. What is meant by Sterilization ?

It is a method of permanent blocking of conception done by vasectomy in man and tubectomy or salpingectomy in women. Recanalisation of the passage is almost impossible but attempts are now being made to devise an operation which will permit the reestablishment of the passage if necessary. This operation does not usually causes an unfavourable physiological effect but some persons may develop some psychological symptoms :

(a) Vasectomy :

It is a simple operation of identifying the vasdferences through skin, incision on either side of the inguinal canal and excising it between two sutures blocking either end of the vase followed by stitching off the skin wound. The person is able to go home after operation and after 2 days' rest can attend to his duties.

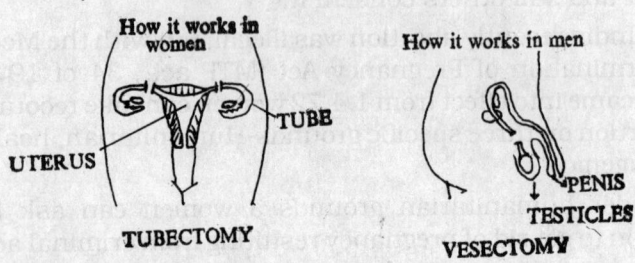

(b) Tubectomy or Salpingectomy :

The usual technique of sterilization of woman involves excision of a segment of both fallopian tubes in the same ways as the vasdeferens is excised. This operation needs opening up of abdomen in the pelvic region, but it may also be easily done through the vaginal route— a few days after delivery when the tissues still remain flexible. It is a more difficult operation than vasectomy and needs the services of a gynecologist in a hospital and it also carries certain operational risk.

Q. 15.17. What is meant by Laparoscopic Sterilization ?

A laparoscope is a long slender tube, provided with a series of lenses along the length of the tube and fibre-optic illumination. Modern laparoscopes use a fibre-optic bundle, to transit 'cold light' from an external source, into the abdominal cavity, directly. Originally laparoscope was used for diagnostic purposes to visualise the interior of the abdominal cavity. In 1837 A.T. Anderson suggested its use for female sterilization. In 1960 the development of 'cold' fiber-optic light sources, and other design improvements, it became an instrument suitable for female sterilization in outpatient clinics. Since 1970 there is world-wide use of this technique in contraceptive programmes.

The patient may be admitted a few hours before the operation. The bladder is emptied, if necessary by catheter. Generally, local anaesthesia is given. Some surgeons prefer one abdominal incision, and others two. There incisions are very small, and used for introduction of the laparoscope and instruments into the abdominal cavity.

The essential step in this operation is production of pneumoperitoneum, which pushes away the intestine from the site of the operation. For such purpose CO_2 is widely used. As absorption of CO_2 slow, some surgeons prefer nitrous oxide, Some surgeons use more readily available air.

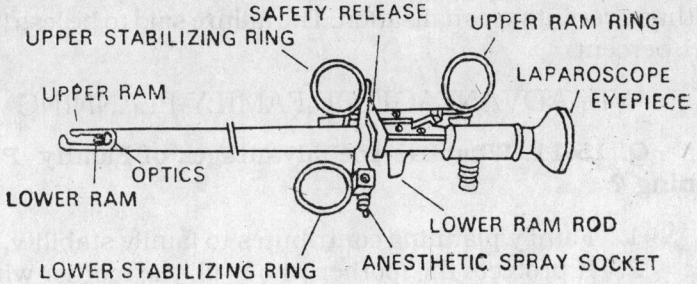

Laparoscope

After producing pneumoperitoneum, the patient is put in an inclined position with head end lowered which pushes the intestine downwards. Then the laparoscope is introduced and by illuminating the pelvic cavity the fallopian tubes are visualised. Simultaneously, the uterus is rotated with the help of a speculum or volselum forceps better location of the tubes. After transillumination of the abdomen by laparoscope, the operating instruments are introduced through another site nearby. There after different techniques are adopted by different surgeons.

Some perform only electro-coagulation of the fallopian tubes, after securing them. A majority of surgeons, however, prefer to divide the tubes after electro-coagulation to reduce the possibility of recanalisation. Some surgeons go a step further and electro-coagulate, divide and remove a section of the tubes.

Though a simple and outdoor operation, laparoscopic sterilization is a sophisticated and complex surgical procedure, requiring good training, experience and skill on the part of the operator.

In more modern techniques, instead of electro-coagulation, self closing clips are applied to the tube, with the help of a laparoscope. This procedure offers better scope for reversing the tubal occlusion later, if necessary.

Dr. Jaroslow Hulka of North Carolina and bio-engineer of Illionis Mr. George Clemens, developed a clip, fitted with spring, which is widely being used now. After application, the clip causes atrophy of about 4 mm. of the fallopian tube and thus prevents recanalisation. The failure said to be less than 1 percent.

VII. ADVANTAGE OF FAMILY PLANNING

Q. 15.11. What are the advantages of Family Planning ?

1. Family planning contributes to family stability.
2. It protects the mother who is ill, the mother who is exhausted from bearing too many children, and the parents who want to postpone having babies until they can give them emotional and material support.
3. It protects the couples who feel, they should have no children at all because one or both carries a hereditary disease.
4. It protects the child so that he will not come into the world without a welcome from the family and proper support for his future.
5. It builds a happier family life. A child's first birth right is to be wanted. When babies come too close together, a mother may be so worn out that she cannot help resenting her whole family. Fear of another exhausting pregnancy may interfere with her emotional relation with her husband, but with suitable spacing of births the mother feel relaxed and happy, she has a better chance of surviving delivery, and each child can have a fair share of his parent's attention.

6. It is also a help to the nation. the growth of population should be up to the level, which the National Economy can sustain, otherwise shortage, proverty and crimes etc. will be increased.

IX. NATIONAL FAMILY PLANNING PROGRAMMES

Q. 15.19. Describe the National Family Welfare Programme in India.

The programme in India has been started from 1975. National Family Welfare Programme was launched in India in 1952. The National Family Eelfare Programme has five components :

 (i) Material and Child Health (MCH) care.
 (ii) Immunization of pregnant women by tetanus toxoid and children (infant and preschool age upto 5 years) by diphtheria-tetanus-pertusis, oral polio, BCG.
 (iii) Nutritional supplement-iron and folic acid to pregnant women and children and Vitamin A in oil to children for prevention of blindness.
 (iv) Contraceptives including voluntary sterilization.
 (v) Health Education particularly motivation to accept contraception.

Medical Termination of Pregnancy (MTP) is also available from 1972 throughout the country as a health measure for protection of woman's health against criminal abortion. This indirectly helps the couples to accept contraception.

The principles of the programme are :

1. To make propaganda and educate the people for the social acceptances of the Family Planning Programme by the married couples.
2. Educate the people that small family is a happy family and family planning programme is really a social welfare programme.
3. There should be easy accessibility to the service agency by the couples.

4. Popularising every known method of Family Planning.

The organisational set up of the Family Welfare Programme at the state and district levels are :

ORGANISATIONAL SET UP FOR FAMILY WELFARE IN A STATE

```
                    State Cabinet Committee
                              |
                Deptt. of Health and Family Welfare
                Minister for Health and Family Welfare
                              |
            Secretary to the Deptt. of Health and Family Welfare
                              |
                   Directorate of Health Services
                     Director of Health Services
                              |
                    State Family Welfare Bureau
          Additional/Joint/Deputy Director of Health Services
                      (Family Welfare & MCH)
                   (State Family Welfare Officer.)
```

Audit party	Operation, planning and training division, Asstt. Director of Health Services.	Education and Information Division Mass Education and Communications officer.
Administrative and Stores Division, Administrative Officer (FW)	Statistics, Demography and Evaluation Division. Demographer.	Construction cell.

Similarly, at the District level has a District Family Welfare Bureau in each district. The District Family Welfare officer heads each District Bureau. There are also Urban Family Welfare Centre, Rural Primary Health Centre and Sub-centres. In each of the Family Welfare Bureau at Centre, State, District, Urban FW centre and PHC levels, there is complements of Medical, Para-medical and Non-medical staff drawn from different specialities, viz. Public Health and MCH, Mass and Extention Education and Demography. At the sub-centre level, however, the staff is the Auxiliary Nurse Midwife.

X. PRESENT ATTITUDE TOWARDS FAMILY PLANNING

Q. 15.20. What is the present attitude towards Family planning ?

Which will be the ideal method to cheek these ideas ?

Those Indian villagers and urban people, are not educated they seem that their male children are their assets as they can give security to the family in future and act as helping hands, so they avoid to go through family planning methods. Many people belive that use of birth control measures are against nature and the use of contraceptives might produce premature sterility among woman and also upset mental conditions. Generally this attitude arises from their ignorance as well as the following social customs and beliefs:

  (i) Children are the gift of God.

  (ii) The number of children is determined by God and there is no responsibility of the parents.

  (iii) Every Hindu must have a son to perform the funeral activities.

  (iv) Children are an asset to which parents can look forward in periods of dependency caused by old age or misfortune.

  (v) Children are a poorman's wealth, as they can give security to the family.

So the problem of family planning is essentially a problem of social changes. Contraceptive technology is not the only solution to the problem. What is more important is to stimulate social changes affecting fertility are :

  (i) Raising the age of marriage.

  (ii) Increasing the status of women, education and employment opportunities.

  (iii) Old age security.

  (iv) Compulsory education of children.

  (v) Accelerating economic changes designed to increase the per capita income.

(vi) The standard of living of the people.
(vii) Industrialisation.

Above all problem of family planning in India can be solved by *mass education* and/or by *conveying its benefits* to the poor and illiterate masses by motivation; so that people may understand the benefits of a small family by adopting family planning methods.

The process of education and motivation should cover the following six stages :

(i) Awareness
(ii) Education
(iii) Acceptance
(iv) Involvement
(v) Trial
(vi) Practice

> "It is a cruel crime thoughtlessly to living more children to existence than could properly be taken care of."
>
> **Rabindranath Tagore**

CHAPTER-XVI

MATERNITY AND CHILD HEALTH (M.C.H)

(For B.H.M.S. and Graded B.H.M.S. Courses only)

DISCUSSION FOR LEARNING

I. Definition, aims and objectives.
II. Antenatal care.
III. 5 Point MCH programmes.
IV. Under Five Clinics.
V. Maternal mortality rate and infant mortality rate.

I. DIFINITION AIMS AND OBJECTIVES

Q. 16.1. What is meant by Maternal and Child Health Programme or MCH programme?

Child is the father of man and future of the nation. The quality, character and health of the child depends on the mother that bears him. So the child care and child health are intimately associated with maternal care and maternal health. Generally the term "maternal and child health" refers to the promotive, preventive, curative and rehabilitative health care for mothers and children. It can also be defines :

"A sepcialised service designed to promote, protect and restore health of mothers and children and provide safe confinement from conception to school age."

Generally MCH programme, includes maternal health, child health, family planning, school health, handicapped children, adolescence and health aspects of care of children in special setting such as day care.

Q. 16.2. What are the main objects of MCH programme ?

Main object of MCH Programme is life long health. The specific objects of MCH Programme are :

(a) reduction of maternal, perinatal, infant and childhood mortality and morbidity.

(b) promotion of reproductive health.

(c) promotion of physical and psychological development of the child and adolescent with the family.

Recently in this programme besides providing normal MCH programme, special emphasis is laid on :

(i) *Immunisation of children against diphtheria, whooping cough and tetanus* : Children under five years of age are given triple vaccine. The unprotected children of 6-11 years of age also being protected against diphtheria and tetanus, by double antigen.

(ii) *Prophylaxis against nutritional anaemia among mothers and children* : To combat the nutritional anaemia in mothers and children, daily requirement of iron and folic acid in tablet form is provided.

(iii) *Prophylaxis against Vitamin 'A' deficiency disease among children*: Under this scheme children in the age group of 1-5 years in rural areas are given 200,000 international units of Vit. A in oil, orally every 6 months.

Q. 16.3. What are the chief components of MCH programme ?

The chief components of MCH programme are :

(A) Maternal Health Care

(B) Infant and Child Health Care.

(A) Maternal health care programme consists of :

(1) Antenatal care through :

(a) home visiting—by Midwife, Health Visitor or Public Health Nurse.

(b) antenatal clinic—by Medical examination, Consultation, Extra-nourishment, Educational classes and Demonstration.

(c) Laboratory service.

(d) Ante-natal beds of treatment in a hospital.

N.B. : *Antenatal care* should be ideally associated with a maternity institution. But, as sufficient hospital beds are not

MATERNITY AND CHILD HEALTH

available in most of the countries, this service has to render through *antenatal clinics*. Moreover, since a vast majority (90%) of pregnancies, end in normal deliveries and a few (10%) develop abnormalities it is imperative to be very watchful, to screen out, this small abnormal group. Inadequate care is worse than no care and therefore regularity in attendance and cheek up in the antenatal period are only too essential.

Generally antenatal clinic is staffed by a :
   (i) *Lady Medical Officer.*
   (ii) *Health Visitor* (recommended for 5000 population).
   (iii) *Midwives* (recommended 25,000 population).
   (iv) *Public Health Nurses* (for 10,000 population).
   (v) *Other Auxiliary Nurses based upon the strength of the antenatal clinic.*

2. International care through :
   (a) *Domiciliary service.*
   (b) *Maternity beds in hospitals and homes.*
   (c) *Care of the premature babies.*

3. Postnatal care through :
   (a) *Home visiting.*
   (b) *Hospital beds for puerperal complications.*

4. Health education of every stage :

(B) Infant and child care consists of :
   (a) *Facilities for the care of premature babies.*
   (b) *Infant and toddler clinic.*
   (c) *Paediatric beds in Children's Hospitals or General Hospitals.*
   (d) *Day nurseries and nursery schools.*
   (e) *Facilities for the care of physically or mentally handicapped children.*

Q. 16.4. What are the main objectives of maternal and child welfare services ?

The objective of maternal health care is to ensure that :
(1) Every expectant and nursing mother maintains good health.
(2) Learns the art of child care.
(3) Has a normal delivery and bears healthy children.
(4) Every child lives and grows up in a family unit with love and security in healthy surroundings, recives adequate nourishment health supervision and efficient medical attention and is taught the elements of healthy living.

** The immediate objective of this is the safe delivery, postnatal care of mother and baby, and maintenance of lactation. But its wide scope is health care of young men and women who are potential parents, guidance in parent craft and in problems associated with infertility and family planning.

II. ANTENATAL CARE

Q. 16.5. What is called Antenatal Care ? and what are its main objectives ?

Antenatal care is the care of the women during pregnancy. It has been defined as that part of maternal care which has its objective the complete supervision of the pregnant women in order to protect the health and preserve the happiness and life of the mother and her child, to prepare her physically and mentally to go through pregnancy and child birth and to teach her hygiene of pregnancy and management of her coming child.

The aims of antenatal care services are :
1. To promote and maintain good physical and mental health during pregnancy.
2. To ensure a mature live birth and healthy infant i.e. to reduce maternal and infant mortality and morbidity.
3. To prepare the women for labour i.e. to remove anxiety and dread associated with delivery.
4. To detect early medical and obstetric conditions that would endanger the life, or impair the health of the mother and baby and treat them appropriately.

5. To teach the mother elements of child care nutrition, personal hygiene, and environmental sanitation.

(II) ANTENATAL CARE

Q. 16.6. Describe the antenantal care in brief ?

Antenatal care is the care of the women during pregnancy. Generally this care begins soon after conception and continue throughout pregnancy. The primary aim of antenatal care is to achieve at the end of a pregnancy a healthy mother and a healthy baby. During the antenatal period the general measures which are commonly adopted to protect maternal and child health are :

1. *Early diagnosis of pregnancy.*
2. *Recording.*
3. *Prenatal advice.*
4. *Specific Health Protection through :*
    (a) *Home visiting.*
    (b) *Antenatal clinic.*
    (c) *Laboratory service.*
    (d) *Antenatal beds in hospital.*
    (e) *Mental preparation.*
    (f) *Family planning.*
    (g) *Paediatric component.*

Procedure

1. Early Diagnosis of Pregnancy

The diagnosis of pregnancy is generally confirmed by after routine history taking. The health status of the mother is established by a complete physical and obstetric examination, including Pelvimetry, Urine examination for albumin, sugar, Blood for Hb%, blood group and Rh factor and VDRL.

2. Recording

Early antenatal registration within 12 weeks of pregnancy is required. When the mother is registered, and antenatal card is prepared. The cards generally contains a

Registration number, identifying data, previous health history and main health events, like age at marriage, marital history, detailed history of past pregnancies, family history of diseases such as hypertension, diabetes, current health condition and history of any specific complain. A link is maintained between the antenatal, postnatal card and under fives card. These records are maintained for evaluation and for the improvement of MCH/FP services.

3. Pre-natal Advice

Generally this advice are mainly concerned with (a) *diet* and (b) *personal hygience* like, i) *Personal cleanliness*, ii) *Rest and sleep*, iii) *Bowels*, iv) *Exercise*, v) *Smoking*, vi) *Sexual intercourse*, vii) *Drugs*, viii) *Radiation*, ix) *Warning signs*, x) *Child care*, xi) *German measles*, xii) *Rh status* etc.

Generally these are main for mother health and her baby.

Advices :

1. Generally recommended diet during pregnancy are 50 gms per day cereals, 25 gm pulse, 125 gms milk, 10 gm sugar to be taken in addition to the normal balanced diet.
2. Personal cleanliness includes everyday bathing, washing of hands and faces etc. and wearing of clean clothes.
3. Eight hours sleep and at least 2 hours rest after midday meal is recommended.
4. Avoidation of constipation by regular intake of green leafy vegetable, fruits and extrafluids is necessary. Purgatives like castor oil should be avoided.
5. Exercise by light household work is advised but normal physical labour during late pregnancy should be avoided as it affects the foetus adversely.
6. Expectant mothers who smoke heavily, they must cut down it to a minimum because it is seen that expectant mother who smoke heavily produce babies much smaller than the average by the influence of nicotine.

7. Sexual intercourse should be restricted, especially during the last trimester.
8. Certain drugs taken by the mother during pregnancy affects the foetus causing foetal malformation due to chromosomal aberration. So a great deal of caution is required in the drug is taken by pregnant women.
9. Generally a X-ray examination of the abdomen during early weeks of pregnancy may cause malformation of the foetus, therefore it should be avoided during the first 4 months of pregnancy.
10. (a) *Swelling of the feet*
    (b) *Fits*
    (c) *Headache*
    (d) *Blurring of the vision*
    (e) *Bleeding or discharge per vagina or any other unusual symptoms are the warning signal of pregnant women*, so the mother should report them immediately to the doctor specific.

*Specific Health Protection—Home Visiting

Generally prenatal advice are given to the mother by doctor at maternity institution. But in the rural area where continuous medical supervision not be possible, home visits by the medical officer or by public health nurses/health visitors and auxiliary nurses or midwives must be made to complete antenatal care.

(a) Home Visit

Generally each mother should be seen as early as possible in her pregnancy and there after once a month either at home or at the clinic, particularly home visits are needed to advise her on diets, cleanliness and exercise etc. and to induce her to come to the clinic (antenatal clinic) for medical check up and necessary medical advice.

Generally as sufficient beds are not available in hospital, antenatal care are rendered through antenatal clinics.

(b) Antenatal Care Through Antenatal Clinic

This care/programme includes examination of the pregnant woman by the doctor and advice, or education to the mother.

At least three medical examinations at the clinic are necessary, the first one being a full medical check up with full maternity history between the 6th and 16th week, the second for diagnosis of presentation and position of the baby between 32nd and 36th week, and the third to detect any disproportion between head and the pelvis, if any, during the last 4 weeks and to instruct her on the preparation for her delivery. In each medical examination a general review, is made of the health of the mother, her diet and mode of life. If also includes careful history, systematic obstetrical and relevant haematological and other laboratory examination. All records are to be maintained and appropriate history sheets and follow up cards, including those of home visiting, natal and post natal services. Generally these clinics are stuffed by a Lady Medical Officer, Home Visitor, Midwives, Primary Health Nurses and other Auxiliary Nurses.

The other antenatal cares are teaching infant feeding and mother craft etc. and to remove ignorance and supertitious belief regarding pregnancy and delivery. Close collaboration between the doctor and the nurse, both in the hospital and in the field, is essential for successful antenatal care.

(c) Laboratory Services

Antenatal care are generally supported by the following laboratory examination, as and when needed :

- (i) Weighing.
- (ii) Examination of urine for specific gravity, albumen, sugar, bile and acetic, and also microscopic character of the centrifuged debries (cells, casts, crystals etc).
- (iii) Examination of blood for haemoglobin, total and differential count, biochemical tests if indicated.
- (iv) Estimation of blood pressure.
- (v) Radiological examination.

MATERNITY AND CHILD HEALTH

(d) Treatment

Prompt and adequate treatment should be given for high anaemia, phosphate, sugar in urine and abnormal position of the foetus.

(e) Immunisation

During pregnancy inoculation of tetanus toxide (absorbed) in 3 doses, first at about 5th or 6th month, second, 4-6 weeks after the first, and in the last in late month, is given to prevent the incidence of the dreadful disease in mother, in her puerperium and also of the baby after birth. Other vaccinations or inoculations may also be given when indicated.

Hospitalisation for treatment of mothers with complications of pregnancy or any diseases can be arranged easily where the antenatal clinic is attached to the maternity hospital, but for clinics attached to health centres, maternity homes and welfare centres all cases requiring admission or special treatment should be referred to a maternity hospital by arrangement.

III. 5 POINT MCH PROGRAMME

Q. 16.7. What is meant by 5-point MCH programme ?

In India a *5-point MCH programme* has been undertaken, as a part of the National Family Welfare Programme. This consists of immunisation of the infant against tuberculosis, smallpox, diphtheria, tetanus, whooping cough and poliomyelitis. Administration of vitamin supplements to prevent deficiency diseases and improve nutritional status in early life is also part of programme.

*Schedule for immunisation of children :

The schedule recommended by the Ministry of Health and Family Welfare Govt. of India is as follows :

At the age of	Immunisation recommended
1. 0-4 weeks	B.C.G. Vaccine
2. *3 months	Smallpox Vaccine

3. 4-9 months   Diphtheria, Pertusis, Tetanus (Triple vaccine)- 2 doses at interval of 6-8 weeks. Polio vaccine 3 doses at intervals of 4-6 weeks (preferably trivalent oral vaccine).

4. 1 year   Cholera Vaccine if required.

N.B. :

If there are cases of smallpox in the locality, smallpox vaccination may be given to an infant within first few days after birth with one insertion only, before BCG Vaccination. If such cases, revaccination against smallpox should be carried out at 3 years of age. Smallpox and B.C.G. vaccination may also be given simultaneously on opposite arms.

IV. UNDER FIVE CLINICS

Q. 16.8. What is meant by Under Five Clinics ?

This is a clinic of infant and child upto the age of five years, after which he starts to attending the school under the supervision of MCH programme/centre.

The need and importance of establishing and organising 'Under Five Clinics' in MCH services was realised from the fact that about 100 million of the total population, 17% children are under 0.5 age group in our country and 28% children are died before five years of age by infantile diarrhoea and dehydration, respiratory infections, malnutrition and infectious diseases like tuberculosis, whooping cough helminthiasis etc. *On the basis of above view WHO (1979) established under five clinics and declared "International years of the child".*

Main aims :

1. To check up the children at regular intervals in an endeavour to maintain their positive health.
2. To detect childhood disorders amongst the group.
3. To carry out the nutrition programme.
4. To provide preventive and curative services to maximum number of children.
5. To cover all these children with timely and successfully immunization programme.

V. MATERNAL MORTALITY RATE AND INFANT MORTALITY RATE

Q. 16.9. What is meant by Maternal Mortality Rate?

The conventional Maternal Mortality Rate is defined as the number of deaths arising from puerperium, during a given year per thousand live births during the same year, among the population of a given geographic area. The formula for the maternal morality rate is:

Annual maternal mortality rate = $\dfrac{\text{Number of deaths from puerperal causes which occurred among the female population of a given geographic area during a given year.}}{\text{Number of live births which occurred among the population of the given geographic area during the same year.}} \times 1000$

Q. 16.10. What are the causes of Maternal deaths?

The direct causes of maternal deaths in developing countries are *anaemia, toxemias, haemorrhages, obstetric shock, puerperal infection* and *accidents of child birth.* The underlying factors are malnutrition, repeated child birth at frequent intervals and lack of adequate medical care during pregnancy and delivery. The general health of the mother per age and the prevalence of diseases in the community are also important factors.

** *Repeated pregnancies* have an important bearing on maternal and perinatal mortality rates. The multigravidas, particularly five and above, have a higher incidence of anemia, hypertensive, cardiovascular disease, pre-eclamptic toxemia, placenta previa, premature births, malposition of foetus, prolapsed cord, ruptured uterus, cephalopelvic disproportion and post partum haemorrhage as compared with those with fewer well-spaced pregnancies. Among the social conditions are the customs at delivery of early age, universality of marriage, child bearing irrespective of fitness, overcrowding, proverty, bad housing conditions and bad management at delivery. Illegitimacy, undesired pregnancy and hard manual labour in industrial employment also induce to increased maternal and infant mortality. Besides death the number of mothers permanently injured or invalidated is not small. It is said that for every maternal deaths there are 20 others who suffer from unfavoured health, toward efficiency and sometimes post delivery complications and morbidities such as, displacement of uterus, anaemia, haemorrhages, varicose veins, thrombophlebitis, prolapse, tears, fistula, pelvic inflammation, liver or kidney damage, sterility and precepitated tuberculosis, heart disease and other disabling ailments. The situation is further aggravated by the *ignorance and unwillingness* in most of the mothers to avail of health supervision during pregnancy and skilled help at the time of delivery, even when it is available.

Q. 16.11. What are the indication of high Mortality Rate of mother ?

A high maternal mortality rate indicates *heavy maternal mobility and high perinatal and infant mortality and morbidity.*

Q. 16.12. What is meant by infant mortality rate ?

Infant mortality rate may be defined as the number of infant deaths that occur per thousand live births among the population of a given geographic area with in a given year.

From the definition, it is seen that for the proper calculation of infant mortality rate the cohot-analysis method has to be adopted, that is to say, one has to follow the cohort of live-borne children among the population of an area in one calender year through their first year of life and record the number of deaths among them during the period. Due to administrative and other difficulties, this procedure has been found difficult to follow, and the so-called "coventional infant mortality rate" has been adopted. The conventional infant mortality rate is defined as the number of infant deaths that occur during a given year per thousand live births during the same year among the population of a given geographic area. This is calculated as follows :

Annual Infant mortality rate = $\dfrac{\text{Number of deaths under one year of age which occurred among the population of a given geographic area during a given year.}}{\text{Number of live births which occurred among the population of the same geographic area during the same year.}} \times 1000$

Deaths of infants below one year of age, per thousand live birth, is probably best single indication of the comparative standard of health enjoyed by the infants in various countries, in terms of standard of living, home enviornment and amount of nutrition and care enjoyed by the infants.

Q. 16.13. What are the causes of Infant Mortality ?

The commonly used Infant Mortality are :

1) *Perinatal mortality*—Perinatal Mortality of two types :
   a) *Still birth* i.e. fatal death of infant at least 28 weeks of gestation, and
   b) *Infant death* with in 7 days of birth, i.e. perinatal death proper.
2) *Neonatal mortality* i.e. deaths of infant with in the first 4 weeks.

**The *commonest cause of still births* are—toxaemia pregnancy, anaemia, syphilis, accidental haemorhage, congenital malformation, difficult and abnormal labour, unsuccessful instrumentation, Rh factor etc.

*** The causes of *neonatal deaths* are—prematurity, asphyxia, birth injuries, tetanus, infections, congenital anomalies and disease inherited or acquired during gestation, (pemphigus, erythroblastosis, smallpox, chickenpox, syphills etc.)

**** *Perinatal deaths* are—largely due to high maternal mortality and morbidity and to poor obstetric service. The main causes are prematurity trauma and stress of labour, neonatal infections including tetanus neonatorum.

Other causes of infant deaths are infections of the respiratory and gastro-intestinal tracts, malnutrition, communicable diseases, like measles, whooping cough, chicken pox, small pox and tuberculosis and accidents in the home and its environs. All these conditions are intimately related to the health of the mother during pregnancy, efficiency of some of the disease during pregnancy like German measles and chicken pox may cause mental and physical defects. But above all the basic causes are *proverty, mal and under nutrition, apathy, fear, ignorance, poor hygiene and lack of medical facilities.*

Q. 16.14. What are the significance of infant mortality rate ?

Infant Mortality is a sensitive index of the total cultural milieu of a community or a country. It reflects the state of public health and hygiene, environmental sanitation, cultural moves, about feeding and clothing, socio-economic development and the price of arts and above all the peoples attitude towards dignity and value of human life."

(Chandrasekhar, 1959).

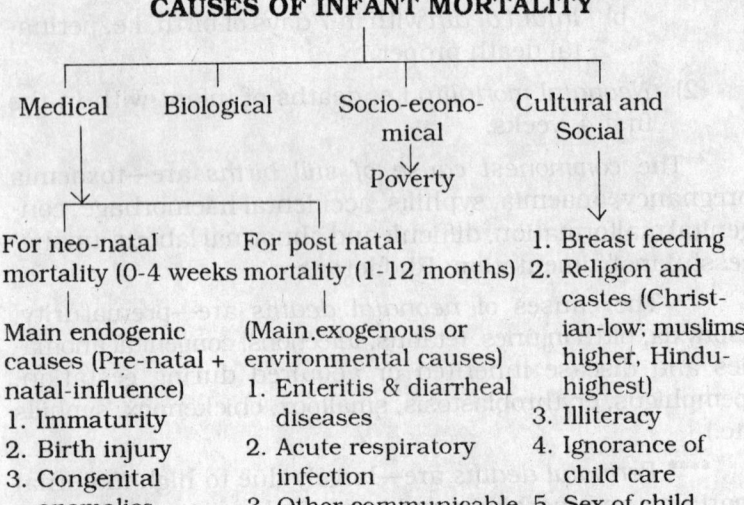

CAUSES OF INFANT MORTALITY

- Medical
- Biological
- Socio-economical → Poverty
- Cultural and Social

For neo-natal mortality (0-4 weeks)

Main endogenic causes (Pre-natal + natal-influence)
1. Immaturity
2. Birth injury
3. Congenital anomalies

For post natal mortality (1-12 months)

(Main exogenous or environmental causes)
1. Enteritis & diarrheal diseases
2. Acute respiratory infection
3. Other communicable

1. Breast feeding
2. Religion and castes (Christian-low; muslims higher, Hindu-highest)
3. Illiteracy
4. Ignorance of child care
5. Sex of child

MATERNITY AND CHILD HEALTH

4. Haemolytic diseases
5. Condition of placenta and cord
6. Enteritis and diarrhoeal diseases
7. Acture respiratory infections

diseas-Whooping cough Influenza, Pneumonia
4. Malnutrition
5. Congenital abnormalities
6. Accidents

6. Broken families
7. Illegitimacy
8. Brutal habit & customs
9. The indigenous dai
10. Lack of trained personnel like midwives, dais, health visitors etc.
11. Bad environtenatal sanitation.

CHAPTER-XVII

SCHOOL HEALTH SERVICE

(For B.H.M.S. and Graded B.H.M.S. Course only)

DISCUSSION FOR LEARNING

I. Its need and main objects.
II. Basic components of School Health Programme.
III. Duties of a Medical Officer as a member of School Or School Board.

I. ITS NEED AND MAIN OBJECTS

Q. 17.1. Why is it necessary ? and what are its main objects ?

A child of today is the future adult citizen and leader of the community and the country life. It is therefore indispensible to underline the needed special care of the health of the school in a over all health programme of any country.

Also in the school the children come in contact with the community of a group of mixed population of children coming from different types of community life, and exposes itself unconsciously to the hazards of an environment which is different in many respects from his own home. So through the School health services a child can protected against various communicable diseases by vaccinations and immunizations, under strict discipline in close community of the school.

The school going age is the crucial period of anatomical and physical development of the children. As such there is an excellent opportunity to detect as well as correct at an early stage, various physical and mental defects of the school going children which might in future ; prevent attainment of full health or vigour, to built ultimately a strong nation with sound physical and mental makeup. So the school service should be provide the school children with a healthy environment at the school. Such as good

SCHOOL HEALTH SERVICE

sanitation, adequate nutrition, health education, proper physical instruction etc. so that they might get an opportunity of health living in their school where they spend six to seven hours of the day from the very beginning of their life and as such, it is very logical to presume that they might practise the same healthy habits at their home.

So the Main Objectives of School Health services are :
1) Health Protection.
2) Health Restoration.
3) Health Promotion.

II. BASIC COMPONENTS OF SCHOOL HEALTH PROGRAMME

Q. 17.2. What are the basic component of school health services programme ?

The ideal health service programme consists of :

1. **Health protection :**
   a) By protecting the child from all kinds of ailments physical and mental, as far as possible, to keep him fit to receive education.
   b) By detecting any thing which amounts to departure from normal health and growth by periodic health examination.
   c) By investigating the causes of such departure.
   d) By preventing communicable diseases by vaccination and inoculation.

2. **Health restoration :**
   a) By arranging measures for treatment and correction of defects.
   b) By maintaining a school health clinic and first aid post with equipments.

3. **Health promotion :**
   a) By improvement of nutritional status by early detection of nutritional deficiency ;
   b) By providing supplementary feeding programme (day-meal programme) ;
   c) By development of good habits by imparting knowledge of personal hygiene and environmental sanita-

tion through integrated health practices and health practices cheeked by health practices in school and maintaining a health practice booklet.

d) By organising physical education in school through regular physical drill and by participating in or out door games.

e) By maintaining ideal standard of sanitation of school premises, class room, hygiene, (good ventilation and lighting), safe drinking water, clear toilet facilities and goody play ground.

f) By organising guidance clinic for problem children.

g) By arranging regular teaching of health and hygiene.

h) By adopting follow up work and organising Parent Teacher Association.

Q. 17.3. What would be the main objects of inspection of a school by a M.O. ?

The main objects of inspection of a school by a Medical Officer should be :

a) *to look after the health of the school children, and*

b) *to look after the sanitation of the school premises.*

III. DUTIES OF MEDICAL OFFICER

Q. 17.4. What would be the duties of a Medical Officer to inspect and to maintain a school health and hygienes ?

Generally the main duties of a Medical Officer of school are :

1) *To look after the health of the school children, and*

2) *To look after the sanitation of the school premises.*

1. For the health of the school children :

He (M.O) should perform the following duties :

i Medical check up :

The Medical Officer arranges for the Medical examination of all the school children. the children are examined twice in the primary school i.e. one in *standard I* and then *standard III.* or *In the secondary school* the new students are examined preferably before registration and there-after every 3 years; and the old students are at least every three years till leaving the school, although the follow up of any defect is done yearly.

With the student's physical examination of the teachers is also necessary for the safty of the scholars; and the routine is similar to those of students. Women teachers are examined by lady doctors, and cooks and other employees are also examined assisted by the usual laboratory tests. In the rural areas, the school health clinics can be arranged in the Government health clinics, at least once a week, so that school going children of the rural areas get health facilities of medical cheek up and treatment when required.

The common defects of school going children are malnutrition, various vitamin deficiencies, caries teeth, enlarged tonsils and adenoid, poor personal hygiene causing scabies, worms, ringworm infestation, visual defects etc.

2. Correction of defects or treatment :

Medical Officer also arranges for the necessary treatment for the ill-health of the students or teachers or employees.

    a) Generally after the consent of the parents, treatment are given. the treatment include removal of tonsils, carious teeth etc. together with other treatments.

    b) The nutritional defects are corrected by supplementing the diet with appropriate food (supplementary food programme) and imparting knowledge of balanced diet and health education measure. The school authorities may provide 'midday meals' or subsidized tiffin to the scholars'.

    c) The ailing children are taken by the school teacher or the Health Nurse to the hospital where treatment is to be given, and brings and children back to their homes.

    d) If necessary the parent are interviewed and explained regarding the ill health of their children.

    e) The medical officer also arranges for the First Aid treatment.

f) He also organies school health week, sports, parent's day etc.

3. Prevention of communicable diseases or immunization.

Medical officer also carries out immunization of the school children :

(a) A children is immunized against smallpox one in 3 years. All new entrants are vaccinated. All the children are also vaccinated against smallpox, if there is an epidemic.

(b) The children are immunized against enteric fever once in every year and plague and cholera if found necessary.

(c) The children are immunized against Diphtheria, Whooping cough and Tetanus by two inoculation at the interval of one month.

(d) They are also immunized by B.C.G. once.

The member of the staff of the school should also be included in the immunization programme if necessary.

(II) Inspection or Examination of school premises or School sanitation.   OR

As a M.O. what will you do to maintain school hygiene ?

The *construction and composition of the school building and maintenance of its sanitation, arrangement of class rooms* are the three most important facts of school sanitation or the main consideration of a Medical Officer.

1. A Primary/Secondary school should be an independent structure with adequate playground and preferably, a ground floor structure of 1,000 sq. yards for a school of 200 children and 1/5 should have structure and 4/5th part playground.

2. The school should away from stables, factory and should be in a hygienic surroundings.

3. If the school has upper floors, then the stair should be board. The height of steps should 6 feet and not more than 15 steps at one stretch.

4. The class room should be well lighted, well ventilated.

SCHOOL HEALTH SERVICE

5. There should not be more than 40 children in each class with 10 sq. ft. space for every children (For Secondary school 16 sq. ft.).
6. There should be some spittoons in the school preferably in the passage so that students not spit indiscriminately. The spittoons can be made of wooden box containing sand and some antiseptic lotions.
7. The benches and tables should be of suitable height according to the age of children in general. The blackboard should be between 7 to 25 feet and the benches should be facing the glare from outside.
8. The sanitary arrangement (Urinals and latrines) should be proper and maintained in clean condition. Generally one water closet (W.C.) for 25 girls, one water closets for 25 boys and 3 water closet for 200 boys with an urinal 10 feet long for every 100 students are necessary. They should be separated for boys and girls. In rural areas septic tank latrines are preferable. There should one urinal for every 50 students (for boys and girls separate).
9. There should be facilities for cool, clean drinking water. Pupils should taught to the separate or clean drinking glass and to keep the class rooms and school premises clean. In the rural area, drinking water should be provided by a tube well. In Urban area drinking water should be supplied from a reservoir which should be cleaned regularly. It should be provided with taps, so that there must be one tap for every 100 students.
10. The school premises should be maintained in a clean and tidy condition, class room should be lighted and good ventilated.

So the duties of Medical Officer are frequent inspection of the school premises and advice to maintain above arrangements.

Q. 17.5. What would be your (as a M.O.) suggestion for the improvement of the health of the pupils and maintenance the proper hygiene of the school ?

To develop good health and habits, the essential steps are :

1. Imparting of knowledge on personal hygiene and environmental sanitation by arranging integrated dietetic teachings and practical demonstrations to all students according to their standard through a School Curriculum by specially trained teachers.

2. **Health practices :**
   (a) By organising health practice through health parade. (From health parade detection of early signs of health disorder can be made).
   b) *Other habits :*
   (i) Going to the bed early and sleeping long hours, windows opened and rising before sunrise.
   (ii) Brushing the teeth at least twice a day preferably after each meal.
   (iii) Habits of regular eating, sleeping going to toilet and taking out door exercises etc.
   (iv) A full bath daily.
   (v) Wearing of clean garments.
   (vi) Drinking of milk as such as possible but not tea or coffee.
   (vii) Drinking at least 4 glass of water.
   (viii) Eating some fresh fruits and green vegetables.
   (ix) Having a clean handkerchief and using it properly.
   (x) Maintaining good posture in standing, sitting and working.
   (xi) Reading books in good light but avoiding direct sunlight on books.
   (xii) Habits of personal cleanliness, especially that of washing hands before meals.
   (xiii) Keeping objects out of mouth (fingers, pencils, pen or books etc.)
   (xiv) Habits of being cheerful.

3. Organising physical education training in the school through regular physical drill or by participating in outdoor games.

SCHOOL HEALTH SERVICE

4. Maintaining ideal standard of sanitation of school premises, class-room hygiene (good ventilation and lighting., safe drinking water, clean toilet facilities and good playground.

5. Organising guidance clinic for problem children.

6. Arranging regular teaching of health and hygiene.

7. Adopting follow up work and organising Parent-Teacher association.

8. *Daily Inspection* :

It is the teacher's duty to take few minutes daily for the inspection of the pupils to check upon habit formation. In this work attention is given to hands, nails, head, eyes, ears, teeth, posture and clothing. It is also important to cheek up on the child's breakfast, since good work cannot be expected from these who do not breakfast adequately. For elder pupils a health monitor is selected by turn every month to held the inspection and report to the teacher the faults of his classmates. These should be corrected with as little delay as possible in a casual manner rather than as punishment or making it conspicuous before others.

Q. 17.6. What would be the duties of a Medical Officer ?

Duties of a Medical Officer should be :

1. *Medical check up* :
   (a) A systemic and periodical physical examination of new and old pupils during their staying at school.
   (b) Physical examination of teachers and employees of the school.

2. *Given up necessary treatments*—for their (pupils, teachers and employees) ill health or correction of defects.

3. *Prevention of communicable diseases*—by immunization of the students against infectious diseases.

4. *Health Education*—Physical education training and health practices.

5. *Maintenance*—of school sanitation.

6. *Dealing with the problem children*—Sometimes some pupils are recognised as a problem children for their less intelligent and delinquency, so they should be given the benefit of investigation and treatment by a children guidance clinic.

Above and all co-operation of teachers, parents and pupils are necessary to make it (the school health services) success.

Notes on :

Q. 17.7. Midday meal programme.

In order to combat malnutrition and improve the health of school children, in 1961 the School Health Committee recommended that school children should be assured of at least one nourishing meal. Those who can afford they may bring their lunch packets from home and during lunch hours take their meals in school. Otherwise, schools should have some arrangement for providing midday meals through their own cafeteria on a 'no profit no loss' basis. In view of the limited finance in India, it is recommended that the school meal should provide at least $1/_3$ of the daily caloric requirement and about half of daily protein requirement of the child.

Generally this supplementary feeding programme are organised by a trained dietitian with the assistance of teachers and senior scholars of the school in choosing the right kind of food. A cheap and nutritious meal is prepared and served daily to children during tiffin recess. For instance, for Primary School children in a morning school a cup of milk along with some solid food like biscuits or a piece of loaf or sandwich or germinated grams or a seasonal fruit (guava, mango slices, banana, orange etc.) or boiled potato or half of a boiled egg can be arranged. Contributions from guardians and the Health the Education Authorities (of Govt.) generally help to cover the overall expenditure. This nutrition programme generally serves two very useful purposes, namely :

    (i) it conserves and improves physical fitness, and

    (ii) provides education on untrition for a healthful living.

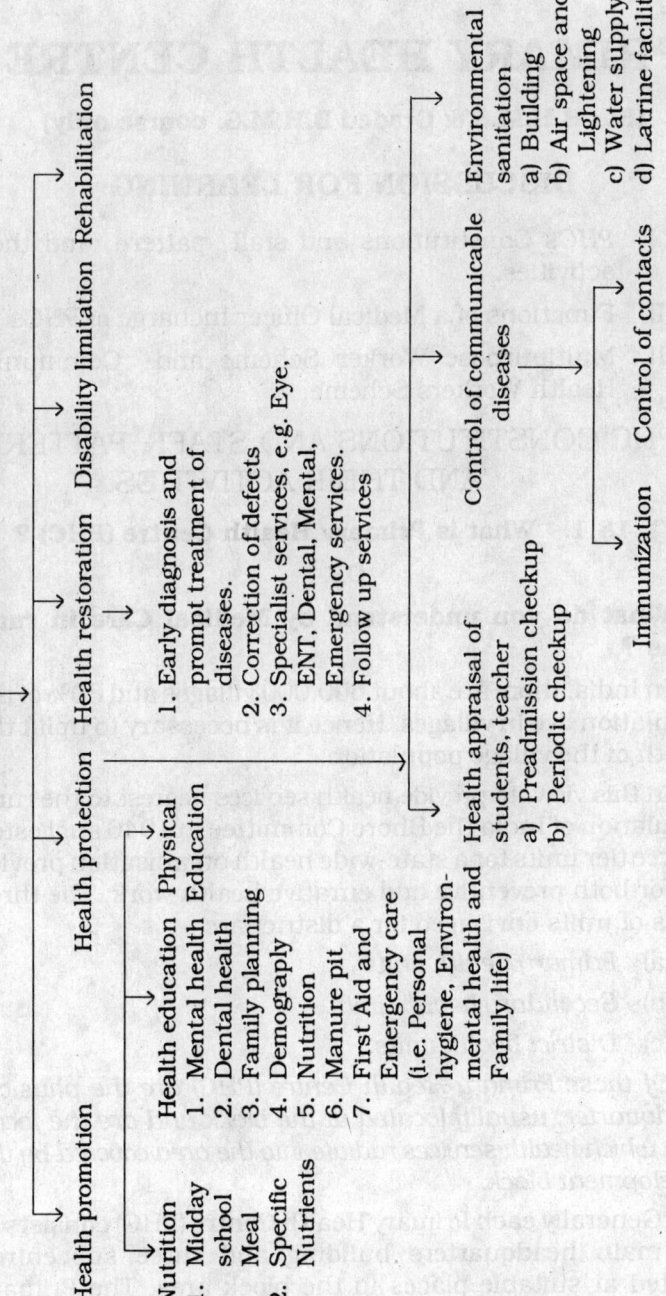

CHAPTER-XVIII

PRIMARY HEALTH CENTRE

(For B.H.M.S & Graded B.H.M.S. course only)

DISCUSSION FOR LEARNING

I. *PHCs* Constitutions and staff pattern, and their activities.

II. Functions of a Medical Officer Incharge of PHCs.

III. Multipurpose Worker Scheme and Community Health Workers Scheme.

I. PHC CONSTITUTIONS AND STAFF PATTERN AND THEIR ACTIVITIES.

Q. 18.1. What is Primary Health Centre (PHC) ?

OR

What do you understand by Medical Care in rural areas ?

In India, there are about 6,00,000 villages and 80% of the population live in villages. Hence it is necessary to uplift the health of the village population.

In this view, to provide health services nearest to the rural population of India the Bhore Committee in 1946 suggested a three tier units for a state-wide health organisation providing for both preventive and curative health work. The three types of units envisaged for a district are :

(a) *Primary health units.*
(b) *Secondary health units.*
(c) *District health units.*

Of these Primary Health Centre (PHC) are the physical headquarter, usually located at the block and are the focus from which health services radiate into the area covered by the development block.

*Generally each Primary Health Centre (PHC) consists of the main headquarters building and three subcentres located at suitable places in the block area. The Primary

Health Centre provides accommodation for an outdoor dispensary, consultation room, maternal and child health care and family planning services, minor surgery, a small laboratory and a ward of at least 6 beds. The subcentres provide maternal and child health care. The W.H.O. provides technical assistance and UNICEF provides vehicles, equipment, drugs, diets and supplements etc. Residential accommodation for all members of health staff and transport are provided for the efficient discharge of their duties.

So the PHC is a multipurpose unit, and renders preventive and curative services in building up the health of the community in the block. The PHC is incharge of a Medical Officer of Health. He is an adviser to the panchayat samiti and at the same time he is a link between the Sanitary Inspector of the Grama Panchayat and District Health Officer of Zila Parishad.

Q. 18.2. What are the aims and objects of PHC ?

The principal aims and objects of PHCs are :
1. To provide medical relief.
2. To control communicable diseases.
3. To provide laboratory services.
4. To organise environmental sanitation with primary emphasis on safe water supply and sanitary disposal of human excreta.
5. To provide maternal and child health services including family planning as an effective measure for population control.
6. To undertake school health services.
7. To organise health education at all levels.
8. To collect vital and health statistics.

Q. 18.3. What are the main activities of PHC ?

I. Routine activities :
1. Food hygiene and sanitation in food, proper nutrition and prevention of adulteration of food.
2. Infectious disease control, and the National Programmes for control or eradication of certain diseases.

3. Registration of births, deaths and infectious diseases and other registrations as required for "Vital statistics"
4. Maternity and Child welfare, and Family planning.
5. Medical care of the public by hospitals, clinics, dispensaries and mobile health units etc.
6. Environmental sanitation i.e. prevention of airpolution, chlorination of water, proper removal and disposal of refuse and excreta.
7. School health services.
8. Health education to the public as to (i) why diseases occur, (ii) how the diseases occur, and (iii) how the diseases can be prevented ?

II. Other Activities

Rural Primary Health Centre also carried out the following health activities as the rural area is vast and the people are of primitive habits, they are often orthodox and finance available is small.

1. Nutritional survey and diet survey.
2. Rural cholera control measures as there is no Infectious disease hospital.
3. Rural maternity and child welfare service. The service is by Auxiliary nurse. Midwives and mostly "Dais".
4. Rural family planning methods.
5. Rural environment sanitation of water. Water is chlorinated by Pot-chlorination method.
6. Rural sanitation of excreta—by latrines of RCA type or other suitable to a particular village.

Q. 18.4. What would be the staff pattern of a Rural Health Centre.

The *Primary health centre* units cover a population ranging from 60,000 to 80,000 population in different districts and states. The staffing pattern also differs in different

PRIMARY HEALTH CENTRE

states depending upon the resources and availability of personnel.

The West Bengal Government have provided some PHC with 10 or 20 bedded and a few with 50 bedded hospitals with necessary augmentation of medical, nursing and general staff, and three subcenters, each with 4 beds or 2 emergency beds. Generally the staff patterns are as follows :

1. One officer/Medical Officer Incharge.
2. One Medical Officer for Dispensary and Family Planning.
3. One Compounder or Pharmacist.
4. One Sanitary Inspector.
5. Seven Auxiliary Nurse Midwives.
6. One Health Visitor.
7. One Leprosy Technician.
8. One Co-ordinator for FP.
9. One Laboratory Technician.
10. One Basic Health worker for 10,000 people with one supervisor for 4 M.H.W.S (Multipurpose Health worker).
11. One Vaccinator for 15,000 people.
12. Four Cholera workers. If the area is an endemic for cholera.
*13. Community Health Workers are most recent additions.
14. Driver for transport vehicle.

For each sub-centre :

1. One Medical Officer.
2. One Compounder or Pharmacist.
3. One Nurse.
4. One Midwife.
5. One Health Assistant.
6. Two class VI staff (including sweeper).

II. FUNCTIONS OF MEDICAL OFFICER

Q. 18.5. What are the main functions of a M.O. of a PHC?

Main functions of M.O. of a PHC are maintained the following *Charts and Graphs* to show the P.H.C's constitution and location.

(A) Charts and Graphs of P.H.C. itself :
1. A chart showing the staff pattern of P.H.C.
2. District Map with location of the P.H.C.
3. Map of the Block showing :
   (a) Location of the P.H.C. in the Block and the 3 sub-centres.
   (b) Location of the 6 Family Planning sub-centres in the Block.
   (c) Location of the SET unit if any, Diespensary. Chest clinics, Rural Hospital etc.

(B) Other Activities :
They should perform and maintain the following activities :

1. Food Sanitation
   (a) No. of food premises inspected and upgraded.
   (b) No. of samples taken under P.F.A. Act.
   (c) Chart of Nutritional survey if this is done.

2. Control of Infectious Diseases
   (a) No. of cases of smallpox and Deaths Vaccination done primary Re.
   (b) No. of cases of Malaria—No of slides taken and No. of positive slides.
   (c) No. of cases of Leprosy—old cases—new cases detected.
   (d) No. of cases of Triple antigen given.
   (e) No. of cases of Tuberculosis and deaths—No. of B.C.G given.
   (f) Special diseases in the P.H.C. if any.

3. **Registration of Births and Deaths**
    (a) M.Y. E.P for 5 years.
    (b) No. of Births and Birth Rate.
    (c) No. of Deaths and Death Rate.
4. **Maternity and Child Welfare and Family Planning**
    (a) No. of Maternal Mortality.
    (b) No. of Infant Mortality.
    (c) No. of Deliversies conducted at the 4 Beds Maternity Home/Home Deliveries.
    (d) Average attendance of A.N.c/P.N.c/Infant welfare centre.
    (e) No. of sterilisation done for males and females.
    (f) No. of loops or other I.U.C.D. inserted.
    (g) No. of couples survey done and number covered up.
5. **Medical Care Clinics, Dispensaries, Hospitals etc.**
    (a) No. of daily attendance.
    (b) Any disease of special importance.
    (c) No. of blood slides, sputum, urine examined.
6. **Environmental Sanitation**
    (a) No. of drinking water wells repaired, chlorinated.
    (b) No. of latrines, urinals, soakage pits constructed.
7. **School Health**
    (a) Total No. of children in primary schools.
    (b) No. of children examined.
    (c) No. of children with defects suffering from deficiency diseases.
    (d) No of children given aids for their defects.
8. **Health Education**
    Health Education is given at every stage on every subject whichever subject is required, through talks, poster, banner, cinemas etc.

III. MULTIPURPOSE WORKER SCHEME

Q. 18.6. Notes on :

1. Basic Health Worker or Multipurpose Worker Scheme :

The *Basic Health Workers* were initially responsible for :
(a) Malaria vigilance.
(b) Health intelligence.
(c) Health education.
(d) Treatment of minor ailments. Later on a Basic Health Worker changed into a Multipurpose Health worker.

In Multipurpose worker scheme, there should be one male and a female worker for every 10,000 population. The Multipurpose worker or Gramsevak works at the village level and thus he is also known as village level worker. Aa a domicilliary worker, he should live in the village, with his place of work or base in the subcentre.

As a link between people and the Government, he should help the village in construction of tube wells, sanitary latrine and takes step to treat minor ailments from local sub-centre, to immunise and educate the villager about Isolation of cases of communicable diseases, and about nutrition of the child, mother and pregnant women.

2. Community Health Worker's Scheme (CHWS)

Under this scheme a community of 1000 population will select a person from among its own residence to work as a *"JANA SWASTHYA RAKSHAK"* (Community Health Protector).

This worker will receive training for 3 months in the fundamentals of health and hygiene at the PHCs before surving his community. His responsibilities will be to take after promotive and preventive aspects of health and will be provided with a Kit Bag to carry elementary medicines of different systems including the Indian system (Allopathy, Homoeopathy, Aurvadya, and Unani). He will also be trained in Yoga and Naturopathy. This Community Health Worker being the man from the community, will be acceptable to the community and the community in turn will supervise his work.

CHAPTER-XIX

MEDICAL STATISTICS

(For Graded B.H.M.S. and B.H.M.S. Courses only)

DISCUSSION FOR LEARNING

I. Vital statistics.
II. Health statistics.
III. Population census.
IV. Vital events.
V. Morbidity statistics.
VI. Indicator of Health.

I. VITAL STATISTICS

Q. 19.1. What is meant by Vital Statistics ?

Vital Statistics is a specialized branch of statistics i.e. application of numerical methods to the subject matter of vital occurrence in the community, e.g. birth, death including foetal and infant deaths, maternal death, longevity, all kinds of sickness and their causes (morbidity and mortality), marriage, separation, divorce, adoption, legislation etc. Vital statistics measure the health of the people and reflect on the hygienic conditions of the environment and also it forms the basis of sanitation, so it is stated as the *barometer of public health*. Recently it may also be defined as the facts, systematically collected and compiled in numerical form, relating to or dervied from records of vital events, namely live births, deaths, foetal deaths, marriages, divorces, adoption, legitimations, recognitions, annulments or legal separations.

Q. 19.2. What are the sources of Vital Statistics ?

The main sources of vital statistics are :
1. Population census,
2. Registration of vital events.
3. Notification of deaths under notifible diseases.
4. Hospital and health centre records.
5. Report of special survey.

Q. 19.3. What are the information we get from the vital Statistics ?

We get following information from vital statistics :
1. The index to the sanitary progress, and the value of the sanitary measures adopted.
2. Mortality of different diseases at different ages, gives us the idea as to what preventive measures are to be adopted.
3. It shows the influence of profession, trade, locality and age, on the well-being of a community.

Q. 19.4. What are the uses of Vital Statistics in community health service ?

1. To measure the state of health of a community and to identify its health problems, their nature, their distribution among the various population groups so that available health and medical care can be used with maximum effect.
2. For planning and administration of health services.
3. For prediction of health trends.
4. For estimating the furture needs of community and to fix suitable targets for achievement.
5. For comparing the health status of one country with that of another.
6. For evaluting the progress, success or failure of health programmes and services already in operation.
7. For research into community health problems.

Q. 19.5. What are the information (data) required for Vital Statistics ?

Data required and recording :
1. *Population according to age and sex.*
2. *Births according to sex.*
3. *Death according to age, sex and the nature of the diseases.*

4. *Recording of the Bio-statistics* i.e. the vital events of life e.g. births, deaths, neonatal deaths, marriages, divorces etc. except morbidity statistics and population data.

5. Health statistics (It includes the vital statistics as well as the morbidity statistics and population)..

N.B. : If the cause of death is not correct, vital statistics will not give the correct picture. Hence WHO in the Manual of International Statistical Classification of diseases has classified causes of deaths under about 500 categories. The cause of death should not only give the disease directly leading to death, but should state the antecedent cause of death also.

6. *Notification of communicalbe disease.* i.e. Notification of infectious diseases or deaths due to small pox, cholera and plague etc.

N.B. : As per act of 1886 the registration of births and deaths are compulsory and as per Epidemic Act of 1897 the notifications of infectious diseases are compulsory. However, except plague, cholera and smallpox, the notifiable diseases in disfferent states varies. Hence the statistical information of notifiable disease cannot be relied upon. Similar is the cause regarding the registration of births and deaths, the birth, death and infant mortality rates show a wide range of variation. On a sample survey of births and deaths, it was revealed that nearly 47% of births and 50% of deaths are not registered. Hence our vital statistical figures are defective.

For the collection of Vital Statistics the Central Government have allocated the responsibility primarily to the Registrar General of India at New Delhi, while the Central Health Ministry has established at Directorate of Health Intelligence in the office of the Director General of Health Services for Collection of health statistics and receiving the reports of notifiable diseases. At the state level there is a "Statistical Bureau of Health Intelligence" or a section for collecting both vital and health statistics for the state. The latter sends the vital statistics data to the Registrar General who transmits them to the Directorate of Health Intelligence, and other health statistical data directly to the Directorate of Health Intelligence of the G.G.H.s. office at New Delhi, in a series of proformas issued by this Directorate. The final compilation of the composite health statistics is made by this Directorate for annual or periodic publication. Correspondingly a similar compilation is made at the state level for the respective states.

II. HEALTH STATISTICS

Q. 19.6. What is meant by Health Statistics ?

Health statistics is a specialized branch of statistics that relates to the application of numerical method to all matters that have direct or indirect influence upon or relationship with health and are required for health planning, services and reporting. It includes not only vital statistics but also population data, mobidity statistics, hospital statistics, statistics of health personal etc.

Q. 19.7. What are the uses of Health Statistics ?

Uses :

1. To describe the level of community health, both static and dynamic (with changing phases), qualitative and quantitative.
2. To diagnose community ills-prevalance of acute and chronic diseases, impairment and disabilities for adoption of proper curative and control measures,
3. To collect information about the utilization and cost of medical care, cost of medicine, bed and staff requirement of different health centres and agencies.
4. To determine priorites of health problems and to discover their solutions and plan for health services.
5. To assess the man-power needs and to arrange for their adequate training and distribution.
6. To assess the results of health measures and control programmes.
7. To suggest lines of medical research and investigation of health problems.

8. To promote health legislation.
9. To disseminate progress and reliable information on health situations.
10. To obtain public support for health work.

Q. 19.8. What are the sources of health statistics ? or What are the present existing organisations for collection of statistics in India ?

Sources :
1. Population statistics—census and other sources.
2. Collected records of vital statistics.
3. Hospital and dispensary statistics—these include statistics from all types of hospitals, clinics, homes, maternal and child health units, medical care programmes such as, Employees State Insurance Scheme, Contributory Health Service Scheme etc.
4. Physician's records.
5. Family Health records.
6. Police records—for accidents, injuries, suicides, homicides etc.
7. Records of notifiable diseases.
8. Morbidity records from industrial and sickness benefit associations.
9. Records of special investigations of disease like T.B., V.D., Leprosy, Cancer, Mental disease etc,
10. Reports of epidemiologial investigations and mass diagnosis and screening of diseases.
11. Mobidity and health surveys.
12. National sample survey data.
13. Census data for disabled and handicapped groups.
14. Climatic and metrological data.
15. Medico-legal work.
16. Health administration statistics.
17. Sea and air port health administration.
19. Records of medical education and research.

III. POPULATION CENSUS

Q. 19.9. What is meant by population census ?

Census is a process of collecting, compiling and publishing demographic, economic and social data pertaining to all persons in a country at a specified time. It was originally used for counting people, recruitment for military service and taxation. The census is now an essential operation for planning the welfare of the people—if administrative needs of the Government planning for development and planning social welfare schemes relating to total food requirements, schools (education), hospital services, housing orphanages, occupation and employment, development of industries, benefit and security schemes, for calculating indices such as birth rates, death rates, sicknes rates, expectation of life, age and sex composite, urban and rural distribution of population, language, place of birth and nationality, amount of durability (blind, paralysed, crippled etc.), fertility data (number of children born and remaining alive), distribbution of population density of population and sex ratio's etc., and rate of increase of population.

In India first census was in 1871-72 and since then, census taking had become a decimial in each year ; ending in 1 i.e., 1881, 1891, 2001, and so on. Generally census can be taken on *de jure basis, or de facto basis.* In the former each individual will be enumerated, according to his legal place of residence, while in the later, individuals are counted, according to the place they happpened to stay on the census date, a date fixed, before hand. For all purposes, operation has a legal standing and by Act of parliament, each individual is obliged to furnish information to the census interviewers, called enumerators truthfully, to the best of his/her recollection and ability.

Consequently, it is also obligatory on the state, to keep the information, furnished by the public highly confidential, and the data supplied by them, cannot be produced in the court of law, as evidence.

Indian Population Enumerated in the Different Census Since 1891 to 1981

Census Year	Population (in millions)	Increase or decrease (in millions)	Percentage variation during the preceding decade.
1891	236.70	—	—
1901	238.33	− 0.4	− 0.20
1911	252.00	+ 15.4	5.73
1921	251.23	− 0.7	− 0.31
1931	278.86	+ 27.6	+ 11.01
1941	318.53	+ 37.7	+ 14.22
1951	360.95	+ 14.4	+ 13.31
1961	439.07	+ 78.1	+ 21.50
1971	547.94	+ 108.2	+ 24.66
1981	685.17	+ 137.0	+ 25.00

Sources : Registrar General and Census Commissioner of India (1981), Census of India 1981. Provisional Population Totals Paper-1 of 1981.

IV. VITAL EVENTS

Q. 19.10. What is meant by Vital Events ?

Vital Events are those events, like live births, deaths, foetal deaths (still births), marriages, divorces, adoption, legitimation annulments etc in short, all the events, which have to do with an individual entrance into and departure from life, together with changes in civil status, which my occur to him during his life time.

V. MORBIDITY STATISTICS

Q. 19.11. What is meant by Morbidity Statistics ?

Morbidity statistics is a specialised part of the vital statistics dealing with numerical description of deviations from health to sickness in the general and specific population group or in respect of specific disease. The sources of its are the same as those of hospital statistics and morbidity and health survey.

Uses :

(a) It is generally use as a guide to administrative planning and evaluation of official and voluntary programmes in the field of health e.g. priority determination, cheeking of control measures, exppenditure needed, planning of new programmes for control etc.

(b) For evaluation of current morbidity experience in relation to the provision of medical and health services in the country e.g., needs for hospital facilities, beds and home care facilities, rehabilitation programme, insurance plans, medical research, manpower problem and civilian defence etc.

(c) For the use of drug firms and appliance manufacture.

(d) For health education programme.

VI. INDICATOR OF HEALTH

19.12. What are the Indicators of Health ?

In measuring or comparing the state of health of a community or a country some relative figures are necessary. These are called rates. A rate may be looked upon as the estimate of the probability that a person exposed to the risk of the vital event will actually experience the event. These rates are regarded as the indices of health of the population.

$$\text{Rate of a vital event} = \frac{\text{Total number of occurrences of particular vital event in a community during a defined time period.}}{\text{Total number of persons exposed to the risk of occurrences of that event in the same time period.}}$$

A rate when multiplied by 1000 gives the rate per thousand or a rate per mille.

MORTALITY RATES

1. Crude Death Rate (CDR) = $\dfrac{\text{Total number of deaths which occurred in an area in a year.}}{\text{Mid year population of the area in the same year.}} \times 1000$

It is the most widely used of vital statistics rates. As it does not take into consideration the important factors like age, sex, cause etc. specific death rates are used.

2. Specific Death Rate = $\dfrac{\text{Total number of deaths which occurred among a specified section of population in an area in a year.}}{\text{Mid year population of the area during the same year.}} \times 1000$

These are the true and best measures mortality.

3. Standardised Death Rate (STDR)

It is a hypothetical figure. It is not the total death rate that actually exists in a locality, but the rate that the locality would have if, while retaining its own age and sex specific death rates it would have the population of some standard region instead of having its own population. There are two methods of its calculation:

a) Direct Method and b) Indirect Method.

In Direct Method, population of some standard region is to be taken and one has to apply the age and sex specific mortality rates of the given community on the standard population.

In Indirect Method, one has to apply the standard age and sex specific mortality rates on the population of the given community in different age and sex groups and then to adjust the crude death rate of the community by applying to it a factor which measures the relative mortality proneness of the population of the community.

4. Infant Mortality Rate = $\dfrac{\text{Total number of infant deaths which occurred in an area during a year.}}{\text{Total number of live births which occurred in the same area during the same year.}} \times 1000$

For its proper calculation, the cohort analysis method has to be adopted. In otherwords, one has to follow the cohort of live born babies in a region during one calendar year through their first year of life and also record the number of deaths among these babies during the same year. But from administrative view point it is very difficult to follow up and the above formula is used. However, the result is almost the same, becaused in a stable community almost the same pattern of births of babies follow.

Infant Mortality comprises of two parts :

i) Deaths occuring in the neo-natal period (i.e. in the first 4 weeks of life), and ii) Those occuring in the rest of the first year, called post neo-natal period. These are given by :

i) Neo-natal Infant Mortality Rate = $\dfrac{\text{Number of death of infants upto 28 days of age which occurred in a region during a year.}}{\text{Total number of live births which occurred in the region during the same year.}} \times 1000$

ii) Post Neonatal Infant Mortality Rate = $\dfrac{\text{Number of deaths of infants after 28 days of age to one year of age.}}{\text{Total number of live births which occurred in the region during the same year.}} \times 1000$

MEDICAL STATISTICS

It is the post neonatal part of infant mortality which is mainly due to exogenous factors that is most susceptible to preventive measures.

Infant Mortality Rate is one of the most sensitive indices of health and level of living of country.

5. Perinatal Mortality Rate = $\dfrac{\text{Late foetal deaths+deaths under one week weighing over 1,000 gm. at birth}}{\text{Total number of live and still births weighing over 1,000 gm. at birth}} \times 1000$

A late foetal death is the death of foetus after 28 completed weeks of gestation. It is a sensitive index of standard of obstetric, paediatric, social and public health measure in a country.

6. (1 - 4) year Mortality Rate = $\dfrac{\text{Number of death of children of age (1 - 4) year in a region during a year}}{\text{Total child population in the same age group of the region during the same year}} \times 1000$

It is an important Index of community health of nutritional status.

7. Maternal Mortality Rate = $\dfrac{\text{Number of deaths from puerperal causes in an area during a given year}}{\text{Total number of live births which occurred in the same area during the same year}} \times 1000$

Deaths from puerperal causes include deaths of mothers due to complications of pregnancy, child birth and the puerperium.

It is an important index of quality of maternity services of a country.

8. Case Fatality Rate = $\dfrac{\text{Number of deaths from a particular disease in an area during a year.}}{\text{Total number of persons attacked by the given disease in the same area during the same year.}} \times 1000$

9. **Proportional Mortality Rate:**

a) Proportional Mortality Rate from a disease = $\dfrac{\text{Total number of deaths due to a given disease i an area during a year.}}{\text{Total deaths from all causes in the area during the same year.}} \times 1000$

b) Proportional Mortality Rate for persons in a particular age group = $\dfrac{\text{Total number of deaths of persons of giv group in an area during a year.}}{\text{Total deaths at all ages which occurred in the area during the same year.}} \times 1000$

10. Still Birth Ratio = $\dfrac{\text{Total number of foetal deaths of 28 or more completed weeks of gestation in an area during a year.}}{\text{Total number of live births which occurred in the same area during the given year.}} \times 1000$

FERTILITY RATE

1. **Crude Birth Rate** = $\dfrac{\text{Total number of live births which occurred in a given region during a given year.}}{\text{Mid-year total population of the region during the same year.}} \times 1000$

Like CDR, it also suffers from many drawbacks as it is calculated without proper regard to the age and sex composition of the population.

2. **General Fertility Rate** = $\dfrac{\text{Total number of live births in a given region during a given year.}}{\text{Mid-year female population in the age group (15-44) year in the region during the same year.}} \times 1000$

15 and 44 are taken to be the lower and upper limit of the child bearing age respectively.

3. **Age Specific Fertility Rate** = $\dfrac{\text{Total number of births to women of a specified age in a given region during a given year.}}{\text{Mid-year female population of the specified age in the same region during the same year}} \times 1000$

Total Fertility Rate

It is the sum of single year age specific fertility rates in the age group 15 to 44 years. It indicates, on average how many children would be born to 1,000 women during their total reproductive period supposing that none of them dies before reaching the end of the reproductive period.

GROWTH RATE

1. Crude Rate of Natural Increase = CBR - CDR

2. Vital Index = $\dfrac{\text{Total number of biths which occurred in a given region during a given year.}}{\text{Total number of deaths which occurred in the same region during the same year.}} \times 1000$

4. Gross Reproduction Rate (G R R)

It is the sum of single year female age specific fertility rates. It indicates the average number of daughters who would be born to a group of girls heginning life together in a population, supposing none of them died before reaching the upper limit of the child bearing age and each was subject to the observed fertility rates.

Thus $G R R = \sqrt{\Sigma^2 f_{ix}}$

Where f_{ix} = single year female age specific fertility

rates = $\dfrac{f_{Bx}}{f_{px}}$

Where $^fB\,x$ is the number of female births to women of age x during a given period in a given community and is the female population in the same community during the same time $^fp\,x$ period.

1 and 2 are the lower and upper limit of child bearing age group.

5. Net Reproduction Rate (N R R)

It indicates the average number of daughters that could be produced by a group of women beginning life together, throughout their total reproductive span if they were exposed at each age to the observed fertility and mortality rates. It also indicates the rate at which the number of births would eventually grow per generation if the observed fertility and mortality rates be in operation in the future.

Thus $NRR = \dfrac{\Sigma f_{tx} \times f_{Lx}}{F_{lo}}$ where f_{tx} is same in GRR

fLx is a life table standard population for females out of the cohort of females in the age interval x to x + 1

f_{tx} is the cohort of female population in the life table and 1,2 are lower and upper limit of reproductive age.

If NRR = 1, then we say that the stationary population has been achieved.

If NRR>1 or <1 we say that a group of females are expected to be replaced by a greater or smaller number of females in the next generation if the current fertility and mortality rates be in operation.

EXPECTATION OF LIFE

It is defined as the average number of years that a group of persons born at the same time is expected to live it they experience at different ages of life the mortality conditions of a specific area during a specific period of time. It is calculated by using the Life Table technique. In life table, it is the $e^0 x$ column.

MORBIDITY RATE

1. Incidence Rate of a disease:

i) (spells of sickness) = $\dfrac{\text{Number of new spells of sickness which occurred in an area during a given time period.}}{\text{Population at risk in the area during the same time period.}} \times 100$

ii) (sick persons) = $\dfrac{\text{Number of persons starting new spells of sickness in an area during a given time period}}{\text{Population at risk in the area during the same time period.}} \times 100$

2. Prevalence Rate of a disease :

i) (a) Period prevalence Rate (spells) = $\dfrac{\text{Number of sicknesses (old+new) current at any time during a given time period in an area.}}{\text{Average number of persons at risk during that period in the same area.}} \times 100$

(b) Period prevalence Rate (sick persons) = $\dfrac{\text{Number of persons sick (old+new) at any time during a given time period in an area.}}{\text{Average number of persons at risk during that period in the same area.}} \times 100$

ii) Point prevalence Rate = $\dfrac{\text{Number of sicknesses in existence at a particular point of time in an area.}}{\text{Population at risk at that time in the same area duration of sickness}} \times 100$

a) Average duration of sickness per sick person = $\dfrac{\text{Total of the entire durations of all spells of sickness which ended during given time period in a given community.}}{\text{Number of persons who experienced at least one spell of sickness during the same time period.}} \times 100$

(b) Average duration of sickness per completed spell. = $\dfrac{\text{Total of the entire durations of all spells of sickness which ended during a given time period in an area.}}{\text{Total number of spells ending during the same time period in the same area.}} \times 100$

11. (a) **Crude Birth Rate, and Crude Death Rates of India** are given in the following table from 1911 to 1971. Obtain the Natural Growth Rates of India for the given years and present the CBR, CDR and NGR on a same graph paper and draw your conclusion.

Year :	1911	1921	1931	1941	1951	1961	1971
Rate per 1000							
CBR :	48.1	46.4	45.2	39.9	41.7	41.1	36.9
CDR :	47.2	36.3	31.2	27.4	22.8	18.9	14.9

(b) **Infant and Neonatal Mortality Rates** in the city of Bombay during 1938-1956 are given below. Present these rates by drawing line diagrams kand give appropriate coments.

Infant and Neonatal Mortality Rates of Bombay per 1000 live births

Year	IMR	NMR	Year	IMR	NMR
1938	268.0	94.3	1948	165.7	75.6
1939	211.7	88.1	1949	174.2	73.6
1940	201.4	78.5	1950	151.7	70.4
1941	211.4	83.2	1951	148.4	66.8
1942	195.4	79.6	1952	141.2	64.6
1943	197.4	81.1	1953	143.5	62.7
1944	203.0	75.7	1954	135.3	60.9
1945	190.3	75.8	1955	118.6	50.9
1946	195.4	76.8	1956	110.3	56.9
1947	166.6	72.7			

(c) A general health survey was conducted in an area. The surveyed population consisted of 5230 males and 4770 females. There were 1200 females in the age group (15-44) years and 1500 children in the age group (0-4) years. During the year there were 343 live births comprising of 175 males and 168 females. During the year there were 125 deaths of which 47 were infant deaths and 107 in the age group (0-4) years 3 mothers died of puerperal causes during the year. Out of the total deaths 31 were due to G.I.T. diseases. It was reported that during the last one year there were in all 508 cases of G.I.T. diseases. On the day of the survey there were 105 cases of G.I.T. diseases in the population and of these 105 cases 75 cases started on the day of survey. Calculate the different health indicators for the area from this report.

CHAPTER-XX

INTERNATIONAL AND NATIONAL ORGANISATIONS

DISCUSSION FOR LEARNING

I. W.H.O.
II. U.N.I.C.E.F.
III. F.A.O.
IV. E.S.I. Scheme.

I. W.H.O.

20.1. W.H.O. (World Health Organisation)

The World Health Organisation (WHO) is an specialised, non-political, health agency of the United Nation. It came in existance on 7 April 1948 and this date is observed as "World Health Day". Its head quarters is at Geneva in Switzerland. At present 127 Nations are its members.

The constitution of the WHO is the most important document concerning international health work ever drawn up, and making the advances on medico-social thought in wide and liberal terms. In 1960 membership of the Executive Board was raised from 18 to 24. It created for the first time a single world wide international health organisation empowered to deal with every aspect of health.

Principles

The constitution declares the following principles which are basic to happiness, harmonious relations and security of peoples.
1. Health is a state of complete, physical, mental and social well being and not merely absence of disease or infirmity.
2. The enjoyment of highest attainable standard of health is one of the fundamental rights of every human being without distinction of race, religion, political belief, economic or social condition.

3. The health of all peoples is fundamental to the attainments of peace and security and is dependent upon the fullest cooperation of individual and states.
4. The achievement of any state in the promotion of health is of value to all. Unequal development in different countries in the promotion of health and control of disease, especially communicable disease, is a common danger.
5. Healthy development of the child is of basic importance, the ability to live harmoniously in a changing total enviornment is essential to such development.
6. The extension to all people of the benefit of medical, psychological and related knowledge is essential to the fullest attainment of health.
7. Informed opinion and active co-operation on the part of the public are of the utmost importance in the improvement of the health of the peoples.
8. Governments have a responsibility for the health of all peoples, which can be fulfiled by the provision of adequate health and social measures.

Article 1 : The object of the World Health Organisations should be the attainment by all peoples of the highest level of health.

Article 2 : Lists 22 functions covering all the successful work of predecessor organisations and many new ones, including that of acting as the directing and co-ordinating authority on international health work.

Membership is open to all states, with nonself governing territories as associate members.

WHO's campaign is for better health.

FUNCTIONS AND FILDS OF WORK :

1. The classical or inherited works are :

(a) Epidemic intelligence.

(b) Quarantine, i.e. Epidemic warning.

(c) Biological standarisation of drugs, vaccines and pesticides.

2. Direct services :

Direct services, includes (to its member governments, mostly advisory) eradication of diseases, like (i) Malaria, (ii) Tuberculosis, (iii) Veneral diseases, and also, others programmes like (iv) Maternal and Child Health, (v) Nutrition, (vi) Environmental Sanitation and (vii) Mental health

*The essence of WHO assitance is to help people to help themselves.

3. Education and information :

This field includes the expert advisory committees and panels which now cover some sixty and thirty six subjects respectively.

The most common are :

(a) Training of doctors, nurses, sanitary engineers and other professional auxillary staff.
(b) Studies and surveys and stimulation of research.
(c) Course, symposia, seminars and other educational meetings.
(d) Large and popular fellowship programmes.
(e) Publication of various types, like
  - i) Monthly chronicle,
  - ii) Bulletin,
  - iii) Monographs,
  - iv) Technical Report Series,
  - v) Public health papers,
  - vi) International Digest of Health Legislation,
  - vii) Weekly, monthly and annual epidemiological records,
  - viii) World Health-a popular news sheet,
  - ix) Report of official activities-central and regional,
  - x) First ten and twenty years of World Health Organisation.

4. Liasion with other International Organisations :

(a) UNICEF (United Nations International Children's Emergency Fund).

(b) ILO (International Labour Organisation).
(c) FAO (Food and Agricultural Organisation).
(d) UNESCO (United National Educational Scientific and Cultural Organisation).
(e) IRO (International Refusee Organisation).
(f) ICAO (International Civic Aviation Organisation).
(g) Voluntary Organisations :
  i) Religious or Missionery,
  ii) Relief societies,
  iii) Medical and Public Medical Organisations like Rockefeller, Milbank, Carnegie Foundations, Common Wealth Fund etc.
  iv) Professional and Technical Association, like W.M.A. (World Medical Association), I.C.N. (International Council of Nurses).
  v) International Non-governmental Organisations about 40 in number.

5. Structural organisation :
1. A world Health Assembly
2. An Executive Board.
3. A Secretariate
4. Divisions :
   (i) Health statistics.
   (ii) Control of Communicable Disease.
   (iii) Publication,
   (iv) Library.
   (v) Quarantine,
   (vi) Epidemiological Intelligence.
   (vii) Administration.

6. For administrative purposes the world has been divided into 6 regions :
(a) South East Asia—Head Quater—New Delhi.
(b) Eastern Mediterranean—Head Quarter—Alexandria.
(c) America—Head Quarter—Washington.

(d) Western Pacific—Head Quarter—Manila.
(e) Africa—Head Quarter—Brazenville.
(f) Europe—Head Quarter—Copenhagen.

U.N.I.C.E.F.

20.2. U.N.I.C.E.F. (United Nations International Children Emergency Fund).

It was established in 1946 with its Head Quarter at New York. It receives contributions from all governments and gives assistance to all governments that work together in harmony to give their children better life.

The Need : Out of 1,000,000,000 children in the world $3/4$ live in the economically backward countries where proverty, hunger and disease are widespread and most children lack adequate food, clothing and protection. They constitute the most vulnerable group and deserve special consideration and treatment.

Basic Aids

This mainly helps for building up better maternal and children's health and control the disease of children.

The Basic Aids :

1. *MCH services* by net work of permanent health centres and training of national personnel to plan and operate these services.
2. *Disease control* by campaigns to control or erradicate diseases such as malaria, tuberculosis, yaws, trachoma and leprosy affecting large number of children, by supplying vehicles, insecticides, sprayers drugs and laboratory equipments.
3. *Nutrition*—by supplementary, child-feeding schemes, milk conservation, and the development of other protein-rich foods as well as the education of families better nurition practices.
4. Schools services for children—by teaching of homcraft and mother-craft.
5. Emergency aid for the relief of mothers in time of disasters such as, earth quake, flood, drought and famine.

6. Training of all categories of personnel from planning and supervisory caders to auxiliary workers.
7. Enviornmental sanitation through improvement of village water supply, sewage and excreta disposal and related community health education as a part of rural improvement programme.
8. Specialised projects such as for physically handicapped children.
9. UNICEF's aid to health centres includes simple technical equipment, midwives and nurse's kits, drugs, milk, vitamins, motor vehicles or bicycles for supervisers travel round their districts.
10. For trainging UNICEF has supplied teaching and demostration equipment for nurses and midwives training schools,

III. F.A.O.

Q. 20.3. F.A.O (The Food and Agriculture Organisation).

The Food and Agriculture Organization (FAO) was formed in 1945 with headquaters in Rome. It was first United Nations Organization specialised agency created to look after several areas of world cooperation. The chief aim of this organization are :

1. to help nations raise living standards,
2. to improve nutrition of the people of all countries,
3. to increase the efficiency of farming, forestry and fisheries,
4. to better the condition of rurual people and, through all these means, to widen the opportunity of all people for productive work.

It is also concerned with the problems of increased food production and banishment of hunger. In 1960 FAO organised a campaign—World Freedom from Hunger Campaign (FFHC) with the objects to combat malnutrition and to disseminate information and education. It workd in close collaboration with other international organisations and with the Ministries of Food and Agriculture and Health in the Government of India. The joint WHO/FAO expert committees have provided the basis for many cooperative activities like nutritional surveys, training courses, seminars and the coordination of research programmes on Brucellosis and other Zoonoses.

IV. E.S.I. SCHEME

Q. 20.4. E.S.I. Scheme (Employee's State Insurance Scheme).

It is an Act passed in 1948 (amended in 1975) to provide for certain benefits to employees in case of sickness, maternity and "*employment injury*" and for certain related matters. The Act extends to the whole of India except Jammu and Kashmir, applies to all factories (both private and public) other than seasonal ones.

'*Employment injury*' means a personal injury to an employee caused by accident or occupational disease arising out of an in the course of his employment in a factory or establishment to which this Act applies.

Administration

The administration is vested on a corporation consisting of 20 members drawn from ministers, government nominees, representatives of employers, employees, medical profession and Parliament. In addition the corporation has a standing committee of 13 members a Medical Benefit Council of 22 members and an Exceutive staff under a Director General of Employee State Insurance Scheme, assisted by an Insurance Commissioner, a Medical Commissioner, a chief Accountant and an Auditor to run the administration. Besides above, there are Regional Boards, Local Committees, Regional and Local Medical Benefit Councils.

Benefit

Subject to the provisions of the Act, the insured persons as the case may be, and their dependents shall be entitled to the following benefits :

I. Sickness benefits (cash) :

If a sickness is duly certified by an Insurance Medical Personnel, sickness benefit consists of 7/12 of his daily average wages for a maximum period of 56 days in a year.

In case of chronic diseases of long duration like :
1) Tuberculosis, 2) Leprosy, 3) Mental diseases, 4) Paraplegia, 5) Malignant disease, 6) Hemiplegia, 7) Chronic congestive failure, 8) Immature cataract with vision 6/60 or less, sickness benefit is payable for 309 days, and other benefit of 124 days is payable for the following diseases :

1) Bronchiectasis and lung absces, 2) Myocaradial infraction, 3) Parkinson's disease, 4) Dislocation and Prolapse of intervertebral disc, 5) (a) Aplastic anaemia, (b) Gangrane 7) Ankylosis, 8) Spondyolitis, 9) Cirrhosis of liver with ascites, 10) Fracture of lower extremities, 11) Detachment of retina.

The insured person normally protected against discharge from his service for a period of 6 months and in case of long term illness like tuberculosis, etc., the period is extended for 18 months.

2) Maternity benefit (cash) :

The benefit is payable in cash to an insured women for confinement/miscarriage or sickness arising out of pregnancy/confinement or premature birth of child or miscarriage.

For (a) *confinement the duration of benefits*—12 week,
(b) *miscarriage the duration of benefits*—6 weeks,
(c) *sickness associated with confinement"*
—30 days.

The benefit is allowed at full wages.

3. Disablement benefit (cash) :

Periodical payment of an insured person (temporary or permanent) for partial or total disablement as a result of employment injury, for the duration of the period of disablement (which may extend to whole life).

The rates are :

for (a) *Temporary disablement*— at full rate i.e. 72 percent of the wages during the period of disablement.

(b) *Partial parmanent disablement*—percentage of full rate according to the extent of disablement.

(c) *Permanent total disablement*—at full rate i.e. 72 per cent of his wages of the worker (life pension).

(d) *Dependent's benefit* (cash)—on the death of the insured due to injury; at the following rates :

   i) Generally pensions are granted at the rate of 25% more than the Standard Benefit rate.
   ii) 3/5th full rate to the widow till death or remarriage;
   iii) At 2/5th full rate to each legitimate or adopted son till 15 years of age.
   iv) At 2/5th full rate to each legitimate unmarried daughter till 18 years of age or marriage which ever is earlier; upto 18 years if the son or daughter continuous studies.
   v) *Funeral Benefits* : An amount not exceding Rs. 500/- is paid with in 15 days after the death of an insured person for funeral, expenses.

N.B. : Total amount of dependent's benefit cannot exceed the full rate of the insured. There are certain rules for other categories of dependents.

4. Medical Benefit (in kind) :

This benefit is given to all insured persons or a member of his family whose condition required medical teatment and attendance either in the form of out patient and inpatient treatment attendance in a hospital, clinic or other institutions etc. or by visits by the insurance doctor to the home of the insurance persons and also of drugs as per approved list. The insured person can enjoy one benefit at a time. While on medical benefit he shall carry out the doctor's instruction and shall not leave the area without prior permission of the doctor.

The corporation employees a panel doctor (private physician) each having a maximum registration of 750 workers or his register or doctors an employed a whole time basis—certain places to give the necessary medical benefit. It also provides, one general bed for every 800 employees, one T.B. bed for every 1600 employees and one maternity bed for every 500 women employees in all centres where the scheme is in force.

MEDICAL BENEFIT COUNCIL (CHAIRMAN)
(DIRECTOR GENERAL OF HEALTH SERVICES)

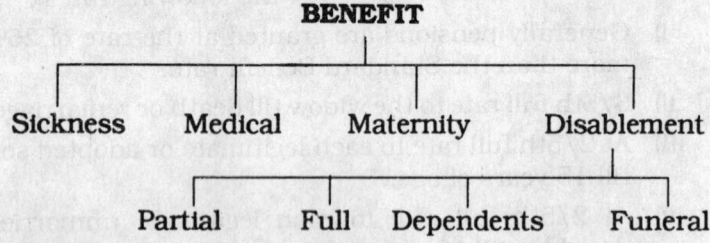

Extra Benefits :
1. Extended Sickness Benefit.
2. Artificial limbs, dentures, family planning etc.
3. Family Medical care.
4. Protection against dismissal or discharges from service, during the period of sickness.

Limitations :
1. The scope is resistricted to certain category of factory employees, seasonal factories, agricultural and other workers are not covered.
2. Benefit to families on restricted.
3. Unemployment is not covered.
4. Old age and retirement benefits have not been included.
5. Medical benefits to clinic attendance is restricted to Rs. 61 to Rs. 81 per insured person.
6. Benefits are primarily curative in character. Prevention and rehabilitation services are not provided in this scheme.

Collection of Finance

The finance is collected by contributors from the Central and State Governments, employers and employees to the central fund known as Employee's State Insurance Fund. The shares are distributed as follows :

(ESI Corporation 7/8th portion)

1. Central Government—annual grant of a sum equivalent to 2/3rd of the administrative expenses, not including cost of benefit for a period of 5 years.
2. State Governments—meets a share of 1th of the total cost of medical treatment and attendance of the insured persons—(West Bengal gives Rs. 8/- per worker per year).
3. Employers—3/4% of total bill and an additional 1/2% i.e. a total of 1/4% from the Employers in areas where the benefit provisions of the Act have been brought into force.

(4% total wage bill in 1975)
4. Employees—No contribution for persons getting below Rs. 1% per day; Rs. 1.25 per week for those receiving wages upto Rs. 8/- per day.

(2.5% wages)

"HEALTH FOR ALL" By the Year 2000 A.D.

Q.1. What is meant by "Health for All"?

"*Health for All*" is meant every individual should have access to Primary Health Care and through it to all levels of comprehensive health system, with the objective of continually improving the state of health of the total population."

But it has defined as attainment of "*a level of health that will enable every individual to lead a socially and economically productive life.*"

Q.2. What is meant by "Health for All" by the year 2000 A.D.?

In 1977, the annual World Health Assembly resolved that the main social target of governments and of WHO in the coming, decades should be "the attainment by all citizens of the world of a level of health that will permit them to lead a socially and economically productive life a goal that is termed as "Health for All" by the year 2000 A.D.

Q. 3. What are the mile stones or intermediate goal have been planned to achieve the goal of "Health for All" by the year 2000 A.D.?

To achive the goal of "Health for All" by the year 2000 A.D. a number of milestones or intermediate goals have been planned in between and they are as follows :

1985	—	Providing right kind of food for all.
1986	—	Providing essential drugs for all.
1990	— a)	Providing adequate basic sanitation for all.
	b)	Providing adequate supply of drinking water for all.
	c)	Immunization of children against six common diseases, viz. measles, whooping cough, tetanus, diphtheria, polio and tuberculosis.

Besides the above, a number of indicators:
e.g.,
i) Health status indicators,
ii) Health care indicators,
iii) Social and economic indicators.
iv) Health policy indicators, have also been developed to enable countries to measure and monitor as they work towards the goal. However, it was felt to each country to decide on its own norms, while suggesting a minimum life expectancy of 60 years and maximum infant mortality rate of 50 per 1000 live births. *(WHO 1979)*

Q.4. What are the National Strategy in India to achieve the goal of Health for All by the year 2000 A.D.?

In the context of achieving the goal of Health for All by the year 2000 A.D., the Ministry of Health and Family Welfare, Government of India; and the Planning Commission, Government of India, formulates the following indicators to monitor the progress achieved from time to time and the Health care delivery to fulfil the main target by the Health Care Services.

Recommended Indicators

1. Reduction of infant mortality from present level of 125 (1978) to below 60 by 2000 A.D.
2. To raise the expectant of life at birth from the present level of 52 years to 64 by A.D.
3. To reduce the crude death rate from the present level of 14 per 1000 population to 9 per 1000 by 2000 A.D.
4. To reduce the crude birth rate from the present level of 33 per 1000 population to 21 by 2000 A.D.
5. To achieve a Net Reproduction Rate of one by 2000 A.D.
6. To provide potable water to the entire rural population by 1990.

So to fulfil the above goals and to deliver proper health care services the followings should be followed :

Assesment of the health status and health problems, (through)

1. Morbidity and mortality statistics.
2. Demographic conditons of the population.
3. Environmental conditions which have a bearing on health.
4. Socio-economic factors which have a direct effect on health.
5. Cultural back ground, attitudes, beliefs and prracties which effect health.
6. Medical and health services available.
7. Other services available.

Resources

1. Health manpower.
2. Money and material, and
3. Time.

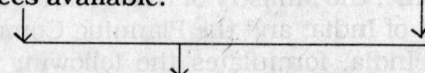

HEALTH CARE SERVICES

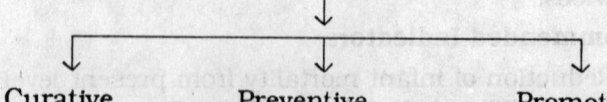

Curative   Preventive   Promotive

(with the agreement that services should be :
    i) comprehensive,
   ii) accessible,
  iii) acceptable,
  iv) provide scope for community participation,
   v) available at a cost the community and country can be afford.

HEALTH CARE SYSTEMS

Public

a) Rural health scheme :
   i) Primary health centres.
   ii) Sub-centres.
b) Hospitals/Health centres :
   i) Community Health centres,
   ii) Rural hospitals,
   iii) Dist. hospital/health centres.
   iv) Specialist hospitals,
   v) Teaching hospitals.
c) Health Insurance schemes :
   i) Employees States Insurance,
   ii) Central Govt. Health Scheme,
d) Other agencies :
   i) Defence services
   ii) Railways.

Private

a) Private hospitals Polyclinics, Nursing homes, and Dispensaries.
b) General Practitioners and clinics.

Voluntary

i) Indian Redcross Society
ii) The Hind Kusht Nivaran Sangha,
iii) Indian Council for Child welfare.
iv) Tuberculosis Association of India
v) Bharat Sevak Samaj,
vi) Central Welfare Board,
vii) The Kasturba Memorial Fund etc.
viii) Family Planning Association of India etc.

Indigenous

i) Ayurvada and siddha
ii) Unani and Tibbi,
iii) Homoeopathy
iv) Unregistered Practitioners Programme.

National health programme

1. National Malaria Eradication Programme
2. National Filaria Control Programme.
3. National T.B. Control Programme.
4. National Leprosy Control Programme.
5. S.T.D. Control Programme.
6. National Goitre Control Programme etc.

PART V

QUICK REFERENCE CHARTS

QUICK REFERENCE CHARTS

1. Select Obstetric dates or Expectant Date of Labour

To ascertain the data upon which labour should take place, add the number of the day of the month on which the last menstruation occurred to the date in the following table placed after the month concerned.

Month in which menstruation occurred	Add day of month to	Month in which menstruation occurred	Add day of month to
January	October 7	July	April 6
February	November 7	August	May 7
March	December 5	September	June 7
April	January 5	October	July 7
May	February 5	November	August 7
June	March 7	December	September 6

Example: If menstruation last occured on December 17, add 17 to September 6 i.e. labour should take place on September 23 ; if June 30 is the date of last menstruation then 30 added to March 7 gives April 6 as the date for labour.

2. What would be the Exjact Weight of Apregnant Mother and Immunization Time

Weight :
   a) Normal Weight—up to 5 months,
   b) 5-7th Months—1/2 lbs/week,
   c) 7-9th Months—1 lbs/week,
   d) After 9th Months may or may not be increases.

Immunization Service :

1st toxoid of Tetanus—at 1st contact with doctor.

2nd toxoid—at least preferably 2 weeks or one week before the expectant date of delivery.

SELECT YOUR BABY'S
3. Developmental Milestones

Age	Weight Kg.	Motor	Mental	Speech
At Birth	3	Suckles, reacts to light, holds head momentarily in prone position.	Grasp reflex on stimulation of palm perceives light.	Cries
6 weeks	4	"Moro Reflex" head movement from side to side.	Follows light from one side to other.	Small throaty noises.
12—14 weeks	4.5	Head lifting can follow the objects with eyes, limb movements.	Shows interest in the surrounding, occasional smile with recognition, concentrates at bright light.	Cooing sounds.
18—24 weeks	6	Can hold the erect. Reaches out his hand for objects. Hand control.	Some recognition of mother.	Turns towards a sound.
6 months	6.5	Site with support. Holds articles in hands.	Tendency for exploring the object with fingers.	Increasing repetion of sounds.
26—30 weeks	7	Can transfar the object from one to the other hand.	Tendency for exploring the object with fingers.	Speaks Monosyllables.

Age	Weight Kg.	Motor	Mental	Speech
30—34 weeks	7.5	Crawling on abdomen, like to stand with	Can play for a length of time with one object.	Imitates the rhythm of the speech heard.
34—38 weeks	8	Sits without support. Leans forward. Progress on all four.	Expresses happiness. Resounds if called by his name.	Says 'Da-Da', 'Ma-Ma' etc.
38—42 weeks	9	Co-ordination of hand and leg movements, Walks with support.	Grips the object with thumb and finger.	Speaks pollysyllables.
42—48 weeks (1 year)	9	Attempts at independent walking.	Claps hands shows more interest in games, toys.	Short words are pronounced.
Upto 52 weeks (14 months)	10	Toddles.	Expresses emotion like joy, fear.	Increase in vocabulary.
18 months to 2 years	12	Slow run, jumps from low height.	Can copy simple lines.	Small sentences.
2½ years	14	Walks on tip-toe.	—	—
3 years	15	Stands on one leg, can climb or run.	Can draw circles.	Nouns and Verbs used can demand, express joy, fear, etc. Can narrate events and stories, Can sing.

4. (a) Eruption of Teeth of your Baby
[Temporary]

Name of the Tooth	Comes	Goes
2 Lower Central Incisors	5 to 8th months	7th year
2 Upper Central Incisors	6 to 9th months	7th year
2 Upper Lateral Incisors	6 to 9th months	8th year
2 Lower Lateral Incisors	12 to 15th months	8th year
2 Lower First Molars	12 to 18th months	10th year
2 Upper First Molars	12 to 15th months	10th year
2 Lower Canines	18 to 24th months	12th year
2 Upper Canines	18 to 24th months	12th year
2 Lower Second Molars	24 to 30th months	11 to 12th"
2 Upper Second Molars	24 to 30th months	11 to 12th"

N.B. : The first, or sixth year molars which make their appearance before the temporary teeth disappear, are permanent and important. These should be mistaken for temporary teeth and they should have special care.

(b) Permanent Teeth

Name of the Tooth	Comes
2 Lower and 2 Upper Molars	6th year
2 Lower and 2 Upper Central Incisors	7th year
2 Lower and 2 Upper Lateral Incisors	8th year
2 lower and 2 Upper First Bicuspids	9th year
2 Lower and 2 Upper Second Bicuspids	10th year
2 Lower and 2 Upper Canines or Cuspids	11th year
2 Lower and 2 Upper Second Molars	12th year
2 Lower and 2 Upper "Wisdom" or Third Molars	17 to 25th year

5. Mean Weights of Indian Children (8)

Age Kilogram	Weights in	
	Boys	Girls
Upto 3 months	4.5	4.2
4-6 months	6.7	5.6
7-9 months	6.9	6.2
10-12 months	7.4	6.6
1 years	8.4	7.8
2 years	10.1	9.6
3 years	11.8	11.2
4 years	13.5	12.9
5 years	14.8	14.5
6 years	16.3	16.0

6. Developmental Milestones in India Infants

Chin slightly off ground	4 weeks
Chin at 45° angle from the ground	8 weeks
Chin at 45-90° angle from ground	12 weeks
Chin at 90° angle from ground	16 weeks
Sitting with support	20.5 weeks
Sitting without support	26 weeks
Standing with support	22 weeks
Crawling on belly	26.3 weeks
Crawling on knees	32.4 weeks
Walking with support	45.1 weeks
Walking without support	52.4 weeks

7. Check up Your Baby's Height and Weight

Height	Weight
1. At birth-50 cm.	1. At birth-2.8 kg (roughly 3 kg)
2. Ist year-75 cm. (50% increase)	2. At 6 month-Double (6 kg)
3. 2nd year-75+12.5 = 87.5 (25% increase from birth)	3. At 12 month-Triple (9 kg)
4. There affter 5-6 cm/ year till adolescence.	4. At 2 years-4 times (12 kg)

8. Check up Your Own Height and Weight

a) Of an Indian Male (Average):

Height (c.m.) Ages	Weight (kg) 20 yrs	25 yrs	30 yrs	35 yrs	40 yrs	45 yrs	50 yrs
148	42.7	44.2	46.2	47.6	48.8	50.0	50.9
150	43.6	44.9	46.9	48.5	49.7	50.8	61.5
153	45.4	47.0	49.0	50.4	51.7	52.3	53.5
155	46.3	48.1	49.9	51.5	52.7	53.5	54.2
158	48.6	50.0	52.0	53.5	54.5	55.7	56.3
160	49.7	51.1	53.1	54.7	55.6	56.6	57.4
163	51.1	52.7	54.9	56.3	57.6	58.5	59.4
165	53.1	54.7	56.9	58.5	59.7	60.6	62.2
168	54.0	56.3	58.1	60.1	61.5	62.4	63.7
170	56.5	57.9	60.3	62.2	63.7	64.7	65.8
173	58.1	60.1	62.2	64.0	65.8	67.0	68.3
175	60.1	62.2	64.2	66.0	68.1	69.7	71.0
178	61.9	64.0	66.3	68.5	70.1	71.9	72.2
180	64.0	66.0	68.5	71.0	73.3	74.4	75.1
183	66.0	68.5	71.0	73.3	75.6	77.1	77.8

QUICK REFERENCE CHARTS

(b) Of an Indian Female (Average):

Ages	Height (c.m.)			Weight (kg)			
	20 yrs	25 yrs	30 yrs	35 yrs	40 yrs	45 yrs	50 yrs
148	38.6	41.0	42.6	44.0	45.1	46.3	47.1
150	38.6	41.6	43.5	44.8	46.0	47.0	47.7
153	41.9	43.5	45.3	46.6	47.9	48.4	49.5
155	42.8	44.3	46.2	47.7	48.8	49.5	50.1
158	44.9	46.3	48.1	49.5	50.4	51.6	52.1
160	46.0	47.3	49.1	50.6	51.5	52.4	53.0
163	47.3	48.8	50.8	52.1	52.2	54.1	54.9
165	49.1	50.6	52.16	54.1	55.3	56.0	57.3
168	50.0	52.1	53.8	55.6	56.8	57.7	59.0

9. Check up your Blood Pressure (Average):

Age (Years)	Systolic B.P. (mm Hg)	Diastolic B.P. (mm Hg)	Age (Years)	Systolic B.P. (mm Hg)	Diastolic B.P. (mm Hg)
6	93	62	31	121	83
7	93	63	32	123	83
8	94	65	33	123	83
9	94	62	34	124	84
10	99	68	35	124	84
11	101	71	36	125	84
12	100	61	37	125	85
13	104	70	38	126	85
14	106	69	39	126	86
15	106	72	40	127	86
16	112	80	41	127	87
17	111	77	42	128	87
18	108	76	43	128	87
19	113	72	44	128	88
20	117	78	45	130	88

Age (Years)	Systolic B.P. (mm Hg)	Diastolic B.P. (mm Hg)	Age (Years)	Systolic B.P. (mm Hg)	Diastolic B.P. (mm Hg)
21	118	78	46	130	89
22	119	79	47	131	89
23	119	79	48	132	89
24	119	89	49	132	90
25	120	86	50	133	90
26	120	80	51	134	90
27	120	81	53	136	91
28	121	81	54	136	91
29	121	82	55	138	92
30	122	82	55	138	92

10. Consumption Unit (C.U.) (6)

Enerfgy needs of in average man doing sedentary work is reckoned as one consumption unit (C.U.)

So 1. C.U. - 2400 Kcal	C.U.
Audit male (sedentary worker)	1.0
Audit male (moderate worker)	1.2
Audit male (heavy worker)	1.6
Audit female (sedentary worker)	0.8
Audit female (moderate worker)	0.9
Audit female (heavy worker)	1.2
12 to 21 years	1.0
9 to 12 years	0.8
7 to 9 years	0.7
5 to 7 years	0.6
3 to 5 years	0.5
1 to 3 years	0.4

11. Nutritive Value of Some Indian Foods (6)

Name of food stuff	Protein (gm)	fat (gm)	Carbo-hydrate (gm)	Calorie (K cal)	Iron (mg)	Caro-tene (mg)
1. Rice par boiled (milled)	6.4	0.4	79.0	346	4.0	—
2. Rice par boiled home (Pounded)	8.5	0.6	77.4	349	2.8	9
3. Wheat (whole)	11.8	1.5	71.2	346	4.9	64
4. Wheat flour (whole)	12.1	1.7	69.4	341	11.5	29
5. Bengal gram dal	20.8	5.6	59.8	372	9.1	129
6. Lentil	25.1	0.7	59.0	343	4.8	270
7. Green gram (Mug) dal	24.5	1.2	59.9	348	8.5	49
8. Horse gram (Kulthi Kalai)	22.0	0.5	57.2	321	8.4	71
9. Khesari Dal	28.2	0.6	56.6	345	6.3	120
10. Cow milk	3.2	4.1	4.4	67	0.2	174
11. Egg (Hen)	13.3	13.3	—	173	2.1	600
12. Egg (Duck)	13.5	13.7	0.8	181	3.0	540
13. Meat (Goat)	21.4	3.6	—	118	—	—
14. Fowl	25.9	0.6	—	109	—	—
15. Fish (Rahu)	16.6	1.4	4.4	97	1.0	—
16. Puti fish	18.1	2.4	3.1	106	1.0	—
17. Cauliflower	2.6	0.4	4.0	30	1.5	30
18. Cabbage	1.8	0.1	4.6	27	0.8	120
19. Tomato (Ripe)	0.9	0.2	3.6	20	0.4	351
20. Onion (big)	1.2	0.1	11.1	50	0.7	0
21. Papaya (green)	0.7	0.2	5.7	27	0.9	0
22. Potato	1.6	0.1	22.6	97	0.7	24
23. Spinanch	2.0	0.7	2.9	26	10.9	5580
24. Ladies Finger	1.9	0.2	6.4	35	1.6	52

Name of food stuff	Protein (gm)	fat (gm)	Carbohydrate (gm)	Calorie (K cal)	Iron (mg)	Carotene (mg)
25. Amarnath (Notya) tender	4	0.5	6.1	45	25.5	5520
26. - do - (Spined)	3	0.3	7.0	43	22.9	3564
27. Mayalu (Poi)	2.8	0.4	4.2	32	10	7440
28. Pumkin	1.4	0.1	4.6	25	0.7	50
39. Cucumber	0.4	0.1	2.5	13	1.5	0
30. Field beans (Sim) tender	3.8	0.7	6.7	48	1.7	187
31. Brinjal	1.4	0.3	4.0	24	0.9	74
32. Banana (ripe)	1.2	0.3	27.2	116	0.9	78
33. Guava (country)	0.9	0.3	11.2	51	1.4	0
34. Papaya (ripe)	0.6	0.1	7.2	32	0.5	666
35. Mango (ripe)	0.6	0.4	16.9	74	1.3	2743
36. Ground nut	25.3	40.1	26.1	567	2.8	37
37. Soya bean	43.2	19.5	20.9	432	11.5	426
38. Drumstick leaves	6.7	1.7	12.5	92	7.0	6780
39. Raddish White	1.7	0.1	3.4	17	0.4	3
40. Raddish Pink	0.6	0.3	6.8	32	0.5	3
41. Drum Stick	2.5	0.1	3.7	26	5.3	110
42. Banana green	1.4	0.2	14.0	64	0.6	30
43. Milk (human)	1.1	3.4	7.4	65	-	137

12. Signs used in Nutritional Survey

Signs known to be of value in nutritional sarveys :

1. Hair — Lack of lustre, Thinness and sparseness, Straightness, Dyspigmentation, Flag sign, Easy pluckability.
2. Face — Diffuse depigmentation Nasolab; al dyssebacea, Moon face,

3.	Eye	Pale conjunctiva, Bitot's Spot, Conjunctival xerosis, Corneal xerosis, keratomalacia, Angular palpebritis.
4.	Lips	Angular stomatitis, Angular scars, Cheilosis.
5.	Tongue	Oedema, Scarlet and raw tongue, Magenta tongue, Atrophic papillae.
6.	Teeth	Mottlod enamel.
7.	Gums	Spongy, bleeding gums.
8.	Glands	Thyroid enlargement, Parotid enlargement.
9.	Skin	Xerosis, Follicular hyperkeratosis types 1 & 2, Petechiae, Pellagrous dermatosis, Flaky paint dermatosis, Scrotal and Vulval dermatosis.
10.	Nails	Kilonychia.
11.	Subcutanious tissue	Oedema, Amount of subcutaneous fat.
12.	Muscular—	Muscle wasting, Craniotabes, Frontal and Parietal bossing epiphyseal & enlargement (tender or painless), Bcading of ribs, Persitently open anterior, Skeletal fontanelle, Knock knees or bow legs, Diffuse or local skeletal deformities, systemic deformities of thorax (selected), Musculo-skeletal haemorrhages.

13. Internal System :

   a) G.I.—Hepatomegaly.

   b) Nervous—Psychomotor change, Mental confusion, Sensory loss, Motor weakness, Loss of position sense, Loss of vibratory sense, Loss of ankle and knee jerk, Calf tenderness.

   c) C.V. System—Cardiac enlargement, Tachycardia.

13. For Practical

(A) Estimation of Total Hardness of Water :

Theory of the test : The hardness test by soap method is based on the titration of a sample with a standard soap solution, till a permanent leather is obtained. This test actually measures the soap consuming power of the water. It is not recommended for accurate determination of hardness procedure.

Procedure :

1. 100 c.c. of sample water was measured and placed in a glass bottle.
2. Burrette was filled with a standard soap solution (1 c.c. = 1 mg. of Hardness).
3. Soap solution from the burrette was added into the bottles in a small portions i.e. 0.5 ml. at each time and bottle was shaken brikly just after addition of soap solution.
4. This addition on the surface was continued till a uniform leather was obtained which would not break on the surface of the liquid for at least 5 minutes. The contents on shaking should also produce a faint dull soft sound and small bubbles of leather should cling to the side of the bottle and descend slowly.
5. When the contents of the bottle did not show the signs mentioned above, more soap solution was added and test was repeated in the above mentioned way.
6. Amount of soap solution was noted and 1 c.c. soap was deducted from that and that multiplied by 10 would be the mg. of Hardness per 1000 c.c.

Example :

16 c.c. soap solution was used for 100c.c. sample water. So 16-1=15 soap solution represent hardness in 100 c.c. of sample.

        As 1 c.c soap sol.=1 mg of hardness

        15 c.c. soap sol.=15 mg. hardness

        So in 100 c.c. there was 15 mg. of hardness

        So in 1000 c.c there was 150 mg. hardness

        or mg/Litre of total hardness as $CaCO_3$

$$= \frac{\text{(ml. soap sol. - ml. leather factor)} \times 1000}{\text{ml. of sample}}$$

(B) Estimation of Nitrite in Water :

Theory : Nitrite is determined through the formation of a reddish purple 'AZO' dye produced at pH 2.0 to 2.5 by the coupling of diazetized sulphanilic acid with α'-Naphthalamine, Copper and Ferric ion interfere.

Procedure :

1. When the sample contained suspended solids and colour 2 ml. of aluminium hydroxide suspension was added to 100 ml. of the samples, stirred thoroughly, allowed to stand for few minutes and filtered.
2. 50 ml. of clear sample was taken in a Nessler's tube.
3. Various amounts of prepared standard Nitrite solution was taken in different Nessler's tube (say 1 c.c. - 0.1 mg. of Nitrites) upto 50 ml.
4. 1 c.c. of sulphanilic acid solution was added in each Nessler's tube (sample as well as standard) and mixed thoroughly and allowed to stand for a few minutes (15 minutes).
5. 1 ml. of $\overline{\alpha}$-Naphthylamine hydrochloride solution was added in each Nessler's tube
6. 1 ml. of Sodium acetate buffer sol. was also added to the sample and standards, mixed and allowed to stand for 10 minutes.
7. Colour produced in the sample was matched with those of standards.

Calculation :

$$\text{mg./litre Nitrite N} = \frac{\text{mg. N} \times 1000}{\text{ml. of sample}}$$

Example : 50 c.c. sample = 0.2 c.c. standard
So, 100 c.c. sample = 0.4 c.c. standard

But since 1 c.c. Pot Nitrite standard = 0.01 mg. of Nitrite.
So 0.4 c.c. Nitrite standard = 0.04 mg. of Nitrite.

Therefore, mg/litre Nitrite N= $\dfrac{.04 \text{ mg.} \times 1000}{100}$ = 0.4 mg/c litre.

(C) Nitrate :

Theory : The basic reaction between nitrate and 1,2,4 phenol disulphonic acid produces 6-nitro 1,2,4-phenol disulphonic acid which upon conversion to alkaline salt yields an yellow colour, which is compared with the standards similarly prepared.

Procedure :

1. 100 ml. of the sample was evaporated to dryness in an evaporating dish, cooled and 2 ml. of phenol disulphonic acid added.
2. It was rubbed thoroughly with the glass rod to dissolve the residue.
3. 20 ml. of distilled water was added continuously to dilute it.
4. KOH solution was added and stirred until the yellow colour developed.
5. Solution was transfered to a Nessler's tube, filtering when necessary and distilled water was added to make the volume 50 ml.
6. It was then compared with standard prepared by adding 2 ml. of phenol of disulphonic acid and a volume of strong KOH solution equal to that used for the sample to various volumes of nitrate solution and diluting then to 50 ml. in Nessler's tube. The standard stays for several days without deterioration.

Calculation :

$$\text{mg./L Nitrate N} = \dfrac{\text{mg. N} \times 1000}{\text{ml. of sample}}$$

(D) Estimation of Chloride in Water :

Theory : Chloride is determined by titration with Silver Nitrate solution in the presence of Potassium Chromate indicator.

Procedure :

1. 100 ml. of the water sample in a white porcelain dish.
2. Add dil. acid or alkali so that it is just colourless to phenophthalein.
3. Add 1 ml. of Potassium chromate indicator and titrate it slowly with standard Silver Nitrate until the colour is changed to red from yellow.
4. An indicator blank has to be determined in the same way by titrating distilled water.
5. This blank is to be placed near the sample to detect the colour changes.

Calculation :

$$\text{mg/Litre Chloride} = \frac{1 \text{ ml. silver nitrate} - \text{ml blank}}{\text{ml of sample}} \times 1000$$

(E) Coliform Count

1. Multiple tube technique :

An estimation of the number of coliform bacilli in a water supply is usually made by adding varying quantities of water (from 1 ml. to 50 ml.) to bile salt lactose peptone water (with an indicator of acidity) or in a chemically defined medium in which the bile salt has been substituted by glutamic acid, known as improved formate lactose glutamate medium, contained in bottles with Durham's tubes, to show formation of gas; acid and gas formation (positive result) indicates the growth of coliform bacilli. In this way it is possible to state the smallest quantity of water containing a coliform bacillus and thus to express the degree of contamination with this group of organisms.

Method : Measured amounts of single and double strength modified MacConkey's fluid medium are sterilised in test tube containing a Durham's tube for indicating gas production. The size of the test tube varies with the quantity of medium and water to be added to it.

With sterile graduated pipettes, the following amounts of water are added :

    One 50 ml. water to 50 ml. double strength medium

    Five 10 ml. water to 10 ml. double strength medium

    Five 1 ml. water to 5 ml. single strength medium

    Five 0.1 ml. water to 5 ml single strength medium.

This range of quantities may be altered according to the likely condition of the water examined. 0.1 ml. (1 ml. diluted 1 : 10) is tested only when the water supply is suspected of being highly contaminated.

The bottles are incubated at 37°C and examined after 48 hours. Those that show acid and sufficient gas to fill the concavity at the top of Durham are considered to be "*Presumptive positve*" as a result of the growth of coliform bacilli. Any remaining negative test tube is incubated for another 24 hours and when acid and gas develop they too will, regarded as being positive. The probable number of coliform bacilli in 100 ml. water is obtained from *McCraday's table*.

PART — VI

MULTIPLE CHOICE OF QUESTIONS INCLUDING ORAL

MULTIPLE CHOICE OF QUESTIONS INCLUDING ORAL

Q. 1. Fill up the gaps :

1. **Levels of prevention are :**
   [Health promotion, specific protection, early diagnosis and treatment, disability, limitation, rehabilitation.]
   (C.U. 1979, 80)

2. **Common arthropod borne diseases in India are :**
   [Malaria, Kala-azar, Filaria etc.]   (C.U. 1979, 80)

3. **Common causses of maternal mortality in India are:**
   [Toxaemias of Pregnancy, Haemorrhage, Sepsis, Anaemia etc.]

4. **Common active immunizations are :**
   [B.C.G. against T.B., TAB against typhoid.] (C.U. 1980)

5. **Sexually transmitted diseases are :**
   [Gonorrhoea, Venereal syphilis etc.]   (C.U. 1979, 80)

6. **Methods of conception control are :**
   [*Permanent*—Vesectomy, Tubectomy ; Temporary- Physiological, Chemical, Mechanical, Safe period, Abstinence during postnatal period, Coitus-interruptas, Condom ; Diaphragm, Jelly, Foam tablet, Sponge, Cervical cap, Oral pill etc.]   (C.U. 1979,Sup.)

7. **Different methods of purification of water are :**
   [Pounding or storage, Oxidation and setllement, Distillation, Boiling, Precipitation, Domestic filtration, Slow and Rapid Sand filtration, Chlorination etc.]
   (C.U. 1979 Sup.)

8. **National Health Programmes in India are :**
   (i) Malaria Eradication Programme.
   (ii) Filaria Control Programme.
   (iii) Smallpox Eradication Programme.

- (iv) Family Welfare Programme.
- (v) Leprosy Control Programme.
- (vi) STD Control Programme.
- (vii) Water Supply and Sanitary Programme.
- (viii) Goitre Control Programme.
- (ix) Prevention of visual impairment and Control of Blindness.
- (x) T.B. Control Programme.
- (xi) Diarrhoeal Diseases Control Programmes,
- (xii) Minimum Needs Programmes.   (C.U. 1979 Sup.)

9. Soil borne diseases are :

Amoebic dysentery, Hookworm, etc. (C.U. 1979 Sup.)

10. Common causes of blindness in India are :

Cataract, Trachoma, Infection of the eye, Smallpox, Malnutrition, Injuries, Glaucoma etc. (C.U. 1979 Sup.)

11. Major benefits in E.S.I. are :

Sickness, Maternity, Disablement, Dependent and Medical.   (C.U. 1980, 81)

12. Social security measures are :

Education, Health, Social security and production.
                                                                 (C.U. 1980)

13. Different methods of adulteration of foods are :

Mixing, substitution, abstraction, concealing the quality, putting up decomposed foods for sale, misbranding falls and additions of poisions etc.]   (C.U. 1980)

14. Deficiency diseases due to lack of vit. A are :

Xerosis, Xerophthalmia, Night blindness, Respiratory infections, etc.   (C.U.1980)

15. Comprehensive health care are :

Provision of integrated preventive, curative and promotional health services from *"Womb to tomb"* to

every individual residing in a defined geographic area.
(C.U., 1980, 1981)

16. Indicators of Health are :
(a) Growth structure i.e. the age and sex distribution (demography).
(b) Amount of death i.e. Mortality-i) Crude Death Rate, ii) Expectation of life, iii) Proportional Mortality Rate, iv) Infant Mortality Rate, vi) Maternal Mortality Rate, vii) Mortality by cause and population characteristics.]
c) Sickness i.e. Morbidity-incidence and Prevalance Rates.
d) Disability Rate.] (C.U, 1980, 81)

17. Determinants of health are :
[1. Human Biology, 2. Enviornment, 3. Ways of living, 4. Socio-economic status, and 5. Health Services]
(C.U. 1982)

18. Statistical average is calculated by :
Vital statistics, Health statistics, Demography etc.
(C.U. 1982)

19. Internationally Quarantinable diseases are :
Smallpox, cholera, plague etc. (C.U.1982)

20. Basic health services mean :
A network of co-ordinated peripheral and intermediate health units capable of performing effectively a selected group of functions essential to the health of an area and assuring the availability of competent professional and auxiliary personel to perform these functions.

21. Primary Health Care means :
The care given to the patient by the health worker who saw him first. It is also known as *First Contact Care*.

ORAL QUESTIONS

22. Range or Spectrum of Health and Sickness are :

	Positive health.
	Better health.
	Freedom from sickness.
	Unrecognised sickness.
	Mild sickness.
	Severe sickness.
	Death.

23. Basic components of the level of living which is identified by 'per capita income' are :

Health, nutrition, housing, education, employment and working conditions, clothing, social security, recreation and human rights.

24. Five giants for backwardness of family welfare are :

Poverty, disease, ignorance, sequalor and idleness.

25. Family Health Programme includes :

   (a) Maternal and Child Health Care.
   (b) Human Reproduction.
   (c) Nutrition.
   (d) Health Education.

26. P.Q.L. I. (Physical Quality of Life Index) indicates :

The level of progress achieved by any country in meeting basic human needs. (In India it was 41 in 1970).

27. P.Q. L.I Indicators are :

Infant mortality, life expectancy at age one and literacy.

28. Basic health problems of India are :

   (a) Communicable Disease problems.
   (b) Nutritional problems.
   (c) Enviornmental Sanitation problems.
   (d) Medical Care problems.
   (e) Population problems.

29. **Rural Health scheme in 1977, based on the principle of :**
"Placing people's health in people's hands."

30. **Criteria of Sanitary Latrine are** : (1) Excreta should not contaminate the ground or surface water.(2) Excreta should not pollute the soil. (3) Excreta should not be accessible to flies, rodents, animals (pigs, dogs, cattle etc.), and other vehicles of transmissions. (4) Excreta should not create a nuisance due to odour or unsightly appearance.

31. **Vital events of life are :** Births, Deaths, Marriages,.

32. **Early clinical manifestation of Vit. 'A' deficiency are :** Night Blindness, Exerophthalmia.

33. **Cardinal features of pellagra are :** Dermatitis, Diarrhoea, Dementia.

34. **Three important air borne viral diseases are :** Measles, Mumps, Chicken-pox.

35. **M.M.R. Stands for :** Maternal Mortality Rate.

36. **Oral dehydration fluid contains :** [(a) Sodium Chloride 3.5g.; (b) Sodium bicarbonate: 2.5 g. ; (c) Potassium chloride 1.5 g. ; (d) Glucose (dextrose) : 20.0 g. ; (e) Potable water; 1 litre.]

37. **Five levels of preventions are :** Health promotion Specific protection, Early diagnosis and treatment, Disability limitation, Rehabilitation.

38. **Dust borne diseases are :** Anthracosis, Silicosis, Siderosis, Cancer lung, Asbestosis, Bagassis, Bissinosis etc.

39. **Components of under Five Clinic are :** Care of illness,Adequate nutrition, Immunization, Family planning, Health teaching.

40. **Three types of carrier are :** Incubatory, Convalescent, Healthy.

41. **Epediological Triads are :** Agent, Host, Environment.

42. **Three mortality indicaters are :** Infant Mortality Rate, Maternal Mortality Rate, Crude Death Rate.

43. **Three important anthropometric measurements are** Height and weight, Arm Circumference, Skinfold thickness.
44. **Two ill effects of Air Pollution :** Chronic bronchitis Primary lungs cancer.
45. **Three diseases transmitted by Mosquito :** (Malaria, Filaria, Dengue.
46. **Two milk-borne diseases :** Typhoid Cholera, Tuberculosis.
47. **Three sites of occupational cancer :** (Skin, Lungs, Bladder).

Q. 2. For each of the following multiple choice questions, choose the most appropriate answer :
(B.H.M.S. Cal. Uni.-1979)

1. Which of the foodstuff has the highest protein content per 100 gms : a) Milk, b) Egg, c) Bengal gram, [Ans. (c)]
2. Active immunization against diphtheria is imported by : a) D.T.P vaccine, b) Tetanus Toxoid, c) ADS. [Ans. (a)]
3. The average expectation of life at birth in India at present is : a) 41-50 years, b) 51-60 years, c) 61-70 years. [Ans.(b)]
4. Mortality rate means : a) Illness rate, b) Birth rate c) Death rate. [Ans. (c)]
5. Residual DDT Spray is for : a) Eradication of Cancer, b) Eradication of cholera, c) Eradication of Malaria. [Ans. (c)]
6. Arthropod borne diseases mean :
   a) Diseases transmitted through water;
   b) Diseases transmitted through insect;
   c) Diseases transmitted through air. [Ans. (b)]
7. Leprosy control programme includes, are : a) DDT spray, b) SET, c) Application of tetracylineonment, d) None of the above, e) DDS. [Ans.(E)]
8. Tuberculosis Control programme includes : a) Radical Treatment, b) Chemo-prophylaxis, c) BCG vaccination, d) None of the above. [Ans.(c)]

9. Malaria Control Programme includes : a) Radical treatment, b) MMR, c) Chlorination of water, d) None of the above. [Ans. (a)]

10. Nutrition to the school children are provided through : a) Enriched food, b) Fortified food, c) Midday meal, d) None of the above. [Ans. (c)]

11. Domiciliary treatment means :
    (a) Treatment provided at hospital.
    (b) Treatment provided at a private clinic.
    (c) Treatment provided at home.
    (d) None of the above. [Ans. (c)]

12. Insecticide means : a) Agent used to kill animals, b) Agent used to kill arthropods, c) Agent used to kill germ, d) None of the above. [Ans. (b)]

[B.H.M.S., Cal. Uni. 1979 (sup).]

13. Which rate is to be used to compare healthiness of two countries : a) Crude Death Rate, b) Standardised, c) Birth Rate. [Ans. (b)]

14. Last Census of India was conducted in : a) 1881; b) 1981; c) 1971. [Ans. (b)]

15. Carotene is precursor of : a) Vit. K, b) Vit. E, c) Vit. A. [Ans. (c)]

16. Fomite means which is : a) Inanimate object for transmission of a disease, b) False positive, c) Media for multiplication of germs. [Ans. (a)]

17. Trenching is done for : a) Disposal of night soil; b) Disposal of refuse; c) Disposal of sewage. [Ans. (a)]

18. Condom is done for : a) Conception control; b) Control of SDT; c) correction of sterility. [Ans. (a)]

19. Carrier means : a) He who carries infection but does not suffer; c) Fomite; d) None of the above. [Ans. (a)]

20. Census means : a) country of number; b) counting of population of a country at a regular interval; c) None of the above. [Ans. (b)]

ORAL QUESTIONS 545

21. Birth registration means : a) To register a birth; b) To register the birth of a new born with the appropriate health authority; c) Registration of birth of a baby in hospital; d) None of the above. [Ans. (b)]

22. Pasteurization of milk means : a) Sterilization of milk; b) Cooling of milk; c) Boiling of milk; d) None of the above. [Ans. (a)]

23. M.T.P. means : a) Medical Termination of Pregnancy; b) Metropolition Transport Project; c) Medical Treatment Plant; d) None of the above. [Ans. (a)]

24. Epidemic means : a) Large number of cases; b) Occurrence of number of cases within a short period; c) Sudden occurrence of large number of cases within a short period in a area; d) None of the above.
[Ans.(c)]

[B.H.M.S, Cal. Uni. 1980]

25. Vegetable protein is rich in : a) Milk; b) Pulses; c) Potato. [Ans. (b)]

26. Statistical averages are calculated by : a) Arithmetic mean ; b) Standard deviation; c) Census. [Ans. (c)]

27. Incubation period means : a) Illness period; b) Safe period; c) Time interval from entry of micro-organisms to the appearance of signs and symptoms. [Ans. (c)]

28. Disinfection means : a) Pasturisation of milk; b) Killing of pathogenic organisms; c) Chlorination of water.
[Ans. (b)]

29. I.U.D. is used for : a) Sterilisation; b) Conception control; c) Correction sterility. [Ans. (b)]

30. Animal source of fat is rich in : a) Ghee; b) Butter; c) Dalda. [Ans. (a)]

31. Vital statistics reveals : a) Beauty of a nation; b) Beauty of an adult; c) Vital events of life. [Ans. (c)]

32. Sanitary Latrine is : a) Bore Hole Latrine; b) R.C.A. Latrine; c) Trench Latrine. [Ans. (b)]

33. Infection means : a) Disease; b) Immunity; c) Entry of micro-organisms and its multiplication. [Ans. (c)]

[B.H.M.S., Cal. Uni. 1980 (Sup)]

34. Incubation period of Trachoma is : a) 5 to 12 hours; b) 2-3 days; c) 7 days. [Ans.]

35. Active immnization against Diphtheria is imparted by:-a) D.T.P.; b) Tetanus Toxiod; c) A.D.S. [Ans. (a)]

36. Which of the foodstuff has the highest protein content per 100 gms. a) Milk; b) Egg; c) Green gram chala.
[Ans. (a)]

37. Residual D.D.T Spray is for : a) Eradication of cancer; b) Eradicatication of cholera; c) Control of Malaria.
[Ans. (c)]

38. Biological transmission of disease is present in: a) Diabetes; b) Measles; c) Plague. [Ans. (c)]

39. Diet survey means : a) To note the quality of the diet; b) To observe the per capita consumption of foodstuff.
[Ans. (b)]

40. Non-service type of latrine is : a) Composting; b) Treching; c) Septic tank. [Ans. (c)]

41. Second level of Prevention of disease is : a) Environmental sanitation; b) Early diagonsis and treatment; c) Specific protection. [Ans. (c)]

42. Endemic means : a) Occurrence of huge number of disease; b) Incidence of no disease; c) Few diseases occuring throughout the year. [Ans. (c)]

[B.H.M.S., Cal. Uni. 1981]

43. Richest source of protein : a) Milk; b) Egg; c) Pulse.
[Ans. (c)]

44. Pellagra is caused due to deficiency of : a) Vit. A; b) Bit B_1; c) Niacin. [Ans.(b)]

45. Definitive host of Malaria parasite : a) Human being; b) Mosquito; c) Water Hyacinth. [Ans. (b)]

46. Pneumocociosis is caused due to inhalation of :
a) Dust particles; b) Perfumes; c) Decomposed organic matter. [Ans. (a)]

47. Residual chlorine in drinking water : a) 0.5p.p.m; b) 1.0 p p.m; c) 1.5 p.p.m. **[B.H.M.S., Cal. Uni. 1982]**

48. Bitot's spot is a sign of deficiency of : a) Vit B_{12}; b) Vit C; c) Vit A. [Ans. (c)]

49. Filaria is transmitted by : a) Flies; b) Tics; c) Mosquitos. [Ans. (c)]

50. Protein content is maximum in : a) Fish; b) Wheat; c) Pulses. [Ans. (c)]

[B.H.M.S., Cal. Uni. 1983]

51. Infant mortality rate is measured 1000 : a) Live birth; b) Still birth; c) Total birth. [Ans. (a)]

52. Daily energy requirement of an adult male of sedentary habits is : a) 1900 cal, b) 2700 cal; c) 3300 cal.

[Ans. (b)]

53. Malaria is transmitted by:-a) Water; b) Roddents; c) Mosquito. [Ans. (c)]

54. Iron contant is maximum in : a) Nuts; b) Rice. [Ans. (a)]

55. Beriberi is caused by deficiency of : (a) **Thiamine**; (b) Pyridoxin; (c) Vit B12.

56. **100 gms of Human milk contains** : (a) 3.60; (b) 3.50; (c) 1.25) gm of protein.

57. Rabies is caused by : (a) **Viral**; (b) Fungal; (c) Bacterial infection.

58. Kala-azar is transmitted by : (a) Fleas; (b) **Sand-flies;** (c) House flies.

59. Demography reveals : (a) **birth and death rate;** (b) Marriages; (c) Divorces.

60. Pellegra is caused by deficiency of : (a) **Niacin;** (b) Vit. C; (c) Vt. D.

61. Cholera is a : (a) **water;** (b) air; (c) Soil borne disease.

62. Birth rate of India at present : (a) 35; (b) 45; (c) 25.

63. Balanced diet means : (a) weighing of food; (b) **adequate quantity of proximate principles of food;** (c) adequate quantity of protein in diet.

64. Protein content is maximum in : (a) **fish;** (b) wheat, (c) pulses.

65. B.C.G. Vaccine is used against : (a) **Tuberculosis,** (b) Rabies, (c) Leprosy.

66. Causative agent of plague is a : (a) virus; (b) **bacteria;** (c) protozoa.

67. Bitot's spot is due to deficiency of : (a) Vit C; (b) Vit. B, (c) **Vit A.**

68. Leprosy is spread by : (a) Water; (b) **contact;** (c) Air.

69. Kwashiorkar is caused due to deficiency of : (a) **protein;** (b) Calorie; (c) Both.

70. Social disease is : (a) **Leprosy;**

    (a) Venereal diseases; (c) all of them.

71. Malaria is a disease caused by a : (a) Virus; (b) Bacteria; (c) **Protozoa;** (d) Helminths.

72. Kala-azar is transmitted by : (a) fleas; (b) mosquitos; (c) **sandfly.**

73. Biological value of protein is maximum in : (a) Fish (b) Pulse; (c) **Egg.**

74. Incubation period of measles is in days : (a) 7; (b) **14;** (c) 21.

N.B. Bold Words are Correct Answer.

PART — VII

PRACTICAL PART

[FOR M.B.B.S., B.H.M.S., GRADED B.H.M.S. & D.H.M.S. COURSES IN ALL INDIAN UNIVERSITIES/BOARDS/COUNCILS]

PRACTICAL PART

(I) DEMONSTRATIONS

1. Visit to Hospital.
2. Visit to Community development block office.
3. Visit to Water purification plant.
4. Visit to Sewage disposal plant.
5. Visit to Milk diary.
6. Visit to Primary health centre.
7. Visit to Rural hospital.
8. Visit to an Industrial organisation.
9. Visit to Rehabilitation centre.
10. Visit to Central combined laboratory, Govt. of West Bengal.
11. Visit to Organisation for control of communicable disease.
12. Visit to see how adulteration of food is detected.
13. Visit to State health intelligence bureau.
14. Visit to Fair.
15. Visit to Others, if any.

Notes : **Demonstrations should be written in the following headings:**

   1. Date of visits.
   2. Title of the visits.
   3. Object of the visits.
   4. Brief history/Introduction.
   5. Description (important observations, public health measures adopted, social aspects, functions etc.)
   6. Conclusion and Remarks.

(II) FOR PRACTICAL NOTE BOOK

Lesson 1

INFORMATION ABOUT COMMUNITY

1. **Define community:**

   * Characteristics of the Community at your charge. **Rural/Urban/Slum.**

2. Total population with sex ratio :

3. Total no. of families - hemlet-wise distribution of families :

4. **Main agricultural products of the Community?**
   (Also mention irrigational and manure facilities, per bigha production of different food-stuff, how many crops are grown in a year etc.)

5. Information on climate, particularly about rainfall, temperature, humidity, drought, chances of flood etc.

6. **Planning of the area** : Well planned/planned/unplanned.
   Remarks, if any :

7. **Lanes and by-lanes** : Pucca/Semi-pucca/Kutcha :
   Recommendation, if any :

8. **Drainage** : Underground/open/no drain/soakage pit.
   Disposal of Excreta and Refuse :

9. Comment on Water Supply :

10. **Recreational places and facilities** :
    Play and play grounds, places of worship, mela, yatra and other social gathering and give your comment:

11. Literacy status and rate of the area :

12. Facilities for Libraries etc.

13. No. of different types of shops in the area :

14. What are the facilities and distance of Primary Health Centre, Hospital, Block Development Office, Police Station, Fire Brigade, Market etc.

PRACTICAL PART 553

15. (a) Health facilities available to the area :
   (include facilities beside Government health facilities)

   (b). Methods of treatment are taken Allopathic/Homoeopathic/Ayurvedic and others.

16. Prognostic evaluation according to the classification or Organon or Medicine. (in case of Homoeopathy)

17. Other facilities, e.g. agencies working for village development etc.

18. Give your comments on family illness :

   Where do Head of the family or their members go to the Private practitioner or P.H.C./S.D. Hospital when they fall sick ?

   Comment on the reasons for attending or not attending the Primary health centre :

   Remarks, if any :

19. School : Total number:

    Types of school Number-wise :

    Primary : Junior High : Madhyamic : Higher Secondary : Madarsha

20. (a). Accommodation facilities : Adequate/Inadequate

    (b) Building

    (c) Source of Water supply : (Mention after observing in detail) specially drinking.

    (d) Facilities for Latrine : Present/Absent - Method of disposal of Sewage

    No.   Types

    (e) Facilities regarding play and recreation, library and health promotion :

    (f) Any other relevant observations such as School Health Service, Midday meal program etc.

21. **Customs and beliefs** : Enquire and observe with a view to find out any correlation with these and the prevalence of different diseases and health status. Student should observe throughout his training period.

22. Remarks :

Lesson 2

FORM 1   **FAMILY & GENERAL HEALTH EXAMINATION SCHEDULE**

Family : Nuclear/Joint   Address :   Per capita monthly income :   Household No :

Head of family: Monthly income of family: Religion & Caste:
(H.O.F.)

Resident Family Members

Sl.No.	Name	Age	Sex	Relation to H.O.F.	Occupation and income	Nature of work	Addiction	Literacy	Marital status	Illness or Health			
										Present illness**	Past illness**	Family illness**	Wt. (Kg.)

*   Fill obstetric sheet, for married women

**   H/o Present, past and family illness, if required, may be written in detail in white sheet

*   Date of birth and month of birth in Case of Pre-school children and if possible, in Case of school children.

FORM—2.

SL. No.	*Height /M.A.C./ HC/C.C	Pulse/ Resp. rate	B.P.	Physical Examination				Immunisation		
				Oedema, jaundice cyanosis, clubbing Anaemia etc.(strictly)	Personal Hygiene (See guidelines)	Exam. of different systems like Resp., C.V.S., gastrointestinal, eye, ear, nose, throat, oral cavity, skin glandular and other systems (Positive findings to be mentioned only. Detail examination to be mentioned in separate white sheet)	Immunisation status- Tripple & double antigen, Polio vaccine tetanus toxoid, B.C.G. Small pox, other (specify with data)	Examine for signs of nutritional deficiency, if any, (see guidelines)	Provisional diagnosis and REMARKS

* M.A.C. = Mid Arm Circumference, He = Head Circumference, C.C. = Chest Circumference (for under fives only).

FORM —3.   OBSTETRIC HISTORY

F.F. Sl No of Mother	Order	Date of birth	Result *	Sex	Age **	If dead, cause of death	Complications			Child Neonatal Period
							Pregnancy	Mother Delivery	Puerperium	

* : L-Live birth   S-Still birth   Ab-Abortion   LL-Live birth(twin)   Add P for Prematurity
** : For dead child encircle the age.
N.B.— It obstetric history of mothers could not be accomodated in this sheet, are may attach separate sheet/sheets.
— F.F. = family folder.

FORM—4

4. Follow-up Advice & Treatment Sheet

F.F. Sl. N	Date	Laboratory exam result	Follow-up finelings	Advice treatment

* F F—Family Folder
* Remarks :

FORM—5

5. Deaths in the Family (Last 5 years):

Date of death	Name of the deceased	Relations to H.O.E.	Age	Sex	Cause of death

NOTES:

1. Give your comments on family illness.

2. Where do Head of the family or their members go when they fall sick?

3. Comment on the reason for attending or not attending the Primary Health Centre.

4. Remarks, if any.

Lesson 3

STUDY OF INDIVIDUAL HOUSING : DISPOSAL OF REFUSE & SEWAGE : WATER SUPPLY

A. HOUSING :

1. Location :

2. Type : Single or multi-storyed; rental if any. Pucca/Semi-pucca/Mud-built/Thatched.

3. Prepare a plan of house (room-wise) :

4. Built up area   5. Set-back   6. No. of living rooms

7. Total area of the living rooms (mention height & floor space)

8. Per-capita floor space : Total floor areas

   (in sq. met.)   No. of members

9. Area other than living rooms utilised for living purpose :

10. Define and comment on overcrowding :

11. Windows and doors (comment) :

12. **Ventilation** : Adequate/Inadequate. **Lighting**: Adequate/Inadequate.

    Cross ventilation : Present/absent (Define with comments).

13. Is the Kitchen located in living room, verandah or in a separate room ?

14. Is there a separate shed for the cattle or they are accommodated in the living room? What are the possible health hazards, if accommodated in the living room? Include your comments :

15. What are the advantages of Community Cattle shed?

16. Comment on latrine facilities or Open-field defecation :

17. Enquire and comment on refuse disposal :

18. Comment on drainage around house, breeding place of mosquitoes, houseflies etc. and presence of rodents etc :

19. Remarks : On housing and sanitation with suggestion:

(B) Water Supply :

1. Sources of water supply :
   a) Drinking purpose : Tubewell/Well/Tap/Pond/River.
   b) Cooking purpose : Tubewell/Well/Tap/Pond/River.
   c) Cleaning, bathing and washing purposes : Tubewell/Well/Tap/Pond/River.
   N.B. and Mention under each : category whether the supply is sanitary/insanitary.
   d) Distance from the house :

   e) Private owned/owned by other family or community.

f) When last cleaned, repaired or chlorinated?

2. Observe how water is drawn, transported and stored in the house for different purposes and give your comment :

3. Is the water for different purposes are given special treatment or not (like boiling, straining, domestic filtration or any other) ?

4. Comment on knowledge of the family on water-borne diseases and its prevention :

5. Remarks, including suggestions for improvement :

Lesson 4

COLLECTION OF WATER FOR CHEMICAL & BACTERIOLOGICAL EXAMINATION

(I). *Collection of water* :

(II). *Chemical examination* :

    1. Hardness of water.

    2. Chloride.

    3. Nitrite.

    4. Nitrate.

(III). *Bacteriological examination* :
Estimate the coliform counts

N.B. : Consult quick reference chart.

Lesson 5

METHODS OF CHLORINATION OR DISINFECTION

1. What is chlorine demand, Break point chlorination and residual chlorine :

2. Find out the requirements of bleaching powder (through Horrock's apparatus) :

3. Methods of chlorination in the community :

4. Estimate the residual chlorine :

PRACTICAL PART

5. Any other methods of disinfection :

6. Remarks :

Lesson 6
NUTRITIONAL ASSESSMENT

In the field following three methods are easy to practise:
(a) Clinical (b) Anthropometric (c) Diet survey By ('Oral questionnaire method with 24 hours recall')

Diet Survey by oral questionnaire method with 24 hours recall:

Foodstuffs	Items	Quantity	Calories Carbohydrate/Fat	Proteins	Iron	Vit A
I. Cereals	1. Rice 2. Wheat 3. Muri 4. Chura					
II. (1) Pulses (2) Moong (3)	1. Munsur					
III. Animal protein A. Fleshfood: specify the names of fish etc.) in the ( )	1. Fish ( ) 2. Meat ( ) 3. Egg ( ) 4.					
B. Milk & Milk products :	1. Cow 2. Buffalow 3. Curd 4.					
IV. Oils & fats :	1. Mustard oil 2. Ghee					
V. Green leafy vegetables (specify)	1. 2.					
VI. Non-leafy vegetables (specify)	1. 2.					
VII. Roots & tubers :	1. Potato 2. Onion 3. Kochu 4.					
VIII. Fruits : (specify) :	1. 2.					
IX.	1. Sugar 2. Jaggery					
X. Spices :	1. Chillies 2. Mustard					
TOTAL QUANTITY						

1. Compute total consumption units in the family (specify):

$$\text{Calories per consumption unit} = \frac{\text{Total calories}}{\text{Total consumption unit}}$$

2. Discuss and give your comments on nutritional assessment as done under A & B (consult Lesson 2):

3. Comment on the diet of the family as a whole with recommendations :

4. Falacies of "Oral questionnaire method with 24 hours recall":

PRACTICAL PART 571

Lesson 7

INFANT AND UNDER-FIVE FEEDING AND REARING

1. Describe (preferably after personal observation) the methods of (a) infant feeding practised in your allotted family with special reference to breast and artificial feeding; and (b) underfive feeding. Note the local practices connected with child rearing :

2. Frequency and type of food given :

3. Age of infant at which solid food was/is given :
   Note the type of solid food :

4. Give your critical comment on infant and underfive feeding and child rearing in the family, with due regard to local customs :

5. Give relevent advice to the family including the good or bad aspects of the existing child rearing customs in the family. Give a chart of low cost weaning food and nutritional requirements of infant and underfive :

6. Advantages and disadvantages of breast and artificial feeding :

Lesson 8

GROWTH AND DEVELOPMENT OF INFANT AND UNDER FIVE
(Take help from Lesson 2)

Name of child :   Family Folder serial No.:

Date of Examination	Age in month	Growth*					Development*			Remarks
		Weight	Height	Anterior frontanell	Dentition	Sphincter control	Others	Physical	Psycho-social	

Remarks :

Growth refers to only physical growth by multiplication of cells while development means functional maturity.

Lesson 9

MATERNAL & CHILD HEALTH & FAMILY WELFARE INCLUDING PLANNING

1. Why the mother and the child are considered as one unit ?

2. Note how far the family is acquainted with Maternal and Child Health (MCH) care and whether their family members receive any instruction in this regard :

3. **Note the sources of information:** Midwives (domiciliary midwifery Sub-centre/ P.H.C./ Govt. Hospital/ Private Practitioner/others (Specify).

4. What care is given (in terms of drugs, medical examination, medication)? Do they realise the signficance of this ?

5. Does the family know, the type of diet one should take during pregnancy ?

6. Do the family members avail M.C.H. clinic/ domiciliary services ?

7. What type of care is available there-in ?

8. Reason for not availing the M.C.H. services :

9. Is there any pregnant woman and underfives in the family ? Yes/No (If yes, take obstetric case history as per Lesson 10 and for underfives refer to Lessons 2 & 8).

PRACTICAL PART 575

10. Define Eligible Couple (E.C.) :

11. Average low birth rate (less than 2.5 kg small for gentational age)

12. Average age in % of the married girls during last 5 years.

13. Visit to Maternal and Child Health and Family Planning clinic of the Primary Health Centre or Sub-Centre or others.

---

* Observe how far the different units (as regard Antenatal, Postnatal and derive care and family planning are carried out). Write a note on it.
  Date of visit
  Note :

14. Give the immunisation schedule followed and immunisation administered in M.C. — clinic with comments :

15 What is 'Road to Health Card'? What are its advantages? Is it followed in the Clinic?

16. Comments on the visit :

Eligible Couple Record

Sl. No. of E.C.	No. of alive children With L.C.B.**	Attitude (for negative attitude, give reasons)	Who is Acceptor	L.M.P.	Methods Used***	Source of Supply	Regularity in use	Problems/ Complications	Advice & Remarks

- For each E.C. put the Serial No. from Family Schedule of Lesson No 2. e.g. 1,2,6,7 ** L.C.B.-Last Child Birth *** For permanent method, give date of operation.

Lesson 10

SOCIO-CLINICAL CASE PRESENTATIONS

Guidelines:

Case presentations are done as followed in clinical medicine. Relevant observations from **Lesson 1 to 9** should be included. A broad outline is given below but certain points have to be stressed or might have to be included in case of certain diseases.

1. Identification :   Name, Age, Sex, Religion, Caste, Occupation, Income, Literacy, Marital Status, Address etc.
2. Chief complaints (with duration of illness of incapacitation):
3. Present illness :

Source of infection aid medical and received so far. Reasons for time lag between onset of illness and treatment, if any. Reasons for discontinuation of treatment (defaulter). Socio-economic problems due to illness - job, rehabilitation, etc.

4. Pathological and rediological findings.
5. History of Past illness ;

a) Chronic illness of the past (b) Other illness (c) Childhood diseases (d) Treatment undertaken.

6. Family history :

a) Joint/Nuclear. Lesson No. with all its relevant portions should be included, example is given below :

b) Earning members. c) Dependent members, d) Deaths, morbidity, etc.

N.B. For females past obstetric history

7. Personal history :
8. Economic aspect of the family :

a) Income of head of the family, b) Income of the patient before illness and at present, c) Total per capita income of the family, d) Expenditure per month in the family on Food, Clothing, Housing, Education, Medical care, Functions or ceremonies, Others (specify). Amount of debt (if any) and how much of it is due to illness or incapacitation, f) Approximate total expenditure (fees, drugs, diet, etc.) for the whole course of illness. Mention also expenditure for different types of medical agencies.

PRACTICAL PART 579

9. Diet : Veg./Non-veg.
   Items   Calories   Proteins   Others(specify)

   Morning   1.
             2.

   Midday   1.
             2.
             3.

   Afternoon 1.
             2.
             3.

   Night   1.
             2.
             3,
                    Total _____

10. Environment :
    a) Housing (note—type, ventilation, overcrowding, etc.),
    b) Water supply, c) Disposal of refuse & excreta

11. General examination: (note immunisation status also)

12. Laboratory findings, if any:

13. Provisonal Diagnosis :

14. Examination of contacts:

15. Summary of the case : Bring out the main points e.g. source of infection, circumstances which led to disease, if the disease is treatable or preventable, reasons for allure and non-compliance, any sequalae.

16. Comprehensive Diagnosis:

17. Advice and Treatment :

18. Levels of Prevention recommended:
    a) In case of the patient
    b) In case of family
    c) In case of community (if danger of spread is there)

Notes on Practical Part

GUIDELINES FOR THE LESSONS

Lesson 1

Information should be collected from the village, village panchayet and Block Development Office, Social organisation.

Lesson 2

Study it throughout your community posting period in your allotted families. History of obste. and gynae. data should be carefully studied, also natural history of diseases in the family Literacy status :- Illiterate, Just literate, Primary, Middle School (Class VIII), Secondary, Higher Secondary, Graduate, Post-graduate, Technical (specify).

Monthly Income : It is ascertained by computing the individual income of the family members plus income from other sources, such as property, agriculture, cattle, etc. Per capita monthly income is calculated in the following way :

$$\frac{\text{Total Monthly Income}}{\text{Total No. of Family Members}}$$

Personal Hygiene : Personal Hygiene means all personal factors which affects the health of an individual e.g. care of the 1) Hair; 2) Teeth; 3) Nail; 4) Body (bathing, hand washing etc); 5) Clothing; 6) Posture and habits like; 7) Smoking; 8) Pating; 9) sleep; 10) Exercise; 11) Attitude towards life conciousness of health.

Note :
Very Good : If all positive.
Good : If first seven positive.
Fair : If first five positive.
Bad : Other than above three; record positive findings.
  *Nutritional deficiency : Consult clinical examination schedule.

PRACTICAL PART 581

Lesson 3

In the remarks one should try to correlate his findings on housing, water supply and sanitation with health and disease.

Lesson 4-5

Consult relevant chapter and laboratory text book.

Lesson 6

Consult Lesson 2 and relevant quick reference chart for nutritional deficiency signs, Anthropometric and food value charts.

Lesson 8

Take the help from Lesson No. 2.

Lesson 9

Write notes from the visit of Maternity & child health clinic/well bay clinic, clinic of P.H.C. or Local private health clinic.

APPENDICES QUESTIONERIES

COUNCIL OF HOMOEOPATHIC MEDICINE WEST BENGAL

D.H.M.S. - 1987.
(JUNE)

PREVENTIVE AND SOCIAL MEDICINE

Full Marks - 100

All questions carry equal marks.

Answer any four questions.

(1) What is balance diet? Draw a balance chart for an adult nonvegetarian male of sedentary habit. *(See page no. 29)*

(2) Define : (i) Preventive Medicine *(P-7)*, (ii) Social Medicine *(P-16)* (iii) Genus epidamicus *(P-288)*.

(3) Short notes (any five) :

(a) Vital statistics-*(P-487)* (b) Maternal mortality rate *(P-465)*, (c) Infant mortality Rate *(P-465)*, (d) Koplik's spot (See measles), (e) Sehick test (see diphtheria), (f) Prevention, (g) Vaccination *(P-360)*

(4) What is a primary health centre? Mention the function of a P.H.C. *(*See page no. 480, 484)*

(5) Discuss the life cycle of mosquito. Name the mosquito borne diseases and its prevention. *(*See page no. 365)*

(6) Define family planning. Briefly discuss the common contraceptive devices. *(See page no. - 437)*

(7) What is 'health education' method *(See page no. 484)*

(8) Mention the causes of diarrhoea. Briefly discuss about 'oral rehydration therapy' in diarrhoeal diseases. *(See page no. 322)*

D.H.M.S. - 1988

PREVENTIVE AND SOCIAL MEDICINE

Full Marks - 100

All questions carry equal marks.

Answer any four questions.

(1) What is 'balance diet'? Prepare a balanced diet chart for you.
(See page no. 29) 5+20.

(2) What is "Infant Mortality Rate"? Mention the important causes of infant mortality in our country and how this rate can be reduced? *(See page no. 465)*
5+20.

(3) Write notes on (any five) :

(i) Level's of prevention of diseases, (ii) Pasteurisation *(P-82)*, (iii) Vital statistics *(P-487)*, (iv) Sanitary latrine *(P-222)*, (v) Air pollution *(P-99)*, (vi) World health day, (vii) Mosquito borne disease, (viii) Personal hygiene *(P-129)*, (ix) Maternal mortality in India *(P-465)*

(4) What are the functions of a Primary Health Centre? *(*See page no. 484)* 25

(5) What are the different Hormonal Contraceptive Methods? Mention their advantages and disadvantages. *(See page no. 441, 450)* 25

(6) Describe with examples, the different modes of transmission of communicable diseases. *(*See page no. 309)*

(7) Name the common childhood viral diseases. How those can be prevented. *(See page no. 335)* 5+20

(8) Name some common water borne diseases. How those can be prevented? *(See page no. 193)* 5+20

D.M.S. FINAL PART - I 1989

HYGIENE

Full Marks - 100

Answer any five question.

(1) Classify Vitamins. Mention the functions, daily requirement and sources of Vitamin A. What are its deficiency signs and symptoms? *(See page no. 48+50)*   5+10+10

(2) What are the general principles of control of communicable diseases? *(See page no. 309)*   20

(3) Name the diseases commonly transmitted by mosquito. How these can be prevented? *(See page no. 365)*   10+10.

(4) Name the importent causes of maternal mortality in our country. Mention the different important components of antenatal care. *(See page no. 465+459)*   10+10

(5) Write Notes on (any four) :

    (i) Rehabilitation,   (ii) Vital statistics,
    (iii) Primary Health Care,   (iv) Chlorination,
    (v) School Health Services,   (vi) Ventilation,
    (vii) Zoonoses,   (vii) Rapid sand filter.

(6) Mention the common water borne diseases, suggest measures for control of diarrhoea. *(See page no. 193+322)*   8+12

(7) What are the objective of Family Welfare Planning Programme in India? Mention the different Mechanical and Chemical contraceptive methods with their advantages and disadvantages. *(See page no. 437+441)*   8+12

APPENDICES QUESTIONERIES

(8) Mention the ideal immunisation schedule of an infant. *(See page no. 418+463)*   20

(9) A case has come to you with history of a street dog bit. How can you manage the problem. *(See page no. 376)*   20

(10) What is the population usually covered by a Primary Health Centre and what are its different functions? *(See page no. 480, 484)*   10+10

(11) Name two important (any ten) :
   i) Sources of Iron in our diet. (**Wheat flour**, Bajra).
   ii) Bacterial diseases common to children. (**Diphtehria**, Pneumonia).
   iii) Diseases transmitted by rat flea. (**Plague**, Murine typhus).
   iv) International Health Organisaion. (**WHO**, UNICEF).
   v) Source of vital statistics. (Population census, Registration of vital events).
   vii) Zoonotic diseases. (Malaria, Filaria).
   vii) Objective of School Health Service. (Health Protection, Health restoration).
   viii) Types of rehabilitation. (Physically Mentaly).
   ix) Vital Vaccines. (Poliovaccine, Smallpox vaccine).
   x) Airborne diseases. (Smallpox, Chickenpox).
   xi) Methods of refuse disposal. (Dumping, Sanitary land filt).
   xii) Hazards of noise pollution. (Deafness, Palpitation).
   xiii) Signs of thiamine deficiency. (Beriberi, Footdrop).
   xiv) Methods of pasteurisation. (Holder process, Flashing method).
   xv) Arthropod borne viral diseases. (Encephalitis, Dengue).
   xvi) Mention the common mineral deficiency diseases in our country. How these can be prevented? *(See page no. 403)*   8+1.

B.H.M.S.(F)-P.S.M.
1985

PREVENIVE AND SOCIAL MEDICINE

GROUP - A

Answer four questions, of which Question No. 3 is compulsory.

(1) Write short notes on any ten of the following : 2 x 10

    i) Blocked Flea ;   ii) Secondary prevention
    iii) Vital layer;   iv) Incubation period;
    v) Quarantine;   vi) Iceberg of disease;
    vii) Primary prevention ;   viii) Flurosis;
    ix) Social Anatomy ;   x) Droplet Infection;
    xi) Epidemiology;   xii) Schick test.

(2) Distinguish between any two of the following : 5 x 4

    i) Disease control and Disease eradication;
    ii) Night Blindness and Xerophthalmia;
    iii) Crude Death Rate and Specific Death Rate;
    iv) Presumptive taliform count and presumptive treatment.

(3) (A) From the following multiple choice questions tick (i/) the most appropriate answer :

    i) Beriberi is caused by deficiency of Thiomine/pyridoxino/Vitamin B.
    ii) 100 gms of Human milk contains 3.60/3.50/1.25 gm of protein;
    iii) Rebies is caused by **Viral**/Fungal/Bacterial infection;
    iv) Kala-azar is transmitted by Fleas/Sandflies/House flios;
    v) Demography reveals birth and **death rate**/Marriages/Diverces.

(B) Fill up the blanks by appropriate words: 1 x 10

    i) Two ill effects of Air Pollution ....
    ii) Three diseasesd transmitted by Mosquito..................
    iii) Two milk-borne diseases..
    iv) Three sites of occupational cancer............................

4. Define Health. What do you understand by UNICEF ? State the activities of it. *(See page no. - 509)* 20

5. What is Primary Health Care ? What are its essential components? *(See page no. 477, 484)* 20

6. What is 'Balanced Diet' ? What are its essential constituents? How will you prescribe a balanced diet for a lactating mother? *(See page no. 29)* 20

7. What are the common water borne diseases? Write down the epidemiology of poliomyelitis. *(See page no. 193 + 335)*

8. What are common methods of disposal of refuse? Describe one such method. *(See page no. 248)* 20

GROUP - B

Answer any one question

9. What is "Genus Epidemicus"? How you will arrive at Genus Epidemicus? Discuss the scope of preventive medicine in Homoeopathy. *(See page no. 288, 425)* 5+5+10

10. Who is the writer of "Friend of Health"? When and where it was published? How many articles are there? In your opinion which one is the best and why? 3+4+4+9

11. Describe the concept of Health and Hygiene. How can you apply your knowledge of Organon of Medicine for prevention of disease. *(See page no. 19)* 5+5+10

B.H.M.S.(FI/Sup)P.S.M.
1986 (December)

PREVENTIVE AND SOCIAL MEDICINE

Full Marks - 80

Answer any four questions of which question No. 7 is compulsory

GROUP-A

1. Mention the mosquito-borne diseases prevalent in our country. Give a brief outline of measures adopted for control of mosquitoes. *(See page no. 365)*   5+15

2. What is a balanced diet? Draw up a balanced diet chart for a lactating woman. *(P. 29)*   8+12

3. Explain with examples different modes of spread of communicable diseases. *(P. 309)*   20

4. Define family planning and name the different contraceptive methods. *(P. 437)*

5. Write short notes on any two of the following :   10+10
   (a) Pasteurisation milk *(P. 82)*
   (b) Over crowding; *(P. 103)*
   (c) Sanitary latrine *(P. 222)*

6. Mention the common water borne disease in our country. Describe measures to be adopted for control of one such disease *(P. 193 + 322)*   5+15

7. (a) Complete the following sentences by choosing the most appropriate answer :   2 + 4

   i) Japanese encephalitis caused by **Viral**/Bacterial/Fungal infection.

ii) 'Night-blindness' is due to deficiency of Vitamin B,/Iron/Vitamin C/**Vitamin A.**

iii) Mosquito is a vector of kala-azar/**Japanese Encephalitis**/Plague.

iv) Leprosy is caused by Virus/**Bacteria**/Protozoa.

(b) Fill up the blank (Any four) : 3 x 4

i) Three types of prevention are ....

ii) Three mortality indices are ....

iii) Epidemiological triade are ....

iv) Three types of carrier are ....

v) Three commonly used live vaccine are ....

vi) Three international health organisations are ....

8. What are common nutritional disorders affecting children in our country? Describe the prevention of one such disorder.
(See page no. 58, 68) 10+10

GROUP - B

Full Marks - 20

Answer any one question

9. What is 'Genus Epidemicus ? How you will arrive at genus epidemicus ? Discuss the scope of preventive medicine in homoeopathy. *(See page no. 288)*
5+5+10

10. Who is the writer of "Friend of Health" ? When and where it was published ? How many articles are there ? In your opinion which one is the best and why ? 3+4+4+9

11. Discuss the concept of health and disease. How can you apply your knowledge of Organon of Medicine for prevention of disease ? *(See page no. 19).*

B.H.M.S. (1) P.S.M.
1986

PREVENTIVE AND SOCIAL MEDICINE

Full Marks 100

GROUP - A

Answer any four questions of which question No. 8 is compulsory.

1. What do you understand by the term 'vital statistics'? What is the procedure for collection of relevant information in West Bengal ? *(See page no. 487)*
   3+15

2. What are mosquito-borne diseases in our country ? What are the measures for control of mosquito ? *(P. 365)*
   3+15

3. Discuss the modes of transmission of diseases. What do you understand by the term 'carrier' ? *(See page no. 292 + 294)*
   15+5

4. How will you organise school health service ? What are its benefits ? *(See page no. 471, 479)* 10+10

5. Define social medicine. Describe the importance of social medicine in our country. *(See page no. 16)*
   5+15

6. How milk is pasteurised. What are the benefits of such a procudure ? *(See page no. 82)* 12+8

7. Write short notes on : 10+10
   i) Flea index.   ii) Sullivan index.

8. (A) A complete the following sentences by choosing the most appropriate answer : 5+2

   i) Scurvy is caused by deficiency of VIT. E/VIT. C/RIBOFLAVIN.

   ii) Endemic goitre is caused by deficiency of Vitamin.Iron/**Iodine**.

   iii) Japanese encephalitis is caused by **Virus**/Bacteria/Fungus.

   iv) Composting is a method for disposal of Refuse/night soil/Both.

   v) Plague is caused by a bacteria/virus/protozon.

(B) Fill up the blank : 5x2

   i) Incubation period of malaria is ....

   ii) Rahses of Chicken pox is .... in distribution.

   iii) Koplik's sport is found in ....

   iv) For prevention of rabies the latest vaccine is being prepared from ....

   v) The commonest mode of transmission Hepatitis B is through..........................

GROUP - B

Answer any one question

9. What is Social Medicine ? What is preventive medicine ? Write the scope of preventive medicine in Homoeopathy. *(See page no. 16)* 3+5+10

10. Discuss prophylaxis and vaccination critically from Homoeopathic point of view. *(See page no. 419)* 20

11. What is immunization ? Describe the scope of immunization in Homoeopathy.*(See page no. 408 + 410 + 411)* 8+12

PREVENTIVE AND SOCIAL MEDICINE
INDEX

A

Abortion - 446

Activated sludge - 245

Active immunity - 402, 403, 405

Active immunization - 411, 412

Adulteration of foods - 88, 89

Aerobic oxidation - 232

Aids - 406

Air - 99

— Changes of - 100

— Composition of - 99

— Conditioning - 112

— expired - 100

— disinfection - 106

— humidity - 118

— inspired - 101

— pollution - 104

— purification - 105

— temperature - 122

Air borne transmission - 160

Aminoacids - 29

Anaerobic digestion - 232

Ancylostomiasis - 328

Antenatal care - 458, 459, 462

Antibodies - 410

Antirabies treatment - 376

Antispetic - 272

Aqua privy - 237

Ariboflavonosis - 57

Artesian well - 175

Arthropod borne disease - 307

Artificial feeding - 44

Ascorbic acid -

INDEX

B

Bacteriological examination of water - 170

Balance diet - 29

Balance diet chart - 36

Basic health service - 509

B. C. G. - 342

Beriberi - 391

Biological carriers - 300

Biochemical oxygen demand-(BOD)-242

Biological filters - 207

Bitot's spots - 51

Bleaching powder -179

Boiling - 201

Borehole latrine - 223

Boxtype - 223

Breast feeding - 86

Broad irrigation - 245

C

Calcium - 42

Calciferol - 53

Calcutta water supply - 185

Carbohydrate - 33

Chickenpox - 349

Chlorination of water - 204

Cholera - 316

Cholera vaccine - 317

Cirrhosis of liver - 97

Clark's process - 214

Cleanliness - 131

Climate - 117

Clothing - 134

Communicable disease - 308

Community health worker scheme - 486

Composting - 256

Comprehensive health care - 507

Condom - 443

Constant water supply - 187

Conservancy system - 220

Contact bed - 243

Contagious disease - 308

Contraception - 441

Contraceptive methods - 441, 443

Controlled tipping - 256

D

Deep well - 178

Demography - 431

— data - 434

— features - 432, 435

Diet - 35

— infant - 44

Dietotherapy - 95

Diabetes - 96

Different methods of disinfection in hospitals - 268

Disablement benefit - 512

Disease - 19

Disinfection - 260

—— concurrent - 261

—— precurrent - 261

—— terminal - 261

Disinfection of

— bedding, occupied room and scrubs of a smallpox case - 269

— furniture beddings, utensils and room of a T.B. patient - 269

— clothing, bedding, stools and vomiting of cholera patient - 269

— stool, urine, bedpan and clothes of typhoid patient - 271

— feeding and cooking utensils of cholera patients - 270

Disinfectants - 262

Disinfestation - 271

Disposal of human excreta - 218

— of refuse - 248

— in rural area - 251

— town refuse - 255

Droplet infection - 312

INDEX

Dual water supply - 188

Dugwell latrine - 225

Dumping - 256

Dysentery - 322

E

Endemic goitre - 389

Environment - 149

Epidemic - 282

— prevention - 287

Epidemology - 282

E.S.I. Scheme - 511

Excreta disposal - 218

Exercises - 138

Expired air - 101

F

Family planning - 437

—advantages - 450

needs - 438

National Programme - 451

— present attitude 451, 453

— various methods - 443, 445

F.A.O - 510

Fats - 31

Fly control - 303, 305

Filaria - 372

Filteration - 203

Five points MCH programme - 463

Fomites

Food - 26

— adulteration - 89

— borne disease - 92

— inspector - 91

— poisoning - 91

Fumigation - 272

G

Gangasagar mela - 279

Gastro-enteritis - 322

Giardia - 333

Genus epidemicus - 425, 288

Germicides - 271

H

Hardwater - 210

Health - 19

— for all by 2000 A.D.- 516

— centre - 480

— education - 485

— services in school - 470

— statistics - 490

— workers -

Healthy carrier - 301

Heat exhaustion

Heat stroke

Heat immunity

Hook worm - 328

Host factors - 22

House fly - 304

Humidity - 118

Hydrological cycle - 216

Hygiene - 14

I

Immunity - 395

— acquired - 399

— artificial - 401

Immunization against

— cholera - 319

— polio - 335, 336,

— rabies - 376

— smallpox - 356

— tuberculosis - 342

Immunization schedule 418

— active - 411

— passive - 411

Immunizing agents - 412

Impurities of water - 190

Incineration - 256

Incubation period - 313

Indicators of health

Infant feeding - 86

Infant mortality rate - 466

INDEX

Infection - 289

—various methods - 292

Infectious disease - 301, 308,

— prevention - 295

Infective hepatitis - 324

Insect borne disease - 311

Insecticides - 265, 311

Inspired air - 101

Intranatal care - 474

Intra uterine devices - 444

Intermittent water supply - 187

Iodized salt - 390

Isolation - 297

K

Keratomatacia - 51

Kwashiorkor - 64

L

Lagooing - 246

Land treatment - 244

Laparoscope - 448

Larvicides - 265

Leprosy - 384

Lighting - 114

Live vaccines - 416

M

Malaria - 362

Malnutrition - 58

Manure pit - 258

Manhole - 246

Marasmus - 64

Maternal mortality rate - 465

Maternity benefit - 512

Mechanical carrier - 300

Medical officer - 472

— function as a M.O. of a PHC - 477, 484

—duties as a member of a school committee-489

Medical benefit - 513

M.C.H. programme - 455

Midday school meal - 478

Milk - 72

Milk borne disease - 77

— prevention - 78

— is a complete food - 75

—humanised - 73

Morbidity statistics - 493

Mosquito borne disease - 362, 372

M.T.P - 446

Multipurpose worker scheme - 486

N

National family planning programme - 445

National malaria eradication programme - 370

National tuberculosis control programme - 347

National cholera control programme - 321

National and International preventive measures in Small pox - 357

Notifible diseases - 296

Notification - 296

Nutritional assessment - 68

Nutritional deficiencies - 46

O

Obesity - 98

Occupancy - 102

Oral contraceptives - 446

Over crowding - 103

Oxidation pond - 246 (o-pond)

P

Passive immunization - 415

Pasteurisation - 72, 82

Pellagra - 392

Peptic ulcer - 97

Percolating filter - 243

Permutit process - 214

Personal hygiene - 129

Pill - 446

Pit type - 222

INDEX

Polio myelitis - 335

Polio - vaccine - 335, 338,

Pollutant - 150

— their effects - 153

— pollution -150

— prevention - 157

Population census - 492

— population control - 432

— growth in India - 433

Porter's clark's process -214

Postnatal care - 462

Potable water - 168

Pot chlorination - 180

Prenatal care - 460

Pressure - 124

Preventive & social medicine - 7

Preservation of food - 87

Primary health centre - 480

Prophylaxis - 420

Protein calories malnutirtion (PCM) - 62

Protein energy malnutrition (PEM) - 62

Proteins - 29

Proximate principle of Food - 28

Q

Quarantine - 298

— domestic - 299

— international - 298

— scholastic - 299

R

Rabies - 374

Rapid sand filter - 207

RCA latrine - 226

Repellantes - 272

Rickets - 54

S

Sabin vaccine - 338

Salk vaccine - 338

Sanitary landfill - 256

Sanitary latrine - 222

Sanitation - 147

—— of a fair or normal - 272

School health service - 470, 479

— components - 471

Scurvey - 56

Septic tank - 228

Sewage - 240

Shallow well - 182

Sleep - 137

Slow sand filter - 206

Smallpox - 349

Smog - 154

Social medicine - 16

Soil borne disease - 333

Solid wastes - 250

Specific dynamic action (SDA) - 33

Sterilization - 447

Sunshine - 115

T

Thiamine deficiency - 391

Trench latrines - 235

Trickling filters - 243

Tubectomy - 448

Transmission of common diseases - 307

U

UNICEF - 509

Under five clinic - 464

V

Vaccination - 360

Vacinosis - 361

Vaccination against
— cholera - 319

— diphtheria - 360

— polio - 338

— rabies - 376

Smallpox - 358

Tuberculosis - 341

Vector - 300

— control - 302

Vesectomy - 447

Ventilation - 106

INDEX

Vital events - 493

Vital statistics - 487

Vitamines - 48

— deficiencies

— Vit A - 52

— Vit B - 57

— Vit C - 56

— Vit D - 54

W

Water - 162

— borne disease - 193

— chemical qualities - 169

— disinfection - 179

— filtration - 203

— hardness - 210

— removal of hardness - 212

— pollution - 190

— purification - 199, 205

— Standards of purity 164

Water carriage system - 220, 239

Water closet - 252

Waste products - 250

Wells - 175

World Health Organisation - 505 (WHO)

X

Xerophthalmia - 51

INDEX

Vital events - 493
Vital statistics - 487
Vitamines - 48
— deficiencies
— Vit A - 52
— Vit B - 57
— Vit C - 58
— VIT D - 54

W

Water - 162
— borne disease - 193
— chemical qualities - 169
— disinfection - 179
— filtration - 205
— Hardness - 210
— removal of hardness - 212
— pollution - 190
— purification - 199, 205
— standards of purity 164
Water carriage system - 220, 239
Water closet - 252
Waste products - 260
wells - 175
World Health Organisation (WHO) - 505

X

Xerophthalmia - 51